Neoplastic Mimics in Thoracic and Cardiovascular Pathology

Pathology of Neoplastic Mimics Series
Mark R. Wick and Peter A. Humphrey

Series Editors

Dermatopathology
Mark R. Wick and James W. Patterson

Thoracic and Cardiovascular Pathology
Mark R. Wick and Henry D. Tazelaar

Genitourinary Pathology
Peter A. Humphrey, Robert H. Young, and Carlos Manivel

Forthcoming Volumes

Breast Pathology

Gastrointestinal and Liver Pathology

Gynecologic Pathology

Head and Neck Pathology

Bone and Soft Tissue Pathology

Neoplastic Mimics in Thoracic and Cardiovascular Pathology

Mark R. Wick, MD
Professor of Pathology
Associate Director of Surgical Pathology
University of Virginia Health System
Charlottesville, Virginia

Henry D. Tazelaar, MD
Chair, Department of Laboratory Medicine and Pathology
Professor of Pathology
College of Medicine
Mayo Clinic
Scottsdale, Arizona

demosMEDICAL
New York

Visit our website at www.demosmedpub.com

ISBN: 978-1-620700-13-6
e-book ISBN: 978-1-617051-77-7

Acquisitions Editor: Rich Winters
Compositor: diacriTech

Library of Congress Cataloging-in-Publication Data

Wick, Mark R., 1952-
Neoplastic mimics in thoracic and cardiovascular pathology / Mark R. Wick, Henry D. Tazelaar.
p. ; cm.
ISBN 978-1-62070-013-6
I. Tazelaar, Henry D. II. Title.
[DNLM: 1. Granuloma, Plasma Cell—pathology. 2. Cardiovascular Diseases—diagnosis. 3. Diagnosis, Differential. 4. Lung Diseases—diagnosis. 5. Neoplasms—pathology. QZ 140]
RB113
615.5—dc23

2013003004

Printed in the United States of America by Bradford & Bigelow.
13 14 15 / 5 4 3 2 1

Thanks to Jane, Robert, Morgan, and Kellyn for giving me their time so that this project could be done. Also, I am grateful to my past mentors in thoracic pathology who are no longer with us, but whose teaching and encouragement is warmly remembered. MRW

This work is dedicated to my wife Peggy and sons Andrew and Jeff without whose unfailing support and understanding, works like this would not be possible. I am also deeply indebted to devoted mentors and friends in cardiac and thoracic pathology, Drs. Margaret Billingham (1930–2009), William D. Edwards, and Thomas V. Colby. Their pioneering work, inquisitive minds, and indefatigability continue to be inspirational and motivating. HDT

Contents

Preface

One of the most humbling aspects of pathology practice is the well-known ability for disparate biological processes to resemble one another morphologically. This capacity for mimicry is shared between nonneoplastic processes and neoplasms alike. More problematically, and with particular reference to this monograph, it is also possible for nonneoplastic proliferations to assume the guises of neoplasms at a macroscopic level, a microscopic one, or both. When that occurs, there is a real danger that pathologists will misinterpret the lesion under study, and do so in such a way that incorrect treatment of the patient takes place as a consequence. This sort of error can have potentially grave ramifications.

All systems of the body serve as possible hosts to the development of pseudoneoplastic proliferations, but, for reasons that are not entirely clear, some do so much more commonly than others. Perhaps because the intrathoracic organs are such key participants in immunological processing, they house a considerable array of nonneoplastic lesions that can simulate autonomous growths. In the following monograph, these are presented in a systematic fashion, according to their lineages of differentiation. Comparisons are made throughout between the neoplasms that are imitated, at clinical, gross, and histologic levels, and points that contribute to differential diagnosis are emphasized.

Many of the clinicopathological entities that are considered herein are uncommon, and an effort has therefore been made to illustrate them as completely as possible. The resulting exposition accordingly has more of the qualities of a supplemented atlas than of an encyclopedic compendium. However, an effort has also been made to supply a reasonable number of key references on each topic, so that interested readers may pursue additional information as they wish.

It is our hope that the contents of this book will be an effective adjunct to the now-existing texts on thoracic pathology, in extending their coverage of the subjects that are presented here. The assembly of this material has been a fascinating learning experience for us.

Acknowledgments

The authors wish to acknowledge the strong support of their colleagues in the Departments of Pathology at the University of Virginia Medical Center, Charlottesville, Virginia, and the Mayo Clinic, Scottsdale, Arizona, during the completion of this project. The patience and help of Mr. Rich Winters, Acquisitions Editor for Demos Publishing, is also gratefully recognized.

1

Neoplastic Mimics: General Considerations

- PHILOSOPHICAL AND PRACTICAL ISSUES
- TOPOGRAPHIC DISTRIBUTION AND BIOLOGIC NATURE OF "PSEUDOTUMORS"
    - *Idiopathic* Pseudoneoplasms
    - *Reparative/Posttraumatic* Pseudoneoplasms
    - *Developmental* Pseudoneoplasms
    - "*Functional*" Pseudoneoplasms
    - *Iatrogenic* Pseudoneoplasms
    - *Infectious* Pseudoneoplasms

"Pseudotumor" is an indefinite term that has typically been used to indicate the presence of a mass which is felt to represent a neoplasm at some level of observation. In most circumstances it is a misnomer, because a mass actually exists; in that situation, the term "pseudoneoplasm" would be more appropriate. However, there may still be circumstances in which the term "pseudotumor" is appropriately used; some of those scenarios are presented below. Nonetheless, this discussion will be directed to those lesions that are best designated as "pseudoneoplasms." They are typically represented by masses that have been biopsied or resected, but the microscopic slides do not show the presence of a neoplastic process.

From whence did the designation of "pseudotumor" arise? Ophthalmology has been cited as the first specialty in which the literature used the descriptor of "pseudotumor" (1); in 1930, Birch-Hirschfeld employed it in discussing orbital lesions that had produced proptosis (2). Thereafter, other authors appended such adjectives as "inflammatory," "lymphoid," "granulomatous," "xanthomatous," and "fibrous," in attempts to subdivide "pseudotumors" into *pathologically* recognizable subgroups (3). The word "pseudotumor" has also been synonymized with such alternatives as "postinflammatory tumor" (4,5), "histiocytoma" (6), "plasma cell granuloma" (7–9), "mast cell granuloma" (10), "xanthoma" (11–14), "xanthogranuloma" (15), "plasma cell/histiocytoma complex" (16), and, in some reports (17), "sclerosing hemangioma" as well.

This brief introductory discussion further considers definitions and presentations of "pseudotumors." Because this discussion is especially aimed at pathologists, it will generally be based on the morphologic characteristics of the lesions being considered.

PHILOSOPHICAL AND PRACTICAL ISSUES

The visual images of the same cases that are seen by internists, surgeons, radiologists, and pathologists are potentially quite dissimilar. For example, the surgeon may believe that he or she has identified a palpable mass in the breast, but the radiologist may see little or nothing on mammogram. Similarly, a pathologist examining a fine needle aspiration biopsy of the putative lesion may find nothing that is abnormal. In this scenario, the second and third physicians may question the claims of the surgeon, but unless they physically examine the patient themselves, they can never really determine whether a "tumor" is actually present at a clinical level of assessment. Nonetheless, the palpable lesion is certainly a potential neoplasm in the mind of the surgeon.

Radiologists and pathologists are subject to the same tricks of nature. For example, it is well known that hemorrhages in hemophiliac patients may simulate neoplasms in radiographs, although none are seen through the microscope after excision (18,19). Comparable comments apply to the roentgenographically-defined images of "tumefactive biliary sludge" (20), duodenal ampullary "mucosal rosettes" (21), tumor-like musculoskeletal variations (22), and pulmonary "rounded atelectasis" (23–26). From the perspective of the pathologist, adnexal nevi of the skin (27–29), cutaneous reactions to Monsel's reagent (a styptic solution) (30,31), and the presence of the organ of Chievitz (a histologic imitator of squamous carcinoma) in biopsies of the oral mucosa (32–36) are singular pseudoneoplastic conditions with no associated clinical or radiographic aberrations. Only by face-to-face collegial interaction can all information on such cases be integrated, to yield a clear delineation of the processes or anatomic variations in question (37). Indeed, practically speaking, interpretative disagreement between specialists—as stressful as that can be—is often the principal clue to the existence of a pseudoneoplastic condition.

A considerable number of "pseudotumors" can simulate neoplasms on all levels of analysis—clinical, radiologic, and pathologic—and they consequently represent particular diagnostic pitfalls which can lead to therapeutic misdirection. Those are the entities to which this book is principally directed. In addition, other pathologic conditions are included that histopathologists alone—and not clinicians or radiologists—may uniquely misinterpret as neoplastic in nature.

Certain caveats must be stated in addressing this general topic. First, the lesions known as "inflammatory pseudotumors" (IPs) are generally recognized as representing true neoplasms ("inflammatory myofibroblastic tumors"), although sometimes considerable difficulty may still be encountered in separating them from selected inflammatory conditions (38). Similar comments are applicable to angiomyolipomas, certain melanocytic nevi, and proliferative but reactive lymphoid lesions ("pseudolymphomas"). After the application of such techniques as immunohistochemistry, cytogenetics, and gene rearrangement analyses, the majority of true neoplasms in these lesional groups can be defined correctly. Furthermore, as more knowledge continues to accrue from those studies, the classification of "pseudoneoplasms" will undoubtedly undergo continuing revision.

TOPOGRAPHIC DISTRIBUTION AND BIOLOGIC NATURE OF "PSEUDOTUMORS"

Virtually all topographic sites in the human body may play host to lesions that simulate neoplasms. Perhaps because they are especially sensitive to etiologic influences that cause pseudotumors, some locations appear to be particularly prone to them. Principal examples are the lungs, urinary tract, and gut. In addition, pseudoneoplastic processes are partially overlapping and partly distinctive as seen in various anatomic sites. That observation may again reflect the relative influences of different pathogenetic factors on different tissues, but other variables probably have an effect as well. The following sections consider "pseudoneoplasms," as related to their putative causal categories.

IDIOPATHIC PSEUDONEOPLASMS

True "IP" has an unknown cause in most cases, and is most commonly seen in the pulmonary parenchyma (38–61). It may conceivably represent a localized remnant of unresolved or organizing pneumonia (62,63).

There are several other IP variants that represent etiologically-heterogeneous entities, with at least one variant of each being idiopathic. Examples include nodular lymphoid hyperplasias of the lung, gut, skin, mucosal surfaces, soft tissue, and lymphoreticular system (64–72); and fibro-osseous lesions of craniofacial and small tubular bones (73–76). In these groups of disorders, some potentially-identifiable pathogenetic factors may include viral infection or autoimmune diseases (71,72); and fibrous dysplasia or familial "cherubism" (75,77). However, other morphologically-identical IPs are associated with no causal explanations and are therefore classified as idiopathic.

Still other conditions are "quasi-neoplastic," in that they feature etiologically unknown, and, to some extent, autonomous, cellular proliferations in various locations without a definable stimulus. Radial scar of the breast (78–81); urethral (prostatic utricular) polyp (82); some "tumefactive fibroinflammatory lesions" of soft tissue (84,85), metaphyseal fibrous defects ("non-ossifying fibromas") of bone (86,87); and aneurysmal bone cysts (88–92) belong to that category. They differ biologically from true neoplasms because they are self-limited or even spontaneously-regressing.

Other pseudoneoplastic processes do have a linkage with underlying disease processes, but the ultimate etiology of the *latter* conditions can be idiopathic. Proliferative Paget's disease of bone (osteitis deformans) (93–96), tumefactive plaques of active multiple sclerosis (97–100), and lymphoma-like Hashimoto's thyroiditis (101,102) are representative examples.

REPARATIVE/POSTTRAUMATIC PSEUDONEOPLASMS

Exaggerated host responses to tissue insults arguably comprise the most common mechanisms underlying the formation of pseudoneoplasms. In many of those instances the injury may have been trivial and subclinical—to wit, unnoticed by the patient—and the resulting reparative process might therefore be regarded initially as idiosyncratic. That situation likely applies to nodular fasciitis (103,104), proliferative fasciitis and myositis (105–108), giant-cell reparative granuloma of bone (109–112), fibrohyaline pleuritis (113,114), and xanthogranulomatous inflammation in several sites (115–120).

Still other pseudoneoplams are caused by documented episodes of injury, but again with an amplified and idiosyncratically robust reparative response. Pseudocarcinomatous ("pseudoepitheliomatous") hyperplasias of the skin (121,122), acroangiodermatitis (123), myositis ossificans (124,125), "atypical (ischemic) decubital fibroplasia" (126–129), tumefactive synovial chondrometaplasia (130), necrotizing sialometaplasia (131–133), gliosis in the central nervous system (134), nephrogenic urothelial metaplasia (135), inflammatory polyps of the anorectal region (136), colitis cystica profunda (137), florid reactive mesothelial proliferations (138–141), tumor-like chronic pancreatitis (142), therapy-induced tissue reactions (143–146) (which are simultaneously reparative and iatrogenic, causally), and polypoid-papillary cystitis (147) are all examples of lesions in this category. Why some individuals develop exaggerated repair mechanisms and others do not is an open question at present.

DEVELOPMENTAL PSEUDONEOPLASMS

The most straightforward group of pseudoneoplasms relates to individual abnormalities in development, or, alternatively, ignorance on the part of pathologists regarding the details of normal organogenesis and embryology. Choristomas (148), hamartomas (149–153), and cutaneous non-melanocytic nevi are members of the first of those categories, because they are classified as flaws of morphogenesis. Tissue remnants or heterotopias relating to embryologic development constitute another large subgroup in the same cluster, including examples of vaginal adenosis (154–156), cervical mesonephric remnants (157), "adenomyoma" ("Brunner's gland hamartoma") of the duodenum (158), and cutaneous "rudimentary meningocele" (159) and glial heterotopias (160,161).

On the other hand, the juxtaoral organ of Chievitz is a normal structure rather than an embryologic vestige or developmental anomaly (32–36). However, it is so uncommonly seen in mucosal biopsies that some observers may fail to recognize it and confuse this inclusion with a malignant neoplasm (squamous carcinoma).

Malformations related to congenital or Mendelian syndromes also may resemble neoplasms. The tumefactive lesions of osseous fibrous dysplasia (94,109,162,163) and the paraventricular glial nodules of tuberous sclerosis (161) are representatives.

"FUNCTIONAL" PSEUDONEOPLASMS

Some pseudoneoplasms are caused by a dysfunctional pathophysiologic state, often relating to endocrine abnormalities. "Dominant" nodules often arise in parenchymal hyperplasias of the thyroid or parathyroid glands (102) and that those lesions can simulate adenoma or even carcinoma microscopically. Comparable comments apply to localized unilateral nodular adrenocortical hyperplasia (164). Other pseudoneoplastic conditions with an endocrine underpinnings include prostatic hyperplasias (165,166), focal nodular hyperplasia of the liver (167–169), ovarian stromal hyperthecosis (170), the Arias-Stella reaction in epithelium of the gynecologic tract (171–173), osteitis fibrosa cystica ("brown tumor" of hyperparathyroidism) (174–178), and uterine cervical microglandular hyperplasia (179).

IATROGENIC PSEUDONEOPLASMS

Several medical procedures may produce subsequent tissue reactions that imitate the appearance of neoplasms. Most are reparative in nature and could also have been included in the corresponding section above. However, because of their clearly iatrogenic nature, they deserve special recognition. Instrumentation or surgery of the genitourinary tract may cause an idiosyncratic tumefaction comprising variably-atypical spindle cells, known simply as "postoperative spindle cell nodule" (180–186). In the same vein, application of the iron salt-based cutaneous styptic, Monsel's solution, has caused idiosyncratic cellular proliferations resembling spindle-cell tumors of the skin and uterine cervix (30,31).

Other pseudoneoplasms in this category may be able to imitate an infiltrative or *in-situ* neoplasm. These include urothelial cytotoxicity caused by cyclophosphamide, simulating in-situ urothelial carcinoma (187); epithelial atypia in the breast after chemotherapy (188); and florid vaginal adenosis in women whose mothers took diethylstilbestrol during pregnancy (155). Iatrogenic pseudoneoplasms are particularly problematic for pathologists (189), because we often are not supplied with pertinent—and sometimes crucial—information concerning prior treatments or interventions.

INFECTIOUS PSEUDONEOPLASMS

Particularly because of Acquired Immunodeficiency Syndrome (AIDS), tissue reactions to several infectious pathogens have been increasingly recognized that are capable of simulating neoplasms. Conjointly cytopathic and reparative responses to infection with cytomegalovirus, Epstein–Barr virus (EBV), papovavirus, selected species of mycobacteria, and other bacilli can produce proliferations in several organ systems with a histological likeness to sarcomas, gliomas, or lymphomas (71,190–194).

That phenomenon is not restricted to individuals with AIDS. It is also the basis for malakoplakia (195–199), "histoid" cutaneous infections caused by *Mycobacterium leprae* (200,201), and florid lymphoid hyperplasia of the terminal ileum in patients infected with *Yersinia* (202).

As outlined in the foregoing material, pseudoneoplastic proliferations are potentially encountered in virtually all the topical areas of anatomic pathology, including cytopathology. Thus, they represent a truly-protean challenge with many possible implications for patient care and case outcome. All pathologists must bear those facts in mind during day-to-day practice, in order to guard against misinterpretations.

Table 1.1 presents a synopsis of this discussion in tabular form, separated into organ systems.

This volume, *Neoplastic Mimics in Thoracic and Cardiovascular Pathology*, provides comprehensive descriptions, discussion, and images of the lesions summarized in the table as pertinent to the lungs, pleural surfaces and mediastinum; and to the heart and blood vessels. For similar coverage of the other systems and categories of lesions shown in the table, the reader is referred to the other volumes of the Neoplastic Mimics series of atlases.

TABLE 1.1 Selected Examples of Pseudoneoplastic Lesions and Related Neoplastic Imitators

SKIN
Cutaneous non-melanocytic nevi & hamartomas (Epithelial & mesenchymal neoplasms)
Lymphoid hyperplasias (Lymphomas)
Reactions to Monsel's solution (Sarcomas; sarcomatoid carcinomas)
Acroangiodermatitis (Kaposi's sarcoma)
Proliferating scars & posttraumatic spindle-cell nodules (Mesenchymal tumors; sarcomatoid carcinomas)
Intravascular papillary endothelial hyperplasia (Masson's lesion) (Vascular neoplasms)
Pseudocarcinomatous epithelial hyperplasia (Squamous cell carcinoma)
"Rudimentary meningocele" (Mesenchymal neoplasms)
Ruptured ganglion cyst (Acral myxoinflammatory sarcoma)
Mycobacterial pseudotumors (Mesenchymal neoplasms)
Bacillary angiomatosis (Hemangiomas)
Kimura disease (Hypereosinophilic syndrome; eosinophilic leukemia)
SOFT TISSUE
Neuromuscular choristoma (Peripheral nerve sheath neoplasms)
Fibrolipomatous hamartoma (Lipomas)
Nodular fasciitis (Sarcomas)
Proliferative myositis (Sarcomas)
Myositis ossificans (Osteosarcoma)
"Tumefactive fibroinflammatory lesions" (Fibromatoses)

(Continued)

TABLE 1.1 Selected Examples of Pseudoneoplastic Lesions and Related Neoplastic Imitators *(Continued)*

Florid (tumefactive/focal) lymphocytic myositis (Lymphoma)
"Atypical decubital" (ischemic) fibroplasia (Sarcomas)
BONES & JOINTS
"Bizarre osteochondromatous proliferations" (Nora's lesion) of digits (Cartilaginous neoplasms)
Synovial chondrometaplasia/chondrocalcinosis (Cartilaginous neoplasms)
Fibrous dysplasia and "fibro-osseous lesions" (Osteosarcoma & fibrosarcoma)
Proliferative-phase Paget's disease of bone (Osteosarcoma)
Aneurysmal bone cyst (Telangiectatic osteosarcoma)
Giant cell reparative granuloma (Giant cell tumor)
Avulsion fractures of ischial tuberosities (Osteosarcoma)
"Brown tumor" of hyperparathyroidism (osteitis fibrosa cystica) (Giant cell tumor)
BREAST
Radial scar (Low-grade ductal adenocarcinoma)
Choristoma (Hamartoma) (Metaplastic carcinoma)
Proliferative adenosis (Low-grade ductal adenocarcinoma)
Extramedullary hematopoiesis (Invasive lobular carcinoma)
Collagenous spherulosis (Adenoid cystic carcinoma or intraductal carcinoma)
Pseudoangiomatous stromal hyperplasia (Angiosarcoma)
NERVOUS SYSTEM
Gliosis (Low-grade gliomas)
Active-phase plaques of multiple sclerosis (Gliomas)
Progressive multifocal leukoencephalopathy (Gliomas)
Paraventricular glial nodules of tuberous sclerosis (Gliomas; Gangliogliomas)
Viral encephalitides (Lymphoma)
ENDOCRINE SYSTEM
Sclerosing & proliferative Hashimoto's thyroiditis (Anaplastic carcinomas & lymphomas)
Nodular thyroid hyperplasia (Thyroid adenomas and differentiated thyroid carcinomas)
Nodular parathyroid hyperplasia (Parathyroid adenoma)
Nodular adrenal hyperplasia (Adrenocortical adenoma)
Adrenal myelolipoma (Liposarcoma)
LYMPHORETICULAR SYSTEM
Selected lymphoid hyperplasias (Lymphomas)
Florid oligoclonal hyperplasia in bone marrow recovery (Myelodysplasia; Leukemia)
Infection-related hemophagocytic syndrome (T-cell lymphoma)
Epstein–Barr virus-related atypical lymphoid hyperplasias (Large-cell lymphoma)
Mycobacterial pseudotumors (Dendritic-cell tumors)

(Continued)

TABLE 1.1 Selected Examples of Pseudoneoplastic Lesions and Related Neoplastic Imitators *(Continued)*

UPPER AIRWAY
Pseudocarcinomatous epithelial hyperplasia (Squamous cell carcinoma)
Oral organ of Chievitz (Low-grade squamous or mucoepidermoid carcinoma)
Necrotizing sialometaplasia (Squamous or mucoepidermoid carcinoma)
Radiation effects on mucosal epithelia (Squamous carcinoma)
Benign lymphoepithelial lesion of salivary gland (Lymphomas)
Traumatized antral/choanal polyps (Polypoid sarcomatoid carcinomas)
Glial heterotopias (Peripheral nerve sheath tumors)
Benign fibro-osseous lesions (Low-grade fibrosarcoma or osteosarcoma)
LOWER AIRWAY
Pseudocarcinomatous epithelial hyperplasia (Squamous cell carcinoma & adenocarcinoma)
Atypical bronchiolar & alveolar epithelial hyperplasia (Carcinomas)
Fibrohyaline plaques of pleura & fibrohyaline pleuritis (Desmoplastic mesothelioma)
Florid mesothelial hyperplasia (Epithelial mesothelioma)
Localized tumefactive organizing pneumonia (Inflammatory sarcomatoid carcinoma)
Selected examples of lymphocytic interstitial pneumonia (Lymphoma)
Pulmonary chondroid/lipomatous/muscular hamartomas (Metaplastic carcinomas)
MEDIASTINUM
Sclerosing mediastinitis (Sclerosing carcinomas, lymphomas, or germ-cell tumors)
Thymic dysplasia (Thymoma)
Proliferating thymic cyst (Thymic squamous carcinoma)
Benign mesothelial inclusions in mediastinal lymph nodes (Metastatic carcinoma)
ALIMENTARY TRACT
Pseudocarcinomatous epithelial hyperplasia (Adenocarcinoma)
Enteritis/colitis cystica profunda (Adenocarcinoma)
"Adenomyoma" of duodenum (Well-differentiated adenocarcinoma)
Tumefactive chronic pancreatitis (Well-differentiated ductal adenocarcinoma or lymphoma)
Mycobacterial pseudotumors (Sarcomas)
Bacillary angiomatosis (Hemangiomas)
Florid lymphoid hyperplasia (Lymphomas)
Hepatic bile duct hamartoma (Metastatic adenocarcinoma)
Hepatic focal nodular hyperplasia (Fibrolamellar hepatocellular carcinoma)
Inflammatory "cloacogenic" polyp (Tubulovillous adenoma)
Chronic tumefactive pancreatitis (Low-grade pancreatic ductal adenocarcinoma)
Xanthogranulomatous cholecystitis (Sarcomatoid carcinoma)

(Continued)

TABLE 1.1 Selected Examples of Pseudoneoplastic Lesions and Related Neoplastic Imitators *(Continued)*

GENITOURINARY TRACT (MALE & FEMALE)

- Pseudocarcinomatous epithelial hyperplasia (Carcinomas)
- Postoperative spindle cell nodules (Sarcomas; Sarcomatoid carcinoma)
- Drug effects (e.g., cytoxan cystitis mimicking carcinoma in situ) (Urothelial carcinoma)
- Proliferative prostatic urethral (utricular) polyp (Adenocarcinoma)
- Paratesticular mycobacterial pseudotumor (Sarcomas)
- Lymphoplasmacytic orchitis (Lymphoma)
- Xanthogranulomatous nephritis/cystitis/orchitis/endometritis/oophoritis (Carcinomas)
- Adenomatous and basal-cell prostatic hyperplasia (Adenocarcinoma)
- Cribriform intraductal prostatic hyperplasia (Adenocarcinoma)
- Nodular stromal prostatic hyperplasia (Low-grade sarcoma)
- Prostatic sclerosing adenosis (Adenocarcinoma)
- Radiation effect on prostatic epithelium (Residual adenocarcinoma)
- Granulomatous prostatitis/orchitis (Sclerosing carcinoma & sclerosing seminoma)
- Vaginal adenosis (Adenocarcinoma)
- Uterine cervical mesonephric remnants (Adenocarcinoma)
- Uterine cervical microglandular adenosis (Adenocarcinoma)
- Ovarian stromal hyperplasia/hyperthecosis (Ovarian stromal neoplasms)
- Nephrogenic metaplasia of bladder and urethra (Adenocarcinoma)
- Endometriosis (Adenocarcinoma)

CARDIOVASCULAR SYSTEM

- Rhabdomyomatous hamartomas of myocardium (True "adult" rhabdomyoma)
- Endodermal choristoma of interatrial cardiac septum (Metastatic adenocarcinoma)
- Lipomatous hypertrophy of the heart (Lipoma)
- Mesothelial-monocytic intracardiac excrescences (Metastatic adenocarcinoma or mesothelioma)
- Endocardial and myocardial lymphocytic infiltrates after transplantation (Lymphomas)
- Florid pericardial mesothelial hypeplasia (Epithelial mesothelioma & metastatic adenocarcinoma)

Part I
Thoracic Pathology

2

Pseudoneoplastic Lesions of the Lung

There are relatively few pathological conditions that are considered pseudoneoplastic lesions of the lungs. Paradoxically, however, they appear to account for more cases in absolute numbers than neoplastic simulators in most other organ systems. As is true of "pseudotumors" elsewhere, some pulmonary lesions under this rubric may eventually prove to have clonal attributes in the final analysis. However, at the present time, only a select few are generally regarded as malformative or reactive tumor-like proliferations. Although they have often been included in the past in discussions of "pseudotumors" (203), nodular amyloidoma, hyalinizing granuloma, and rounded atelectasis ("shrinking pleuritis") are likely to be confused with neoplasms only by clinicians and radiologists, rather than pathologists. Hence, those lesions are not considered here.

BRONCHOPULMONARY HAMARTOMAS

The term "hamartoma" was first coined in 1904 by Albrecht (204) to designate a tumor-like malformation that was composed of an abnormal admixture of "appropriate" tissue components. This concept, however, is still not universally embraced and should therefore be considered in evolution. Synonyms and related names for pulmonary hamartoma (PH) include "benign mesenchymoma," "fibroma," "chondroma," "fibrochondrolipoma," "fibrolipomyochondroma," "hamartoma-chondroma," "cartilage-containing tumor of the lung," "adenochondroma," "lipochondroadenoma," "adenofibrolipochondromyxoma," and "mixed tumor."

In an autopsy series, McDonald et al. (205) reported that the incidence of PHs was that of 20 in 7,972 cases, representing 0.25%. Bronchial hamartoma exists in two forms: central and peripheral. The latter type is 2 to 3 times more common in men than in women, but the central variant shows no gender difference (206,207). On chest radiographs, these lesions are found as asymptomatic nodules, usually during the fifth or sixth decade of life (**Figure 2.1**). However, several have been reported in teenagers, and the youngest patient on record was 9 years at diagnosis (208). Hamartomas of the lung have never been documented as congenital lesions. Rarely, they may be multifocal.

Carney et al. have described a complex in young women wherein chondroid intrapulmonary masses are part of a triad of lesions including extraadrenal paraganglioma and gastric epithelioid stromal tumors (209,210). Although they were formerly grouped with PHs, current thought holds that "Carney

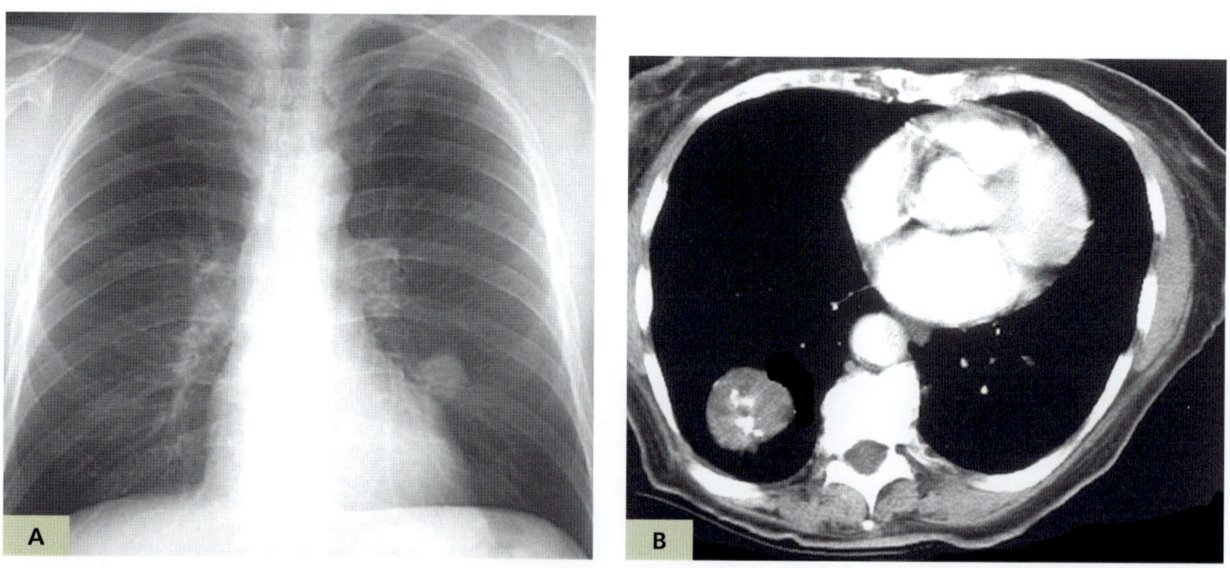

FIGURE 2.1 Plain chest films (A) and computed tomograms of the thorax (B) show well-demarcated and often-calcified peripheral masses in typical cases of pulmonary harmartoma.

chondromas" of the lungs are separate and distinct from them because of reproducible histological differences (**Figure 2.2**). To date, no studies have been done to assess the possible clonality of syndromic pulmonary chondroid masses in the context of "Carney's triad."

Table 2.1 summarizes the general clinical and pathologic features of PHs as seen in several published series (211–214). Grossly, most lesions of this type are found in the peripheral aspects of the parenchyma, sometimes in association with small bronchi or bronchioles. They are exquisitely well circumscribed and vary in diameter from several millimeters to 20 cm. The more uncommon

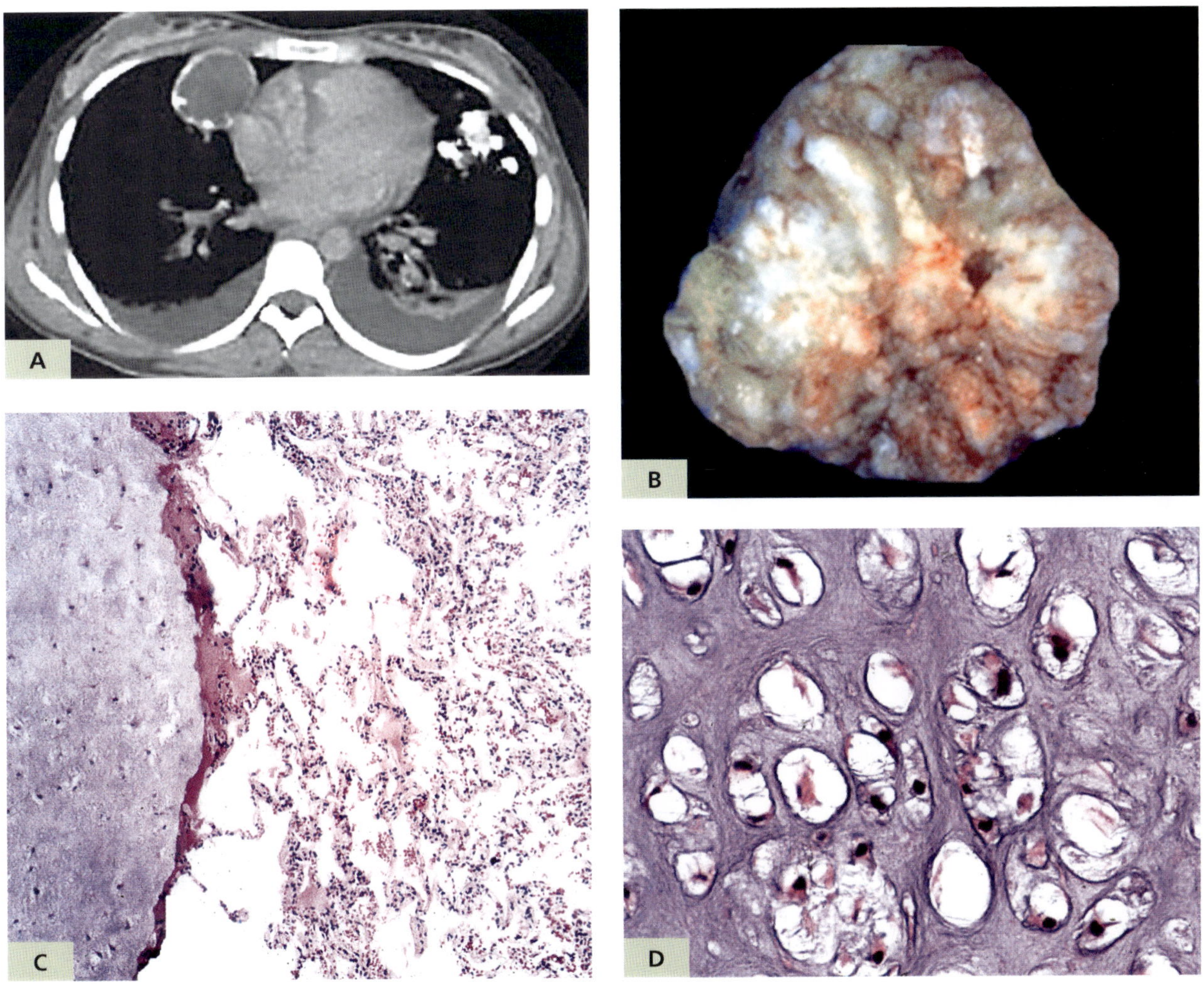

FIGURE 2.2 "Carney"-type chondromas (CTCs) are true neoplasms of the lung that differ from chondroid hamartoma in several respects, although they may be similar in imaging studies (A, this particular patient also has unrelated pleural effusions). CTCs show sharp circumscription, allowing for their "shelling-out" by the surgeon (B). However, they do not exhibit entrapped and proliferating small airways at their peripheral aspects (C), as true of hamartomas. The substance of CTCs is uniformly cartilaginous (D), and does not show an admixture of other tissues as do hamartomas.

central type of hamartoma arises in large bronchi and grows as an endobronchial polypoid mass that is covered by respiratory mucosa. All these lesions—regardless of whether they are central or peripheral—are lobulated with a consistency on cut sections that varies according to histologic constituency (**Figure 2.3**). Most contain substantial cartilaginous tissue and are therefore hard or resilient.

At a histologic level, both central and peripheral PHs are composed of a disorganized proliferation of mature mesenchymal tissues. These, most typically, are represented by cartilage but may also include fibrous tissue, smooth muscle,

TABLE 2.1 Clinical and Pathologic Features of Pulmonary Hamartomas

FEATURE	VAN DEN BOSCH ET AL. (1987) (211)	SALMINEN (1990) (212)	HANSEN ET AL. (1992) (213)	WANG SC ET AL. (1992) (214)
Number of cases	154	77	89	507
Male/female	116:38	43:34	51:38	1.74:1
Mean age (y)	51	ND	57.5	41.4
Range	14–74	ND	14–76	-67
Mean transverse diameter (cm)	2.1	2.27	2.17 + 1.62	3.0
Range	0.8–7.0	1–8	—	—
Pulmonary symptoms (%)	11/154	ND	39	55.7
Peripheral type (parenchymal)	12	ND	ND	30
Central type (endobronchial)	142	ND	ND	467
Recurrence	2	ND	ND	ND

Abbreviation: ND, not described.

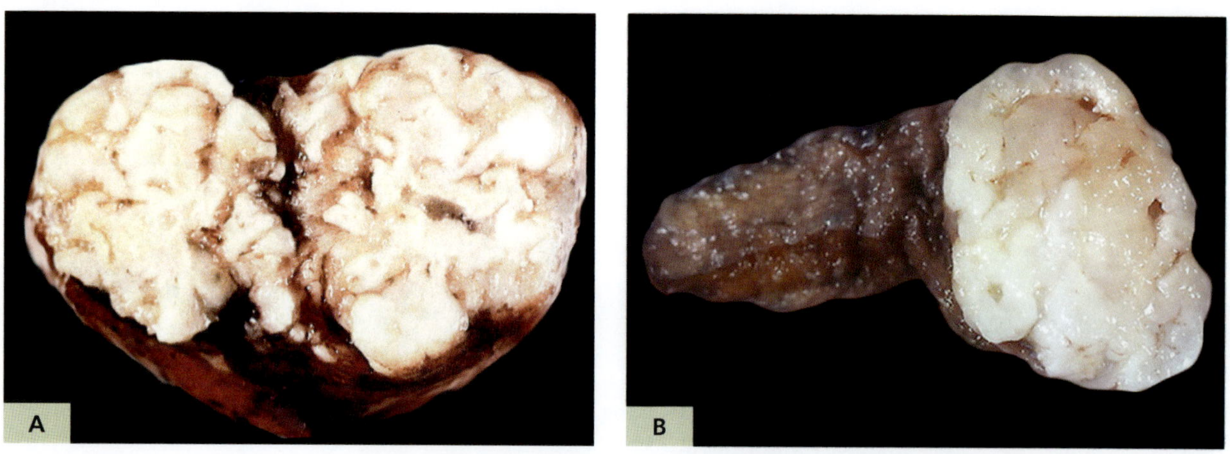

FIGURE 2.3 A & B: Pulmonary chondroid hamartomas bulge away from the cut lung parenchyma and have a lobulated appearance.

or adipocytic elements **(Figure 2.4).** When the lesions lack cartilage, they have been called intrabronchial lipoma, myxoma, leiomyoma, or fibroadenoma in the prior literature, depending on the microscopically predominant elements. As PH expands, the mesenchymal proliferation surrounds and entraps adjacent airways, and it therefore appears to include tubular structures that are lined by respiratory epithelium **(Figure 2.5)**. The latter tissue may be cuboidal or low columnar; in addition, metaplasia, hyperplasia, and papillary change may be observed in entrapped airway elements. Transthoracic fine-needle aspiration biopsy has become a popular and reliable method for the diagnosis of pulmonary mass lesions, and Hamper et al. were able to secure a diagnosis of PH by such means in 12 of 14 patients (215). Indeed, when this lesion is favored diagnostically by

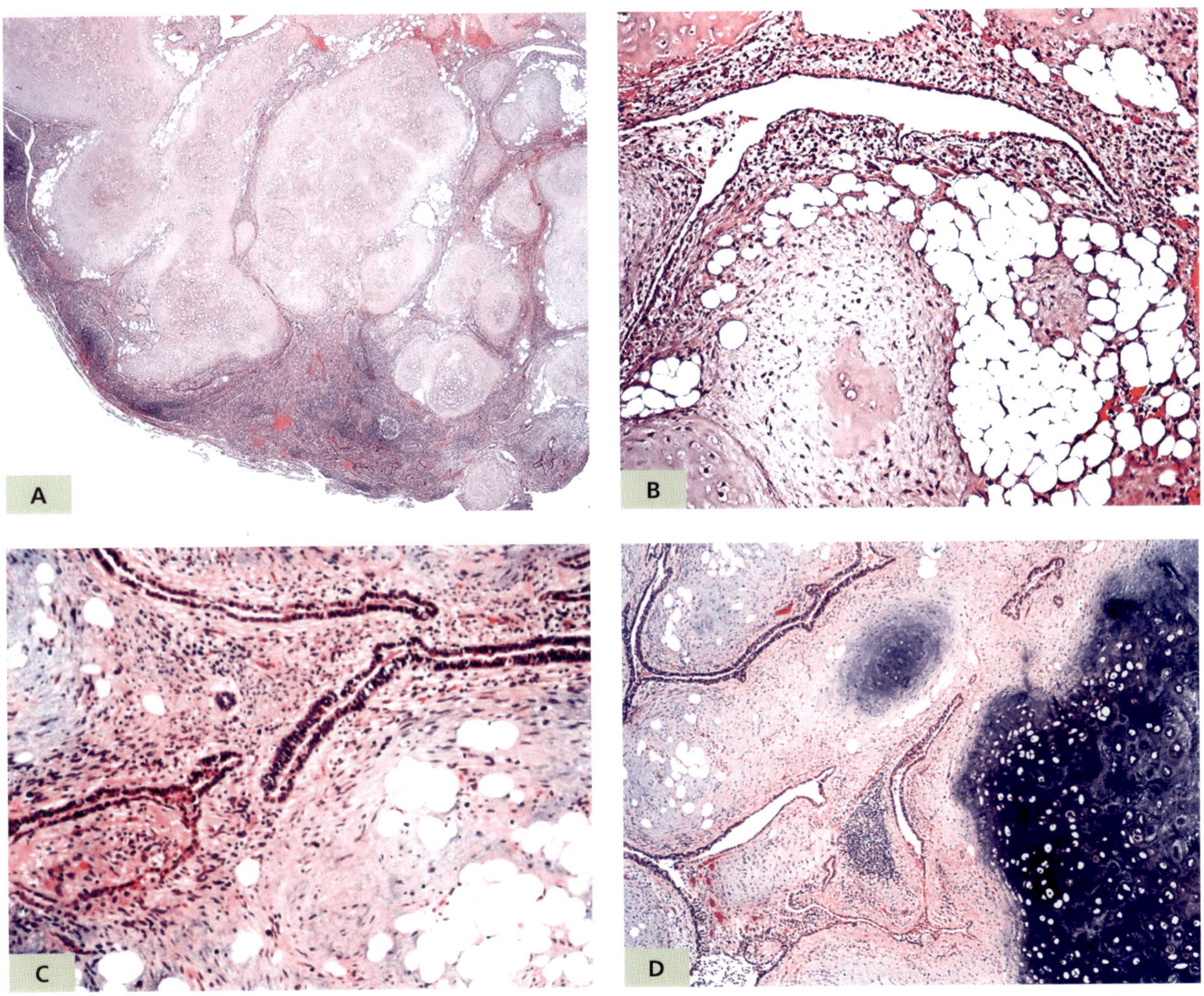

FIGURE 2.4 A–D: In keeping with the macroscopic appearance of pulmonary hamartomas, they are lobulated lesions at a histological level as well. Admixtures of fatty and cartilaginous elements are common in such masses.

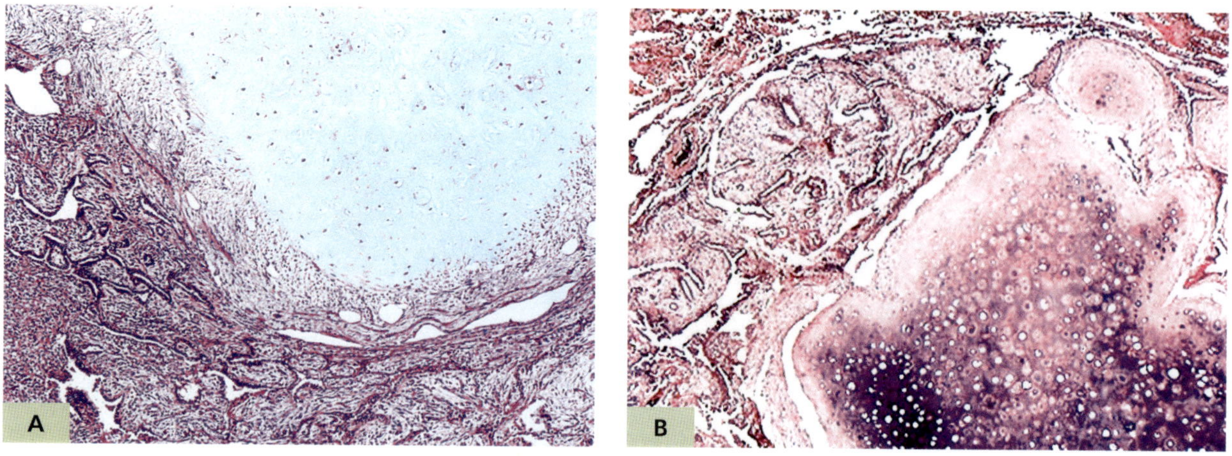

FIGURE 2.5 A & B: Entrapped and proliferating small airways are consistent findings at the peripheral aspects of pulmonary hamartomas.

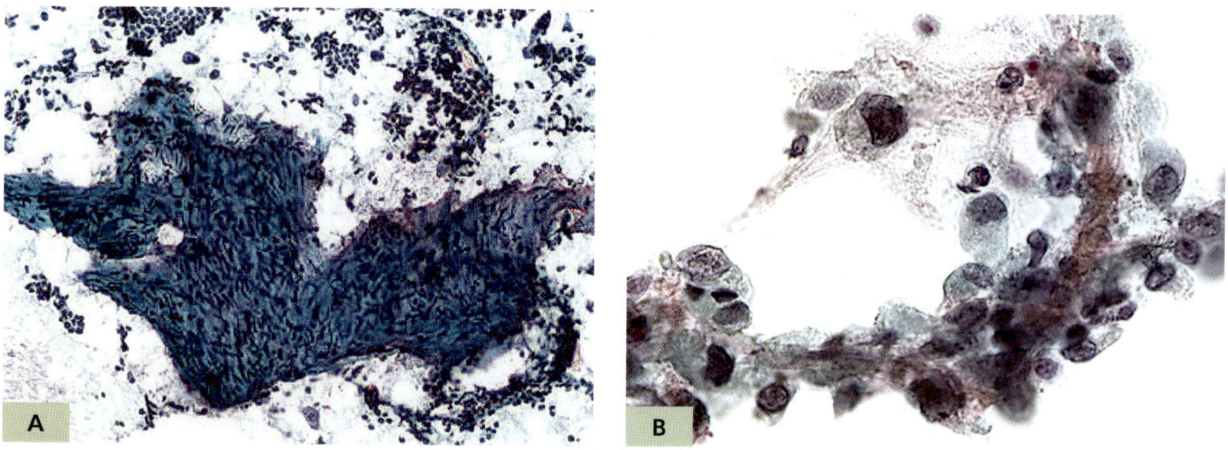

FIGURE 2.6 Pulmonary hamartoma usually is dominated by its mesenchymal components on fine-needle aspiration biopsy (A). However, the trapped epithelial elements in such lesions may demonstrate nuclear atypicality (B), potentially causing a misdiagnosis of malignancy.

the radiologist (a common occurrence), aspiration biopsy **(Figure 2.6)** can be pursued in hopes of avoiding a thoracotomy to establish the nature of the mass.

In the past, the epithelial component in PH has been considered to represent an integral part of the lesion from its inception. However, the studies of Bateson (216–218) have established that it is merely entrapped by the mesenchymal components. Surfactant-containing intranuclear inclusions are sometimes observed in the epithelium (219), in likeness to those seen in bronchioalveolar carcinomas that are composed of type 2 pneumocytic elements. In regard to the mesenchymal components of PH, ultrastructural studies have shown that primitive stellate cells may demonstrate zones of transition to cartilage (220,221). Cytogenetic analysis of cells from PH in short-term culture has also revealed an abnormal karyotype in several instances (222). The most characteristic aberration is an exchange of chromosomal material between 6p21 and 14q24 (223). Break points in this region appear to be related to those seen in uterine leiomyomas. Hence, such information reopens the question of whether pulmonary "hamartomas" are neoplastic rather than malformative, and that issue is still unsettled.

PHs should be distinguished from *primary or metastatic sarcomas of the lung* (**Figure 2.7**) as well as *biphasic sarcomatoid carcinomas* (**Figure 2.8**).

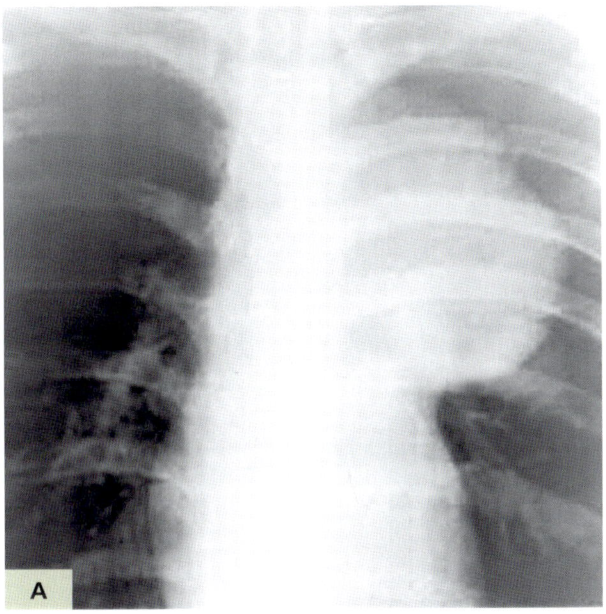

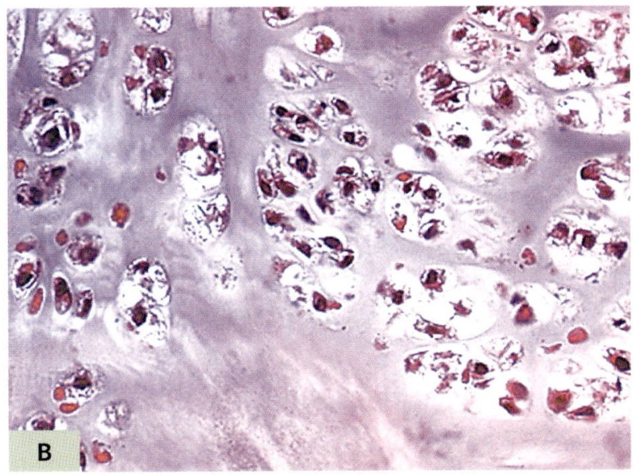

FIGURE 2.7 Primary intrapulmonary chondrosarcoma (PICS) enters the differential diagnosis of chondroid hamartoma. However, PICS shows a bulkier profile in imaging studies (A), and typically manifests hypercellular and cytologically-atypical areas, at least focally (B).

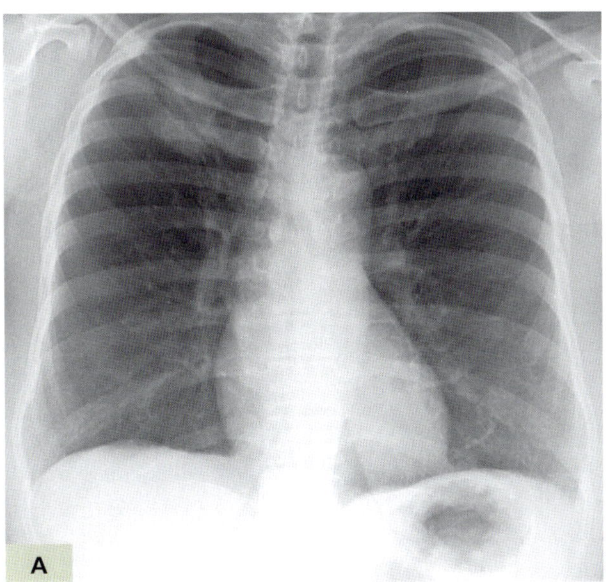

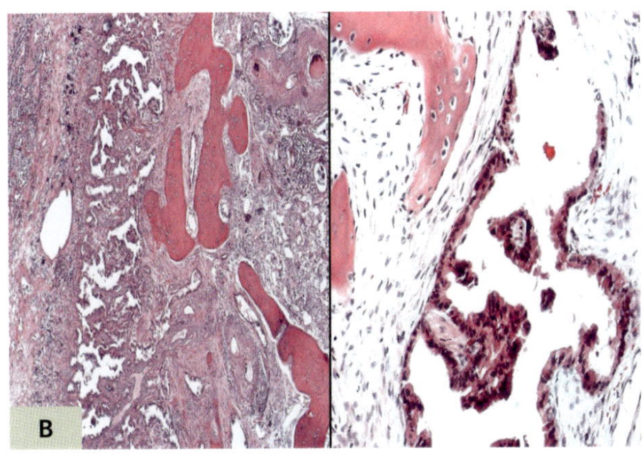

FIGURE 2.8 A & B: Another true pulmonary neoplasm that may contain an admixture of glandular and mesenchymal-like tissue, potentially simulating a hamartoma, is represented by adenocarcinoma with metaplastic elements.

Multinucleated cells, cellular pleomorphism, and nuclear atypia—as expected in both sarcomas and carcinomas—are rarely, if ever, seen in PH, and mitotic activity and spontaneous necrosis are similarly absent. In regard to sarcomatoid carcinomas, keratin immunoreactivity is expected in both their mesenchymal-like and overtly epithelial elements (if present), whereas PH demonstrates epithelial markers only in entrapped alveolar and bronchial epithelium (224). Liebow made a distinction between "true" bronchial chondroma and PH based on whether there was lesional continuity with bronchial cartilage plates (225). Moreover, in retrospect, that separation seems arbitrary.

PHs continue to increase in size if left to their own devices, but they do so only very slowly and rarely cause significant morbidity. Generally, simple conservative excision of the lesions constitutes adequate therapy.

Advances in endoscopic equipment and laser technology have expanded the role of thoracoscopy to include video-assisted thoracoscopic excision of peripheral pulmonary masses, including PH (226). Yttrium Aluminum Garnet (YAG) laser treatment has likewise been undertaken successfully for patients with central hamartomas of the lung (227).

INFLAMMATORY PSEUDOTUMOR/PLASMA CELL GRANULOMA OF THE LUNG

The proliferative spindle-cell lesion known as "inflammatory pseudotumor" (IPT) of the lung has undergone much scrutiny in the past two decades. Most proliferations in that category are now generally regarded as true neoplasms that are composed of myofibroblasts (228,229). Those particular entities had previously been called the "fibrohistiocytic" subtype of pulmonary pseudotumor (230–232) but have now been renamed "inflammatory myofibroblastic tumors (IMTs)" (229). The lesion known as "calcifying fibrous pseudotumor" (233–236) debatably represents a related moiety, because at least some cases of both lesions have manifested a t(2;17) chromosomal translocation (237–239). Other pulmonary proliferations that were also formerly included in the category of IPT—namely, "plasma cell granulomas" and "tumefactive organizing pneumonia" (238–246)—probably do represent nonneoplastic masses with variable etiologies. Both of them are composed of inflammatory and mesenchymal cells, potentially including mature lymphocytes, plasma cells, mast cells, macrophages, eosinophils, fibroblasts, and myofibroblasts. There is also likely overlap between some of those lesions and others described in association with IgG4 sclerosing disease of the lungs.

As just defined, the true number of pulmonary IPTs that are *not* IMTs is unclear. Some observers have used "IPT" very broadly to describe circumscribed nodules, large irregular inflammatory masses, and segmental or lobar consolidations (247). Other observers have essentially abandoned the term altogether, preferring to give purely descriptive diagnoses.

The lesion in question shows no sex predilection and occurs over a broad age range, from 1 to 77 years, with a mean between 27 and 50 years **(Table 2.2)** (242). Approximately 50% complain of cough, hemoptysis, shortness of breath, chest pain, or combinations thereof. Chest radiographs usually show a single, sharply marginated, round or oval mass **(Figure 2.9)**, but the edges of large lesions may be more ill-defined (248,249). Some IPTs involve the pleural surface and retract it as seen on computed tomography (CT) of the thorax (259); as expected, those findings may falsely suggest the possibility of malignancy.

Pulmonary IPTs range in size from 0.5 to >30 cm (231,232). Most have well-defined margins macroscopically but do not show true fibrous capsules; the color and texture of such lesions on cut section is variable. Those that contain numerous inflammatory cells are tan-white and fleshy **(Figure 2.10)**, and those with a predominance of mesenchymal tissue are gray and firm. IPTs with secondary xanthomatization may be bright yellow and can also be friable. A few of these masses also exhibit areas of hemorrhage, necrosis, or calcification. Occasionally, IPTs may be sessile intrabronchial lesions, and they can

TABLE 2.2 Clinicopathologic Features of Pulmonary Inflammatory Pseudotumors

	BAHADORI AND LIEBOW (1973) (238)	SPENCER (1984) (230)	MATSUBARA ET AL. (1988) (231)	PETTINATO ET AL. (1990) (232)
Number of cases	40	27	32	19[a]
Mean age (y)	29	36	50	27
Age range (y)	1–68	4–76	2–77	2–72
Male/female	15:25	16:11	14:15	9:10
Symptoms present (%)	40	56	40	60
Previous respiratory infection (%)	5	37	25	21
Right/left lung	21/18	13/12	9/18	1/19
Size (cm)	0.8–1.2	ND	1–15	1.2–15
Follow-up:				
Well (%)	90	ND	100	91
Recurrence (%)	5	ND	7	9

Abbreviation: ND, not described.
[a]Original reports described 20 cases, but 1 case was of esophageal origin.

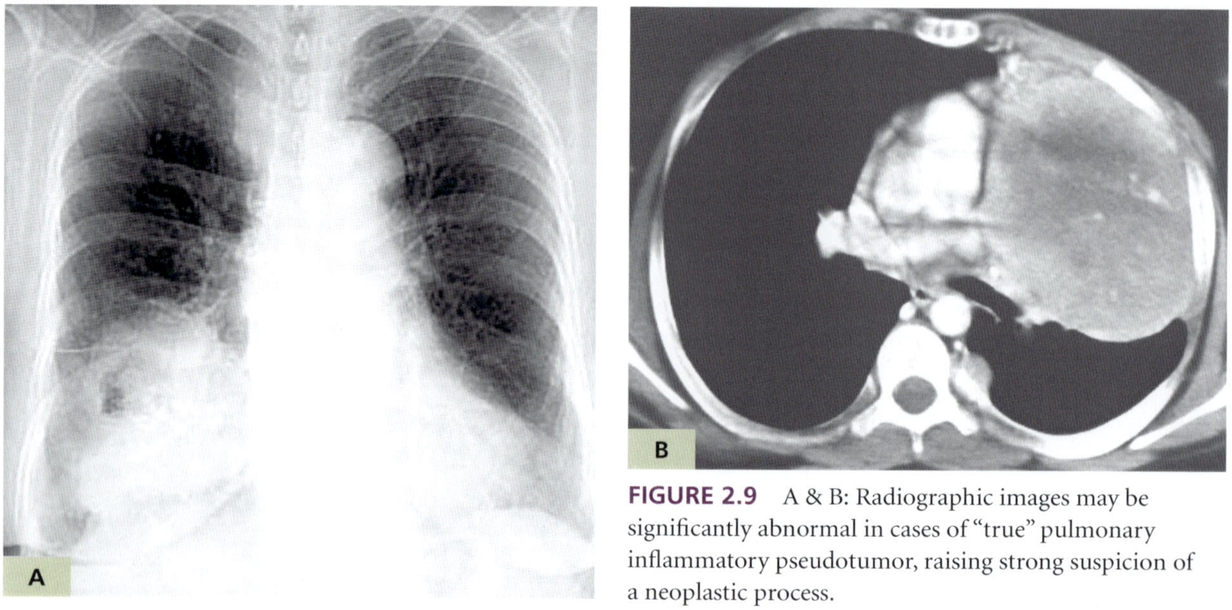

FIGURE 2.9 A & B: Radiographic images may be significantly abnormal in cases of "true" pulmonary inflammatory pseudotumor, raising strong suspicion of a neoplastic process.

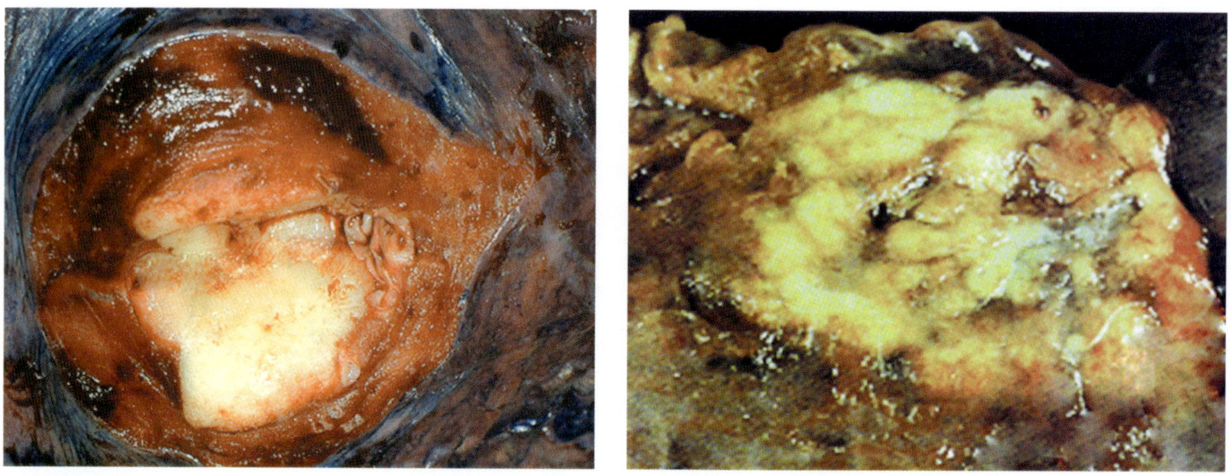

FIGURE 2.10 True inflammatory pseudotumors of the lung demonstrate mass-forming consolidation of the pulmonary parenchyma, and strongly suggest the possible presence of a neoplasm on gross examination.

also be attached to the pleura. In typical pulmonary IPT, the microscopic architecture of the lung is replaced by the lesional fibroinflammatory proliferation. Depending on their dominant cellular elements and major growth patterns, they may be subclassified into two types: "tumefactive organizing pneumonia-like" and "lymphoplasmacytic" (formerly "plasma-cell granuloma") variants (231). These may simply represent different stages in the evolution of IPT, but recent publications suggest that lymphoplasmacytic IPT (LPIPT) may belong to the family of systemic fibrosing autoimmune disorders that feature the presence of numerous IgG4-producing plasma cells (250–253).

The "organizing pneumonia-like" form of IPT shows intra-alveolar lymphohistiocytic inflammation and peripheral as well as central fibrosis **(Figure 2.11)**. Fibroblastic proliferation is admixed

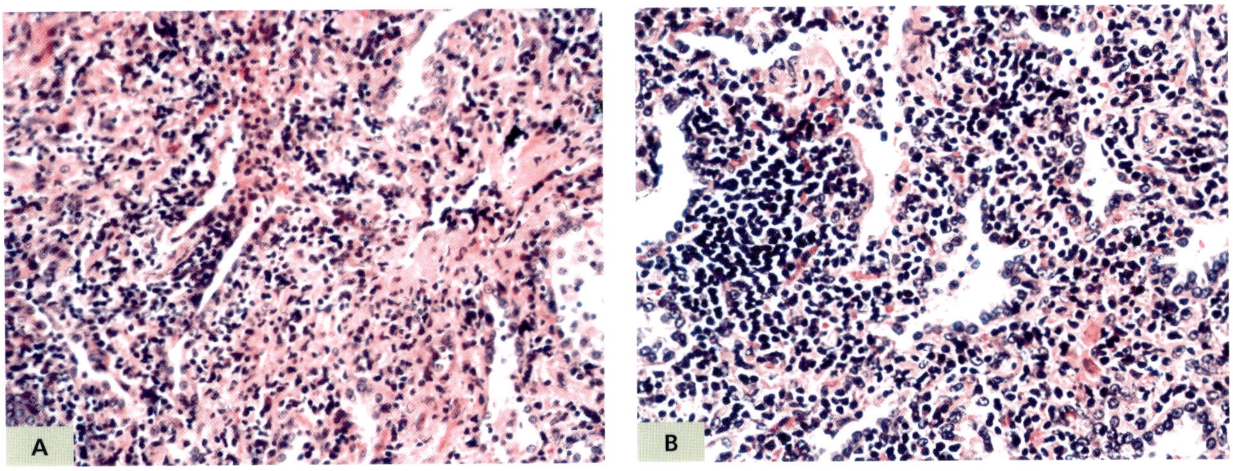

FIGURE 2.11 A & B: Inflammatory infiltration of the interstitium, with or without fibroblastic proliferation, is the basic histologic finding in true inflammatory pseudotumor of the lung.

with fibrino-inflammatory exudate in alveoli, alveolar ducts, and bronchioles. The alveolar architecture is preserved in early lesions and the peripheral portions of "mature" IPT, but it is obscured by superimposed fibrous tissue that tends to assume a whorled configuration. Neutrophils are sometimes interspersed with the lymphocytes and plasma cells, and they may form intralesional microabscesses that result in small areas of cavitation. Alveoli bordering IPTs are often filled with foamy macrophages and mantled by hyperplastic pneumocytes. Multinucleated cells of the Touton type are sometimes apparent within the masses, sometimes with foci of dystrophic calcification, osseous metaplasia, or myxomatous change. Lipoid pneumonia may develop in parenchymal areas where IPT has caused bronchial obstruction by intraluminal proliferation or impingement on the airway. Late in the evolution of IPTs, the lung tissue is replaced by deposition of mature collagen in broad bundles that transect the lesion **(Figure 2.12)**, sometimes with a keloidal appearance.

In the LPIPT, aggregates of plasma cells and lymphocytes constitute most of the lesion; germinal centers and a mature collagenous matrix may also be prominent **(Figure 2.13)** (250–253). Fibroblasts and xanthoma cells are usually relatively scant. The two histologic subtypes of IPT do overlap to some degree. As mentioned earlier, the immunohistological presence of IgG4-positive plasmacytes favors a diagnosis of LPIPT. Other findings that suggest this interpretation are the presence of endothelialitis; lymphangitic inflammatory infiltrates that are rich in plasma cells and histiocytes; and fibrinous pleuritis. Prominently dilated lymphatic spaces may be present, which contain histiocytes showing lymphemperipolesis; that feature is reminiscent of Rosai–Dorfman disease (RDD).

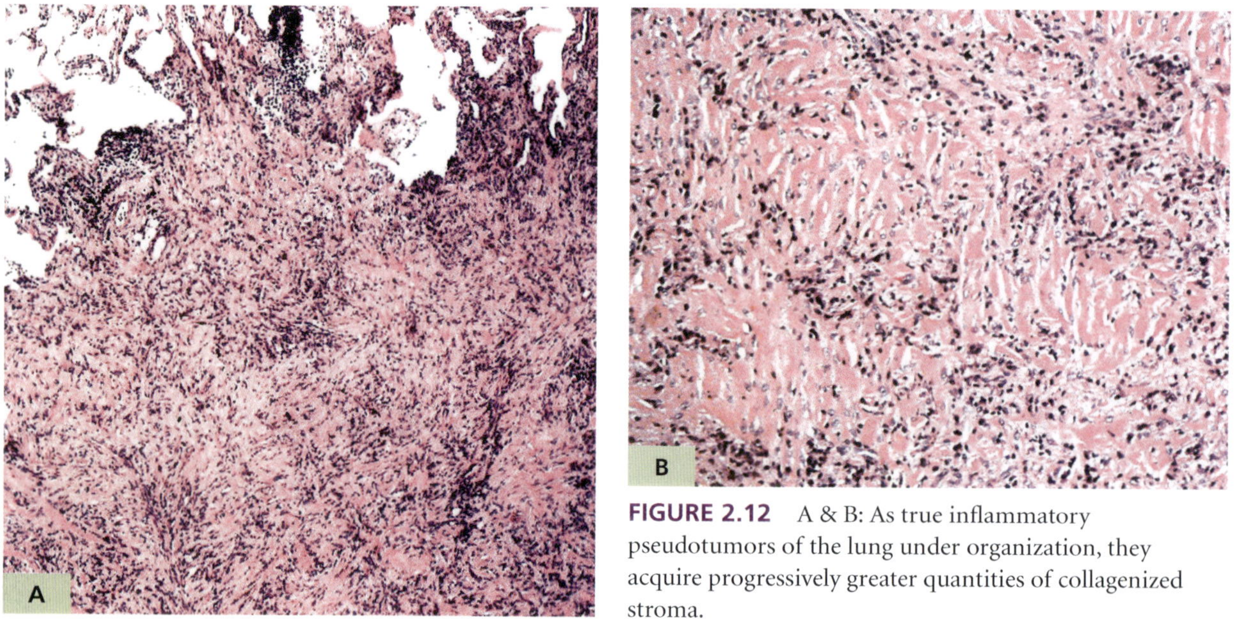

FIGURE 2.12 A & B: As true inflammatory pseudotumors of the lung under organization, they acquire progressively greater quantities of collagenized stroma.

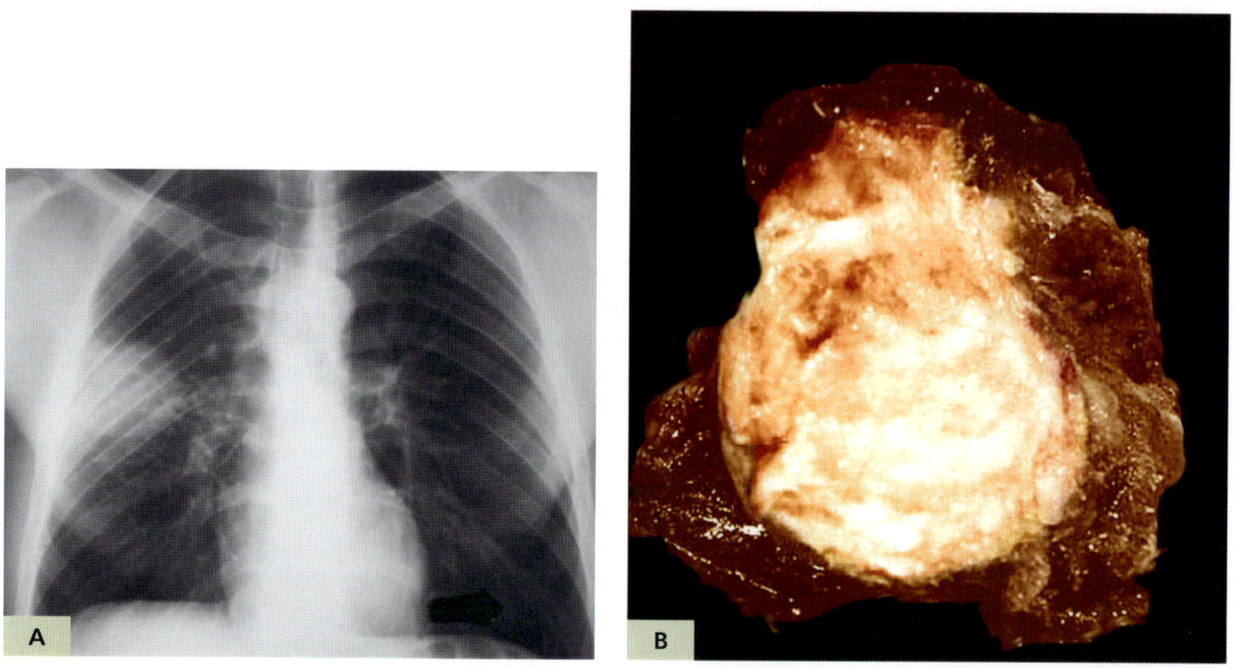

FIGURE 2.13 A–D: A particular subset of true inflammatory pseudotumors of the lungs appears to be mediated by an excess of IgG4-producing plasma cells, and it has been termed the "lymphoplasmacytic" variant of those lesions. (*Continued*)

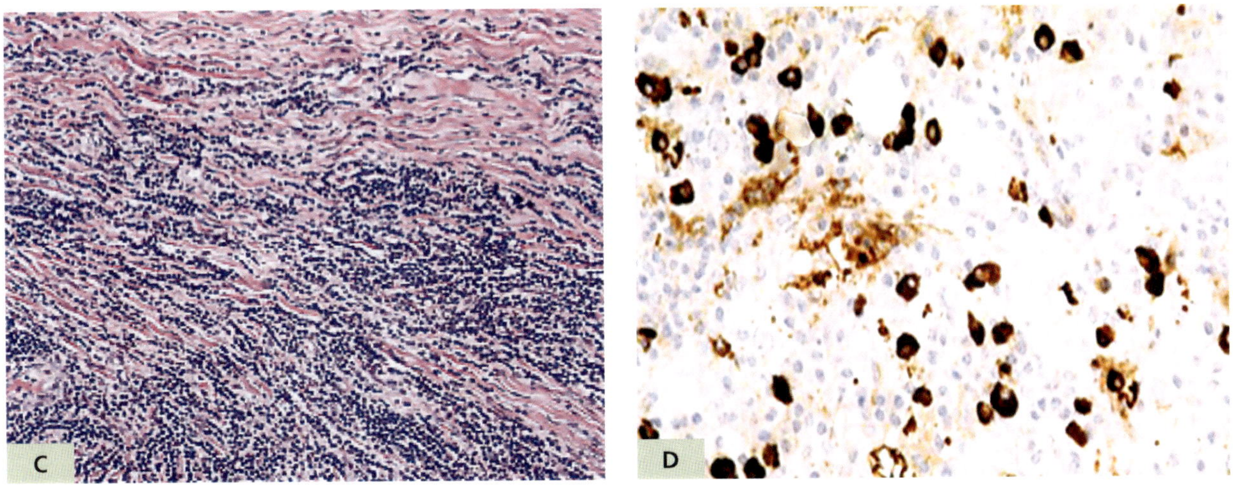

FIGURE 2.13 (*Continued*)

Neither form of IPT manifests solid sheets of lymphocytes or plasma cells, usually preventing diagnostic confusion with lymphoma or plasmacytoma. Nevertheless, Kojima et al. have reported rearrangement of the immunoglobulin heavy chain genes in a subset of LPIPT cases, raising the question of whether those particular lesions might be neoplastic or preneoplastic (254). Usually, however, both kappa and lambda light chain immunoglobulins are detectable immunohistologically in the lesional plasma cells, indicating a polytypic population (243). Lymphocyte-subset markers similarly show an admixture of B cells and T cells (229).

Matsubara et al. (231) found lymphocytic infiltration and scarring of vascular walls in several examples of IPT, often in association with organizing thrombi. These changes were thought to be secondary features rather than reflecting a primary vasculitic process.

The etiological factors for pulmonary IPTs are largely unknown. The idea that some represent peculiar forms of localized pneumonia has support from a history of a previous febrile illness and respiratory complaints in up to 40% of cases. Selected case reports have suggested that a morphologic similarity exists between IPT and tumefactive pulmonary infections with *Aspergillus*, rickettsiae, mycoplasma, various viruses, mycobacteria, *Cryptococcus*, corynebacteria, and other microorganisms (247–249,255–261). Rare examples have also been documented after trauma to the lung (262) and some were related to prior aspiration. As stated earlier, current hypotheses hold that LPIPT is probably part of a systemic autoimmune process (250–253).

The differential diagnosis of pulmonary IPT has been partially cited above. It includes *plasmacytoma* (263), *malignant lymphoma* (264,265) and *lymphoid hyperplasia* **(Figure 2.14)** (266), selected examples of "sclerosing hemangioma"

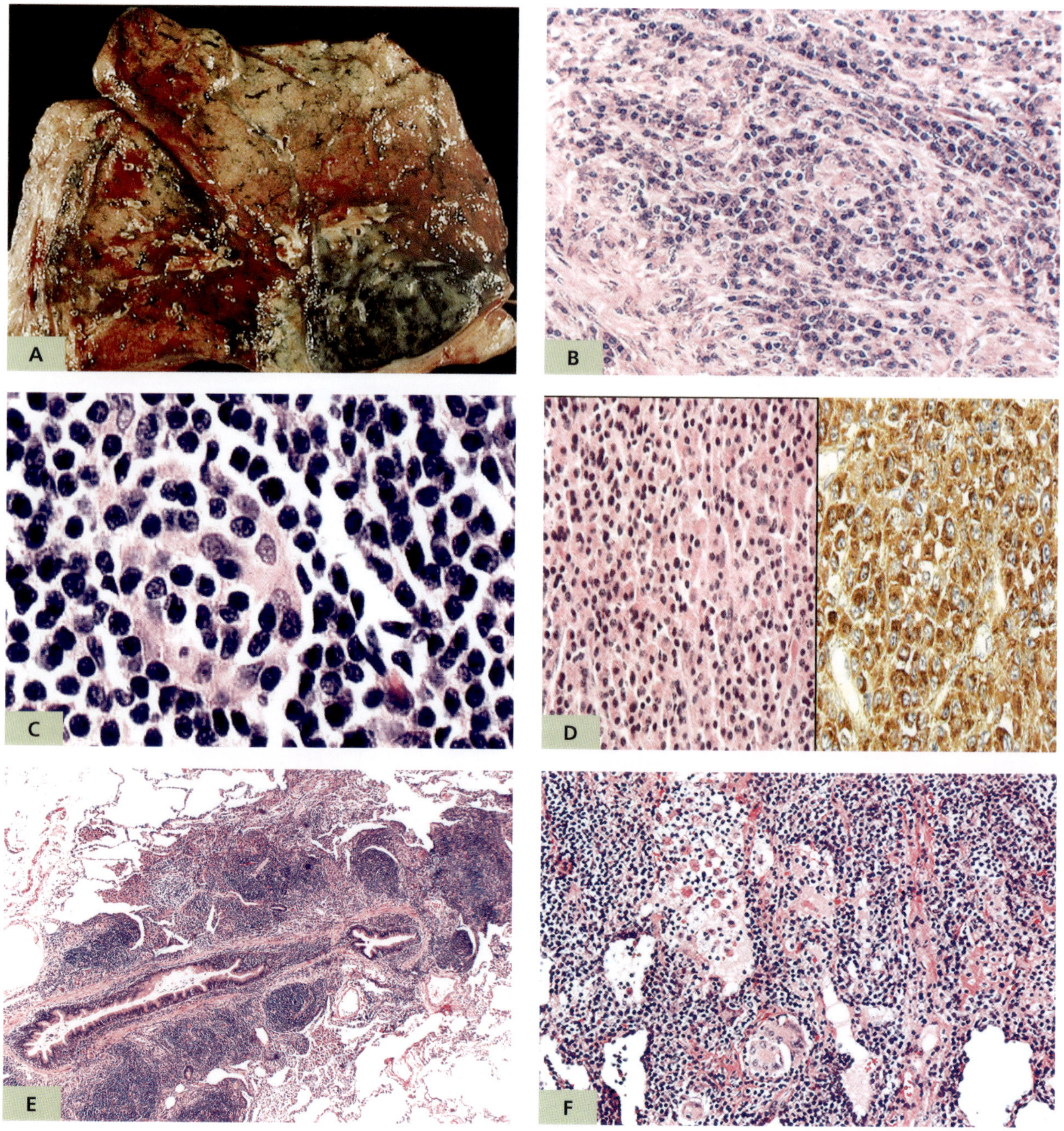

FIGURE 2.14 (A) All lymphoplasmacytic lesions of the lung are potentially comparable at a gross level. (B) They also may show histological similarities, including lymphoplasmacytic inflammatory pseudotumor; marginal zone lymphoma (C); plasmacytoma with monotypism for a light chain immunoglobulin (D); nodular pulmonary lymphoid hyperplasia (E); and lymphoid interstitial pneumonia (F). Correlation of clinical, radiographic, morphological, immunohistochemical, and molecular data is needed for definitive diagnosis in this group of disorders.

(SH) of the lung **(Figure 2.15)** (called "epithelial-plasma cell granuloma-like tumors" by Michal & Mukensnabl [267]), the peculiar variant of lung cancer

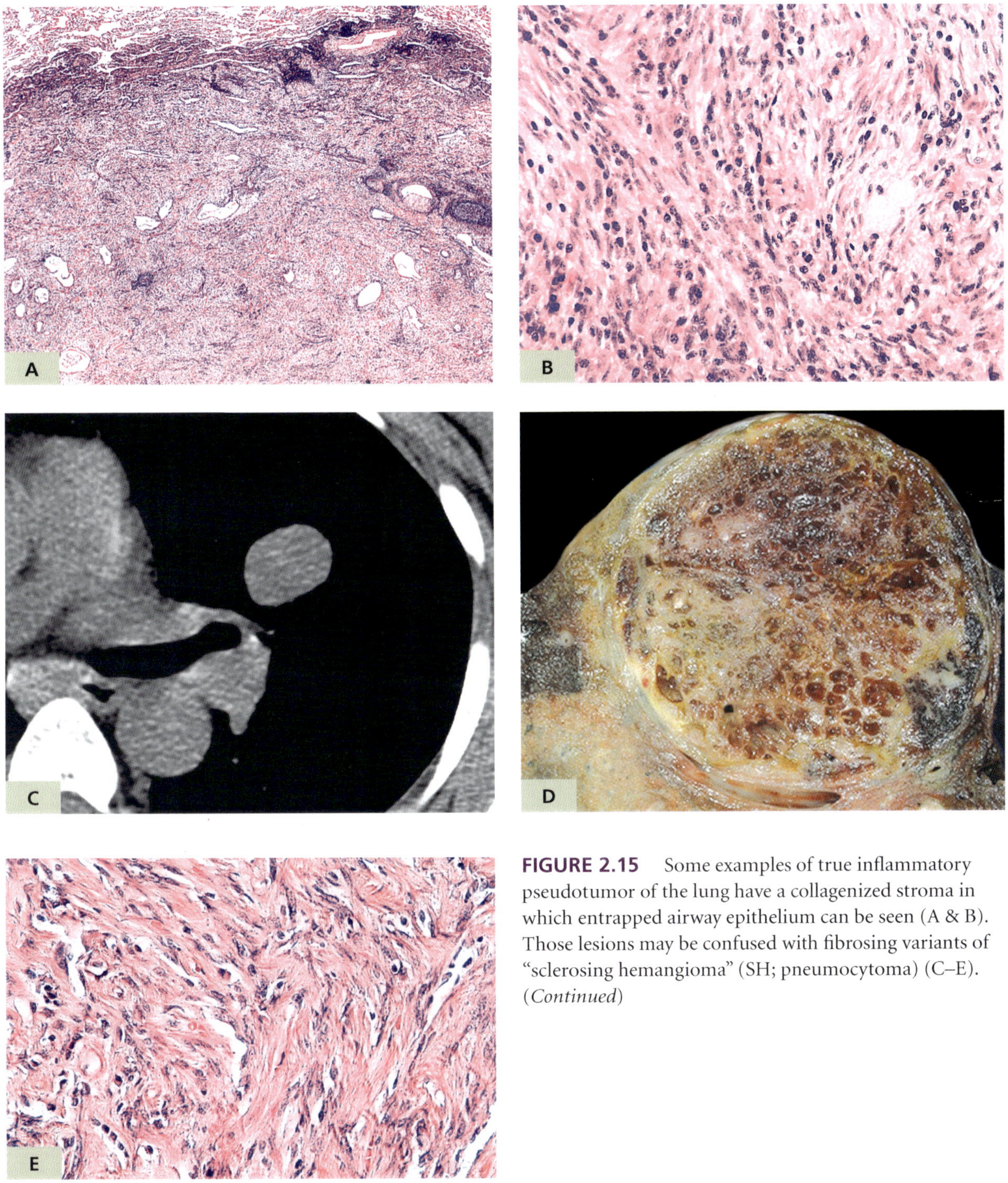

FIGURE 2.15 Some examples of true inflammatory pseudotumor of the lung have a collagenized stroma in which entrapped airway epithelium can be seen (A & B). Those lesions may be confused with fibrosing variants of "sclerosing hemangioma" (SH; pneumocytoma) (C–E). (*Continued*)

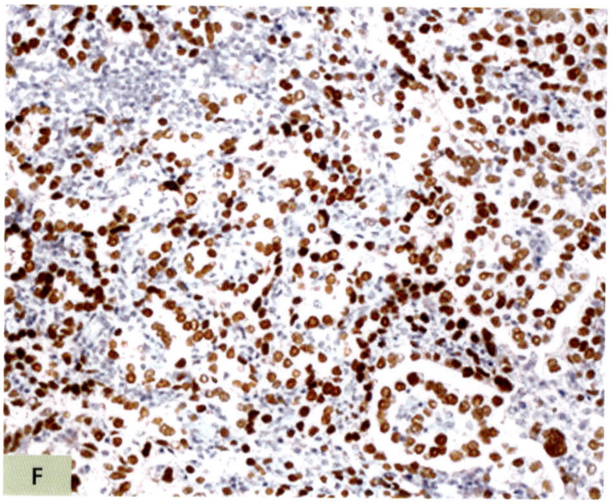

FIGURE 2.15 (*Continued*) A pulmonary neoplasm that contains epithelial cells with alveolar-pneumocytic differentiation, as shown by immunoreactivity for thyroid transcription factor-1 (TTF1) (F). The pattern of TTF1-positivity in SH is not seen in inflammatory pseudotumors.

known as "inflammatory sarcomatoid carcinoma" (268) (ISC) **(Figure 2.16)**, and *IMT* **(Figure 2.17)** (228,229). Among those conditions, plasmacytomas are singularly monotypic for cytoplasmic immunoglobulin, and selected lymphomas may also demonstrate that characteristic. Furthermore, malignant lymphomas are generally less well-circumscribed than IPTs, with more monotonous infiltrates of atypical lymphoid cells. Localized and diffuse forms of pulmonary lymphoid hyperplasia are composed predominantly of mature lymphocytes, in contrast to the heterogeneity of IPT. ISC can be separated from inflammatory mimics by its diffuse immunoreactivity for keratin. IMT contains significantly fewer IgG4-positive cells than those seen in IPT and may be immunoreactive for *ALK*-1 (258).

A minor difference of opinion exists as to whether or not "pulmonary hyalinizing granuloma" (PHG) (269) is a part of the spectrum of IPT or IMT in the lung. In our opinion, PHG shows more lamellar hyalinized collagen than is seen in classical IPT **(Figure 2.18)**. Moreover, hyalinizing granulomas of the lung are commonly multifocal, whereas IPT usually is not (269). SHs (270) were once considered to be related to IPT, but the former of those lesions is now known to be an epithelial neoplasm with pneumocytic differentiation (271). SH may be sclerotic in part, but it also contains aggregates of bland cuboidal cells as well as micropapillary and angiomatoid areas. Inflammation is absent or scanty in SH, and its constituent cells express thyroid transcription factor-1 (271); those of IPT do not. Ledet et al. (272) have examined the utility of immunostains for mutant p53 protein in the diagnostic separation of IPTs from low-grade intrapulmonary sarcomas. In their hands, p53-immunoreactivity was confined to malignant lesions but was not seen in all of them.

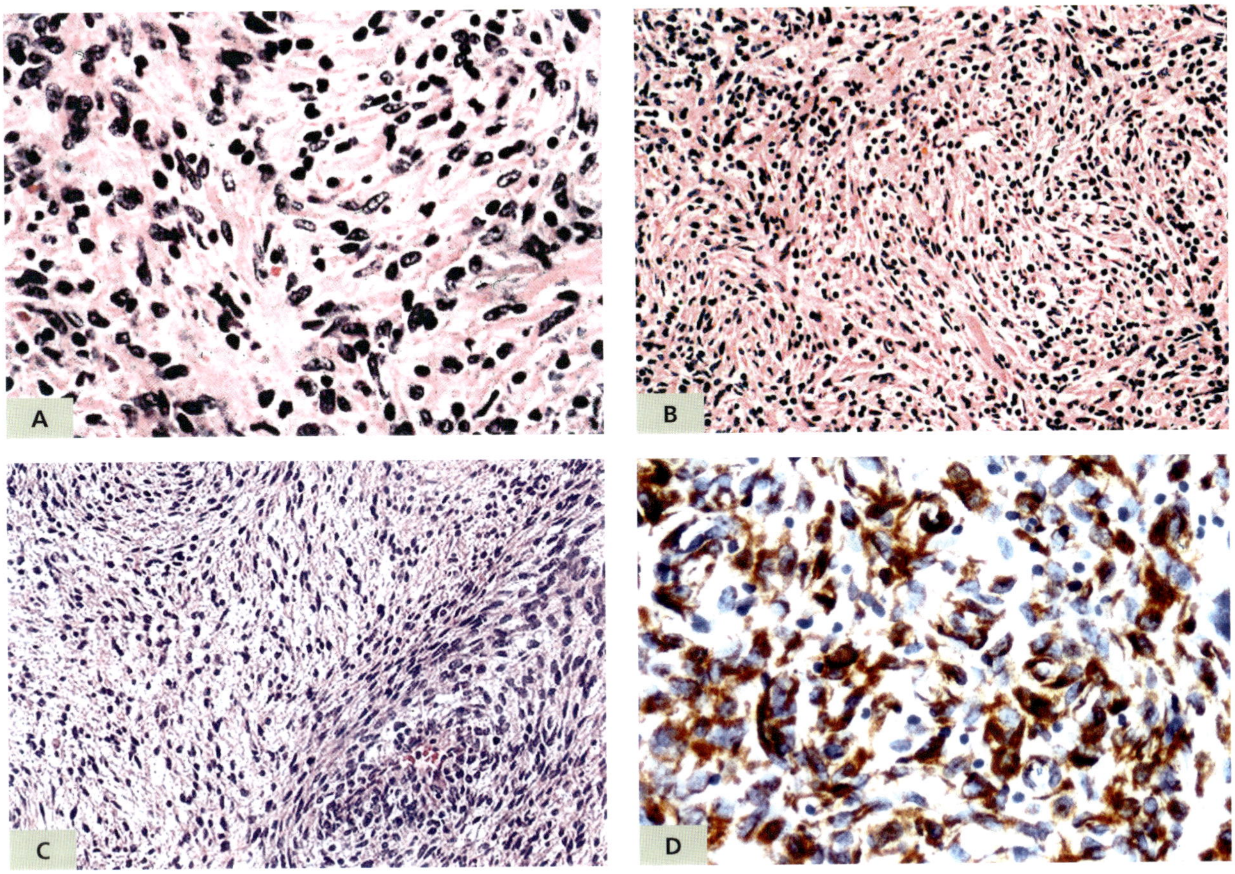

FIGURE 2.16 Another pertinent differential diagnosis for true inflammatory pseudotumor (TIP) (A & B) concerns inflammatory sarcomatoid carcinoma (ISC). That lesion shows more nuclear atypia in proliferating spindle cells (C) and is immunoreactive for pankeratin (D), unlike TIP.

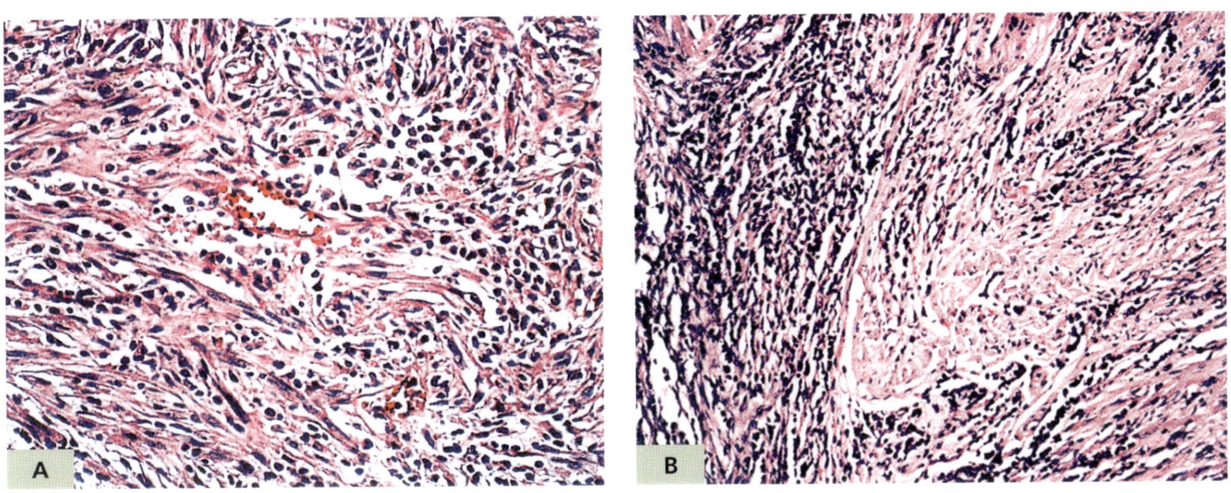

FIGURE 2.17 A particularly difficult diagnostic challenge is the separation of true inflammatory pseudotumor (TIP) (A & B) from inflammatory myofibroblastic tumor (IMT) (*Continued*)

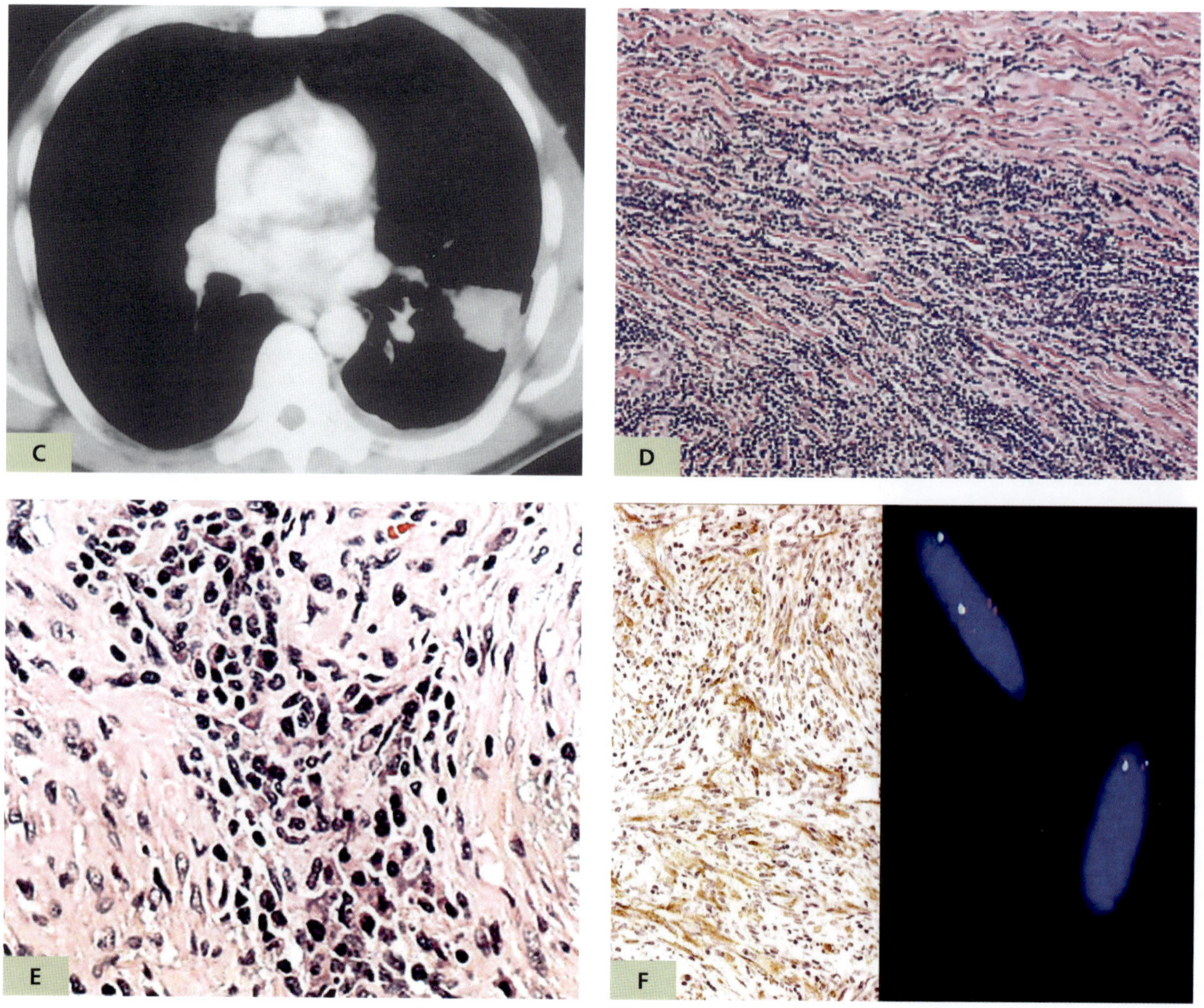

FIGURE 2.17 (*Continued*) (C–E). Those two lesions are closely similar morphologically, and a dispositive distinction between them can only be achieved by observing immunoreactivity for *ALK-1* protein (F, left) or rearrangement of the 2p23 gene complex by in-situ hybridization (F, right) in IMT.

Some examples of pulmonary IPT have been monitored for extended periods of time before excision or examination at autopsy (273–275). Information from such cases indicates that the lesions tend to grow very slowly. Spontaneous resolution has also been documented; a few lesions have regressed after incisional biopsies were done, or after systemic corticosteroids or irradiation were administered (273–275). Surgical removal is usually necessary to establish a definitive diagnosis of IPT, and, if the lesion has been completely excised, no further therapy is needed (248). Long-term follow-up of patients with pulmonary IPTs has shown no untoward clinical events in such cases.

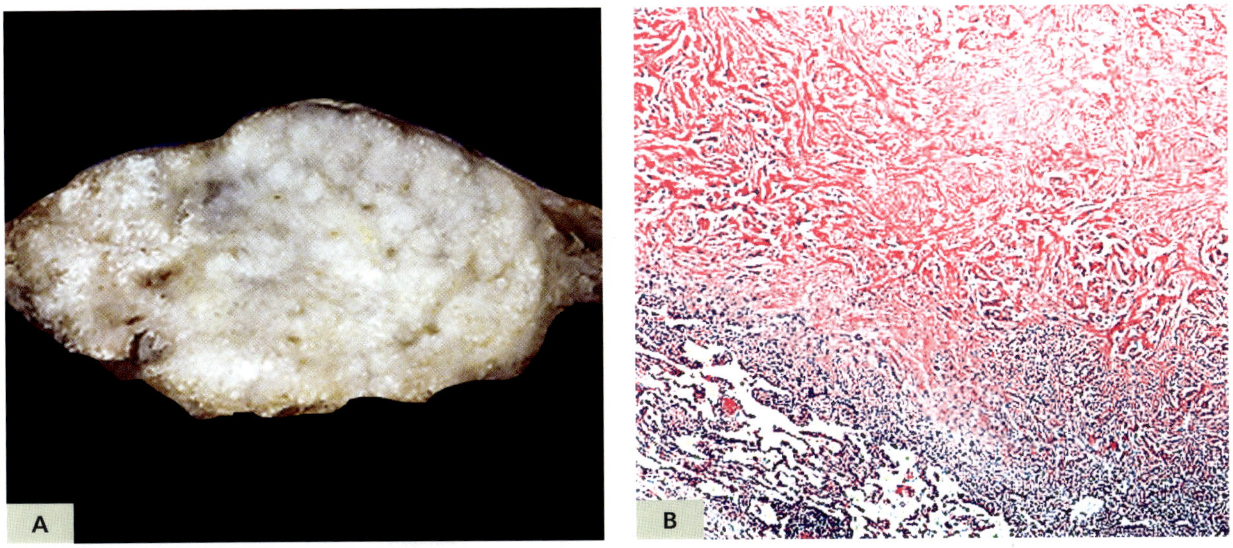

FIGURES 2.18 A & B: Pulmonary hyalinizing granuloma is probably a sclerotic form of lymphoplasmacytic inflammatory pseudotumor. It is typified by internal whorled profiles of mature collagen, and therefore may simulate sclerotic pneumocytoma (see Figure 2.15).

MYCOBACTERIAL SPINDLE-CELL PSEUDOTUMORS

Spindle-cell pseudotumors arising as a reaction to mycobacterial infection have been described in the skin, bone marrow, lungs, and lymph nodes in immunosuppressed subjects (276–279). These lesions closely resemble the histoid variant of leprosy (280), and the majority is caused by "atypical" mycobacteria (276–279).

Pulmonary mycobacterial pseudotumors (MPTs) are typified by multiple firm yellow–gray nodules, some of which are centered on small bronchi. Histologic sections show that these lesions consist of a rather uniform spindle-cell population with a fascicular growth pattern. Significant nuclear atypia and mitotic activity are generally not appreciated. Scattered lymphocytes and plasma cells are seen in the lesions, but there are no overt granulomas (**Figure 2.19**). The cytoplasm of the fusiform elements is usually "foamy," and hemosiderin can be present in the stroma. These features are similar to those of mycobacterial pseudotumors as reported in other locations. The proliferating cells are immunoreactive for lysozyme and CD68, with no reactivity for S100 protein, keratin, actin, CD34, podoplanin, or human herpesvirus-8 latent nuclear antigen-1 (HHV8-LNA). Ziehl–Neelsen or Fite stains typically demonstrate innumerable acid-fast bacilli in the lesions.

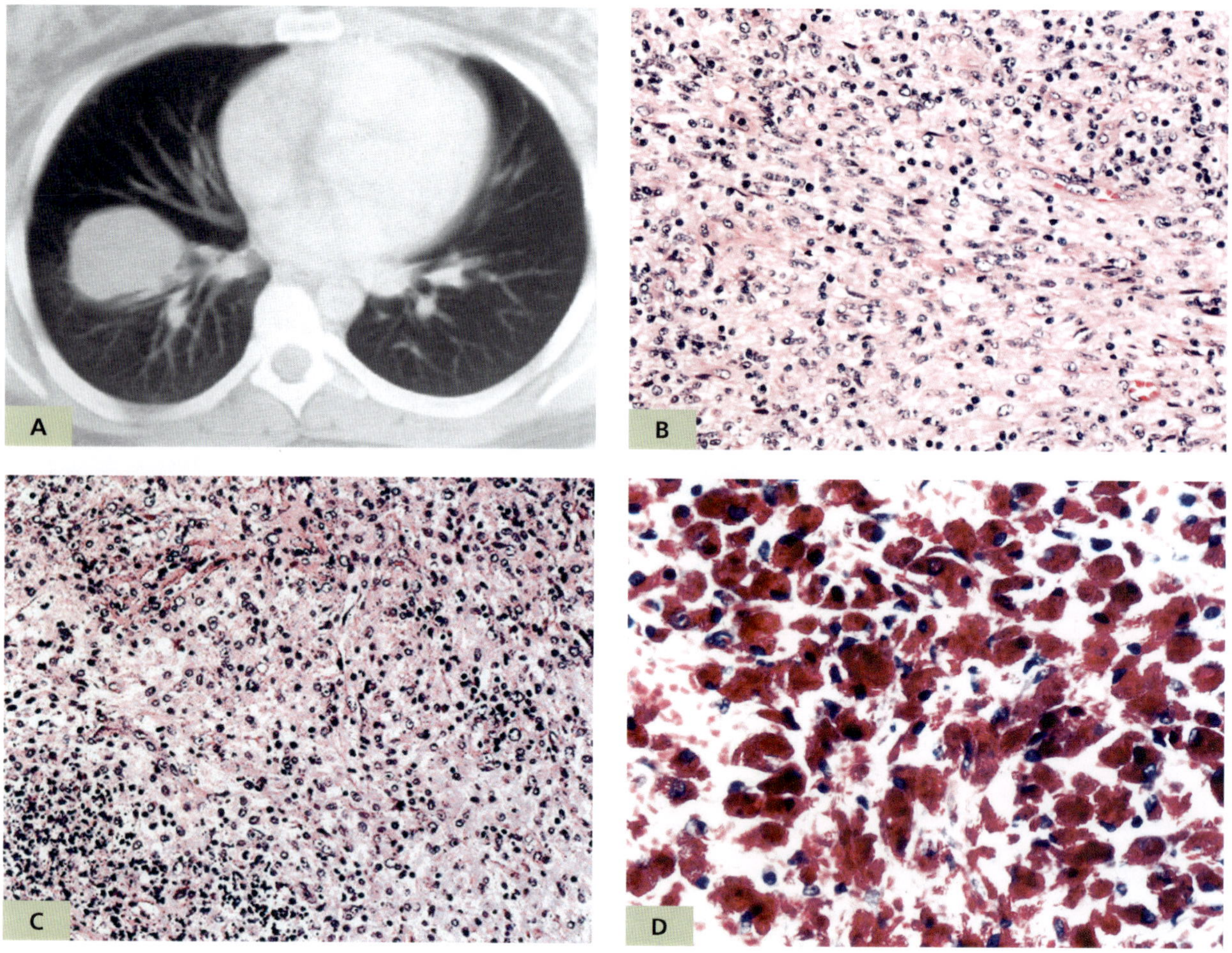

FIGURE 2.19 Tumefactive masses (A) comprising admixtures of inflammatory cells, histiocytes, and fibroblasts (B & C) may be caused by mycobacterial infections of the lung parenchyma in immunocompromised individuals. These may lead to diagnostic consideration of inflammatory myofibroblastic tumor and other spindle-cell neoplasms. Nonetheless, histochemical stains for acid-fast bacteria, such as the Ziehl–Neelsen method (D) are floridly positive in such cases.

Most examples of this entity in other anatomic sites have been associated with *Mycobacterium avium-intracellulare* or *Mycobacterium kansasii* (278). However, pulmonary MPTs have been linked to infection with *Mycobacterium tuberculosis* as well, as proven by culture results (281).

Another reported immunohistological feature of these lesions represents a potential source of diagnostic confusion. That is, there has been a reproducible cross-reaction of certain desmin antibodies with mycobacteria, erroneously suggesting the presence of a myogenic lesion (278). This is particularly problematic in the context under discussion here because *myogenic tumors* do indeed enter the differential diagnosis of MPTs. However, there is no concurrent immunostaining for actin isoforms, and ultrastructural features support histiocytic rather than myogenous differentiation in the lesions (281). Other processes that may be potentially imitated by MPTs include *Kaposi's sarcoma*, *malignant fibrous histiocytoma*, *ISC*, and *metastatic spindle-cell melanoma* (281) (**Figure 2.20**). A clinical history of immunosuppression should always raise the conceptual possibility of MPT in regard to a pulmonary spindle-cell lesion, and acid-fast stains will be confirmatory of the same. Features of malignancy, such as tumoral necrosis, marked nuclear atypia, and a high mitotic rate, are absent in mycobacteria-driven proliferations.

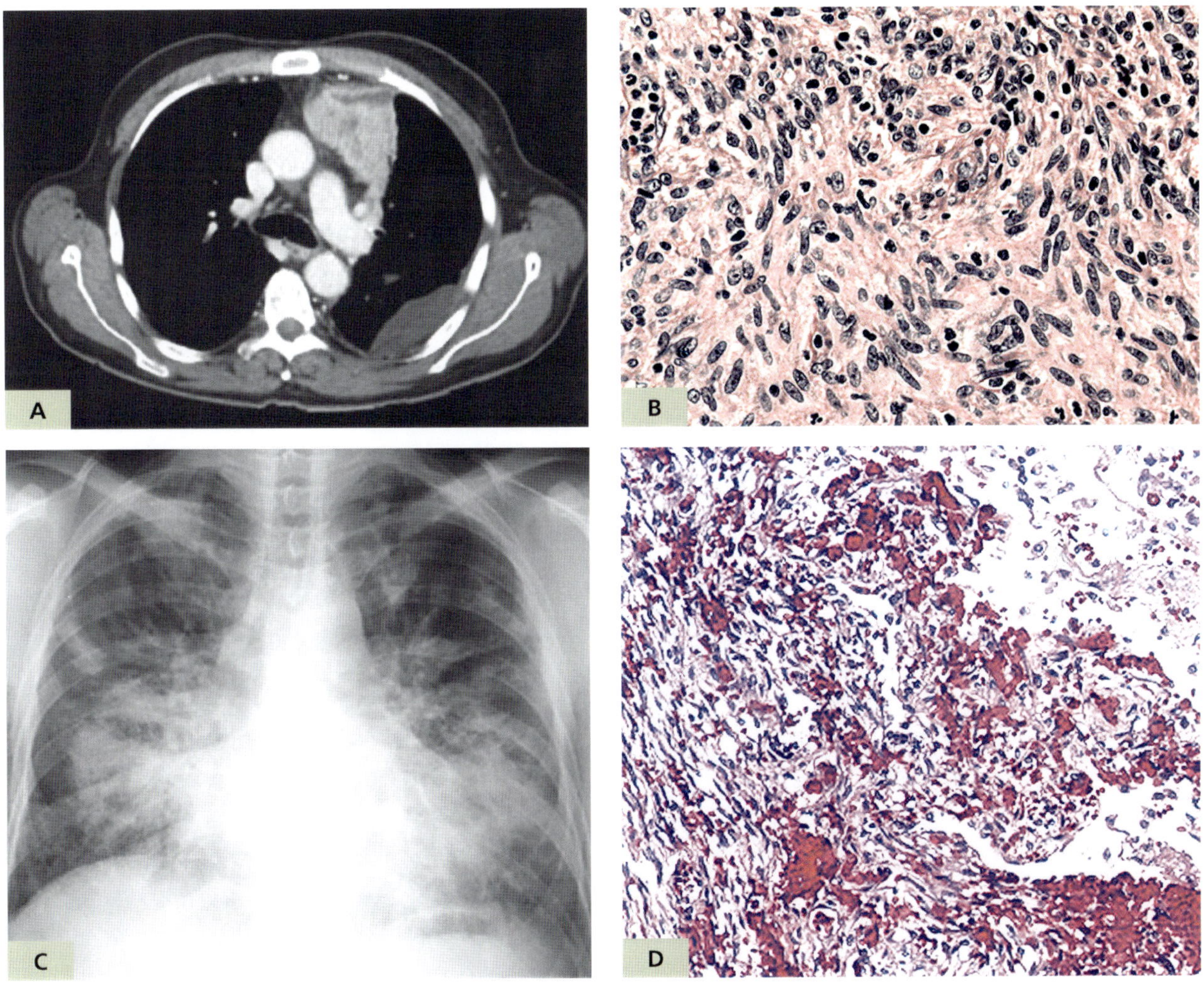

FIGURE 2.20 The differential diagnosis of pulmonary mycobacterial pseudotumor (A & B) includes Kaposi's sarcoma (C–F, immunostained for human herpesvirus-9-8 latent nuclear antigen-1); (*Continued*)

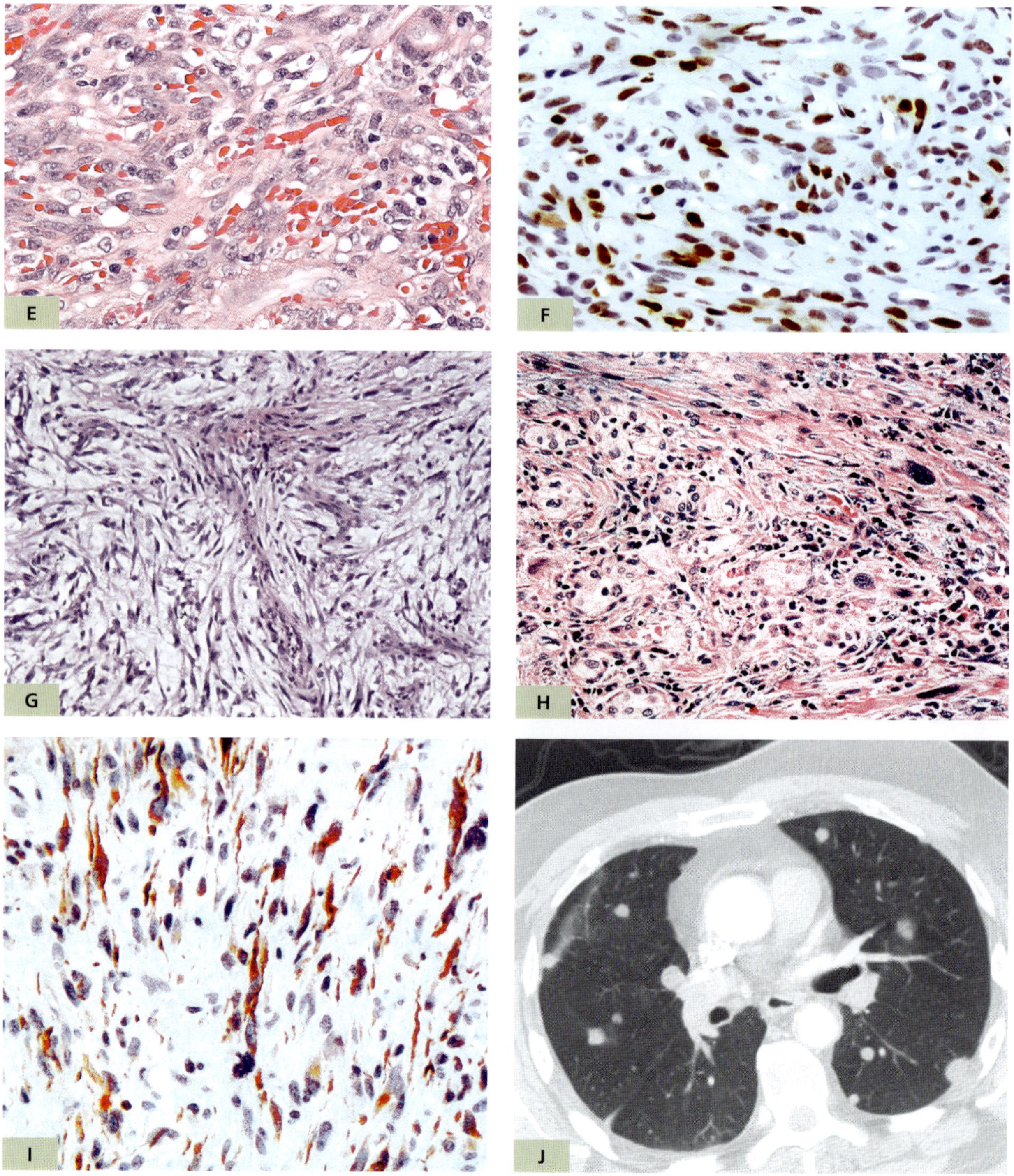

FIGURE 2.20 (*Continued*) malignant fibrous histiocytoma of the lung (G); inflammatory sarcomatoid carcinoma (H & I, immunostained for pankeratin); and metastatic sarcomatoid melanoma (J–L, immunostained for S100 protein).

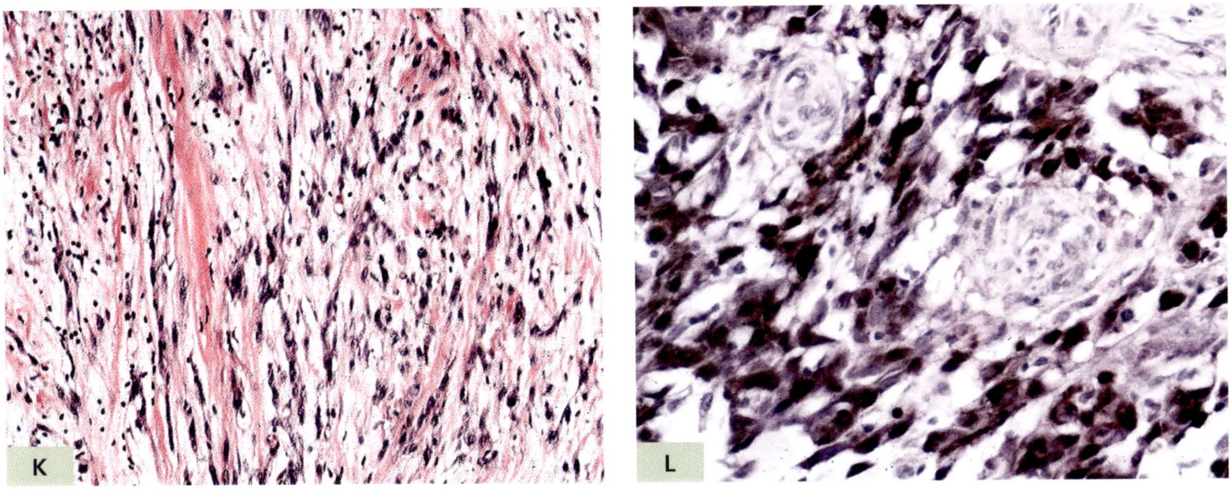

FIGURE 2.20 (*Continued*)

PULMONARY LYMPHOID HYPERPLASIAS

Controversy is still attached to the diagnosis of lymphoid infiltrates in the lungs, and it is associated with the use of such diagnostic terms as "lymphoid interstitial pneumonia (LIP)," "lymphoplasmocytic pneumonia," "plasmacytic interstitial pneumonia," and "pseudolymphoma." Our belief is that some of the latter entities—in particular, many examples of LIP and most cases of "pseudolymphoma"—are, in fact, low-grade *malignant lymphomas of the bronchus-associated lymphoid tissue* (so-called BALTomas) **(Figure 2.21)** (282,283). We shall here focus on examples of LIP that appear to ***lack*** evidence of clonality

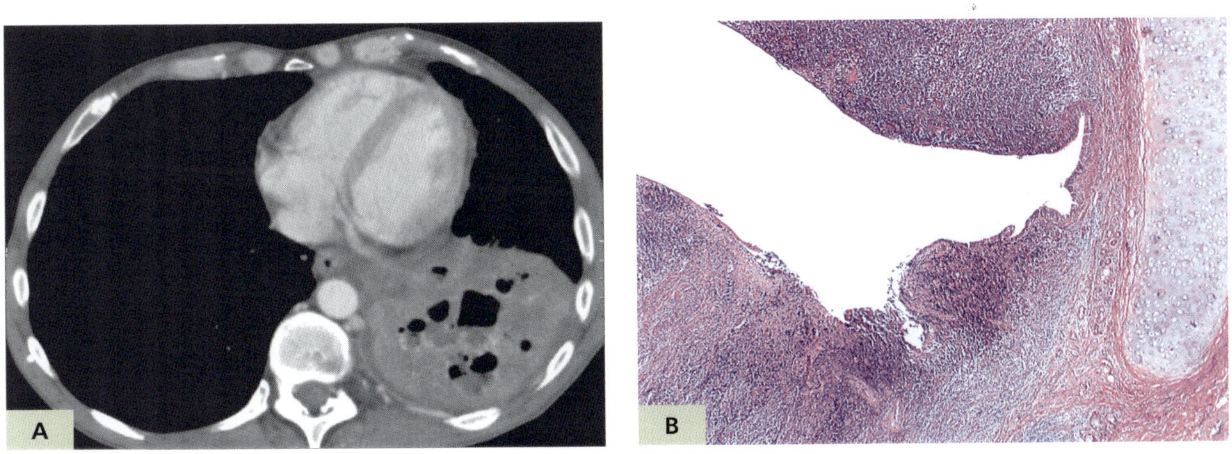

FIGURE 2.21 Marginal-zone lymphoma of the lung is often represented by a single mass (A). Histologic study shows a bulky infiltrate of small lymphocytes affecting the airways as well as the parenchyma (B & C); *(Continued)*

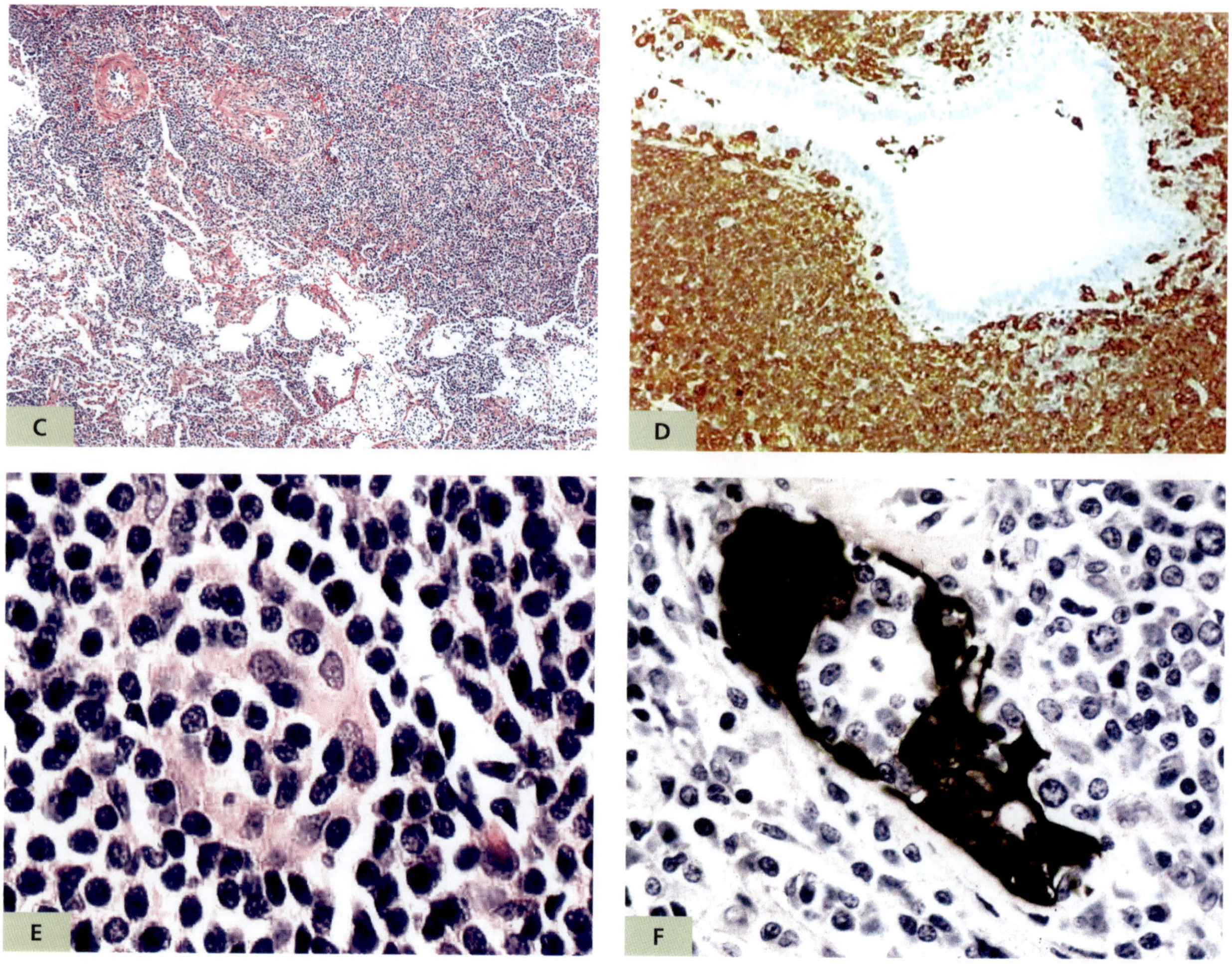

FIGURE 2.21 *(Continued)* the cells are predominantly reactive for B-lymphocyte determinants such as CD20 (D). "Lymphoepithelial lesions" (E) are apparent in which lesional lymphocytes permeate epithelial structures in the lung; these can be highlighted with pankeratin immunostains (F).

by genotypic analysis and therefore seem to qualify as peculiar tumefactive lymphoid hyperplasias. A portion of such lesions is related to infection with the human immunodeficiency virus (HIV) (284). We agree entirely with Koss (285) in saying that LIP (and, perhaps, other forms of pulmonary lymphoid hyperplasia) "*is not a single etiological or pathogenetic entity, but rather a morphological expression in the lung of a variety of diseases.*"

The potential clinical manifestations of LIP are many. They include cough, dyspnea, weight loss, fever, hemoptysis, chest pain, and joint pain. The last of these symptoms may also be associated with laboratory manifestations of an autoimmune disorder, including rheumatoid arthritis and its variants, lupus crythematosus, or myasthenia gravis. Other conditions in which immunity is disturbed—such as primary biliary cirrhosis, Blackfan–Diamond syndrome, "lupoid" chronic hepatitis, and the acquired immunodeficiency syndrome (AIDS)—also have been associated with pulmonary lymphoid hyperplasia (285–287). Paraproteinemias are common in patients with LIP, particularly polyclonal hypergammaglobulinemia (288). In a small minority of cases, however, ***hypo***gammaglobulinemia may be evident as well (286).

Radiographic abnormalities in LIP cases are somewhat variable. They potentially include diffuse interstitial densities throughout one or both lung fields; randomly dispersed nodular lesions of different sizes; or a combination of those findings **(Figure 2.22)** (286,289,290). Importantly, roughly 50% of cases present with a localized single mass (285), raising the suspicion of a carcinoma on radiologic grounds. As noted by Liebow and Carrington (289), mediastinal lymphadenopathy and pleural effusions are rare in cases of LIP and should suggest another diagnosis.

The biological behavior of pulmonary lymphoid hyperplasias is difficult to predict. As many patients die as others who have stable disease or improvement, and overall mortality approximates 50% at 5 years after diagnosis (286,287). Exogenous steroids or DNA-alkylating drugs have been employed to treat LIP, with random success (285,291). Using current technologies, it should be

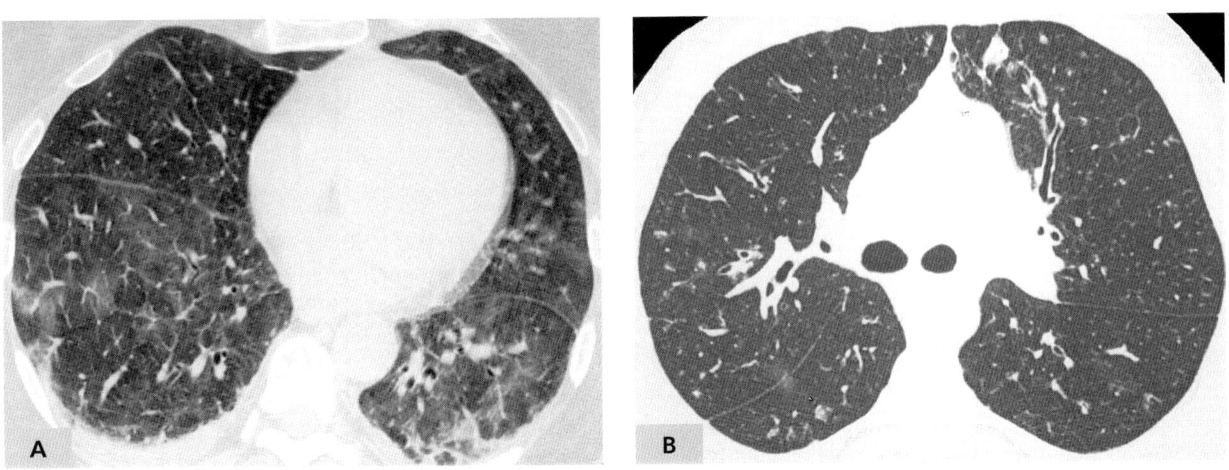

FIGURE 2.22 Lymphocytic interstitial pneumonia (LIP) may assume a variety of appearances in chest radiographs (A–C) or gross examination of the lung (D). Especially in immunocompromised individuals, the lymphoid infiltrates in LIP may be very dense and a distinction from marginal zone lymphoma may depend largely on molecular determinations of possible clonality. *(Continued)*

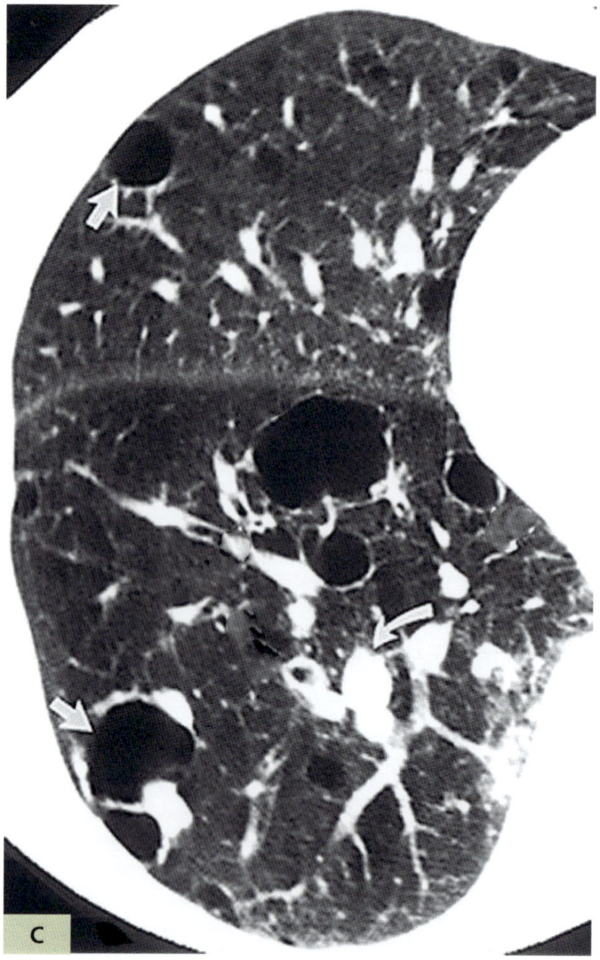

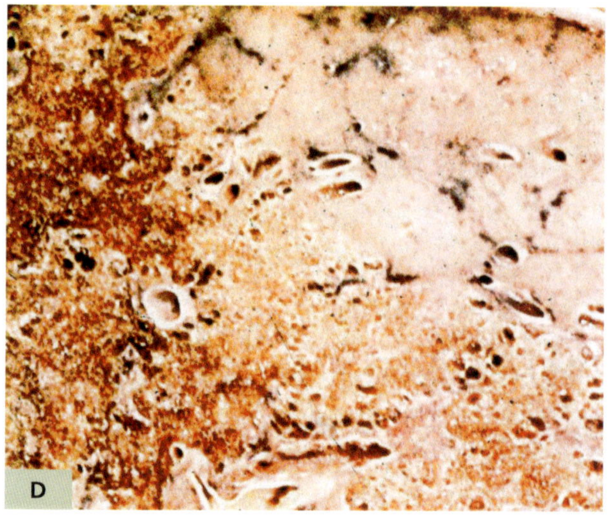

FIGURE 2.22 *(Continued)*

possible to define those lymphoid infiltrates of the lung that show unequivocal evidence of monotypism and therefore are malignant lymphomas. Better prospective identification of such lesions and their exclusion from series of LIP cases will improve our understanding of the behavioral spectrum of the latter disorder. In that specific context, it is noteworthy that 5% to 10% of patients in prior reports on "LIP" have ultimately developed systemic lymphoma (292,293).

The morphological distribution of cells in LIP and other pulmonary lymphocytic infiltrates tends to follow the routes of lymphatic drainage in the lung. Accordingly, they are centered on blood vessels and tubular airways with a "coat sleeve" distribution, or as nodular aggregates **(Figure 2.23)** (285,286,289,290,292). Diffuse permeation into the interalveolar septa is also potentially seen in these conditions. The constituent cells are polymorphous but principally composed of small mature lymphocytes. "Transformed"

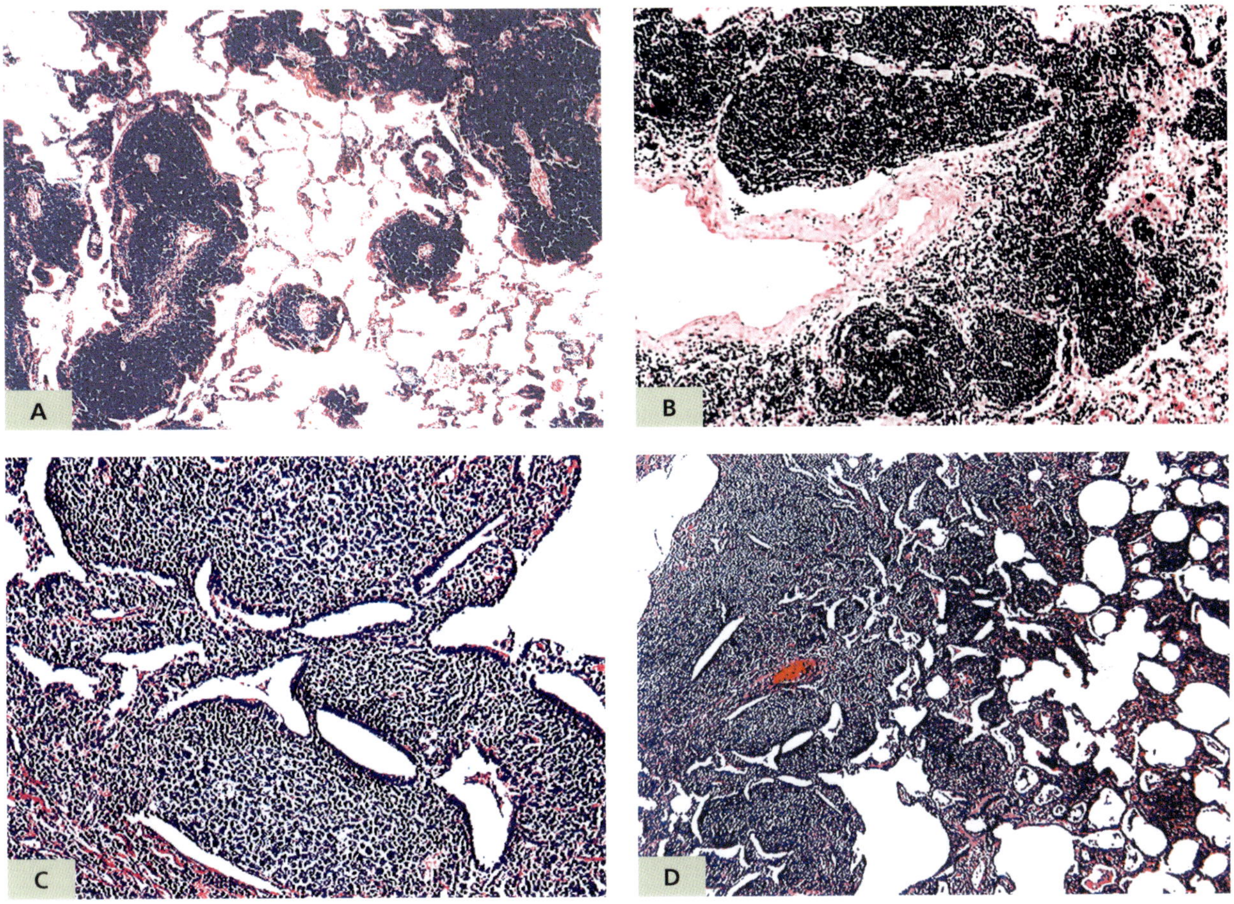

FIGURE 2.23 A–D: Lymphocytic infiltrates in lymphoid interstitial pneumonia principally affect the pulmonary interstitium and are reticulonodular in character.

lymphocytes with larger, more irregular nuclear contours as well as immunoblast-like elements are also commonly present **(Figure 2.24)**, along with scattered plasma cells, macrophages, and neutrophils (285). Germinal centers are evident in approximately 20% to 30% of cases, and primarily those in which the lymphoid infiltrate is nodular (288,289). Unlike follicular lymphomas, the germinal centers contain a heterogeneous population of immunoblasts and phagocytic "tingible body" macrophages. The central aspects of these structures may contain amorphous hyalinized matrical material around blood vessels, recalling the attributes of Castleman's disease.

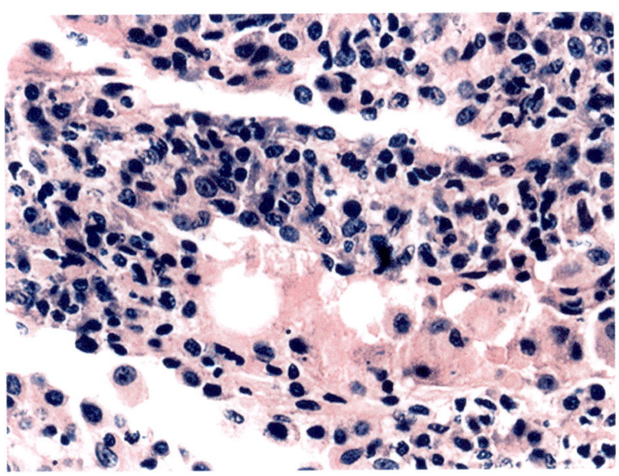

FIGURE 2.24 Large "transformed" lymphoid cells may be evident in the interstitial infiltrates of lymphoid interstitial pneumonia.

Stromal amyloid sometimes has been observed focally in pulmonary lymphoid hyperplasias, as have epithelioid granulomas (285). However, neither of the latter two features is reliable in separating LIP from low-grade lymphoid neoplasia. More useful markers of the latter include cellular monomorphism, subendothelial aggregates of lymphocytes in pulmonary blood vessels, permeation by lymphoid cells of bronchiolar epithelium **(Figure 2.25)**, abundant apoptosis, mitotic activity, and significant irregularity of nuclear contours (291,292).

Malignant lymphoproliferative diseases are characterized either immunophenotypically—with monotypism for light chain immunoglobulins or deletion of "pan-B" or "pan-T" cell antigens (282,283)—or by rearrangement of immunoglobulin genes or T-cell receptor genes using Southern blot methodology or the polymerase chain reaction (293,294). If only formalin-fixed, paraffin-embedded specimens are available for evaluation, our unpublished experience also has shown that a dominance (≥75%) of CD20+ lymphocytes argues in favor of a neoplastic infiltrate, as does coexpression of CD20 and CD43 by the same cells.

Several theories have focused on the potential causes for pulmonary lymphoid hyperplasia. These principally concern two major pathogenetic mechanisms, namely, dysregulation of immunity and virally-driven reactive lymphoproliferation (285,286,290,295–297). These factors are not necessarily mutually exclusive. In favor of the former explanation, many patients with LIP have clinical and serologic evidence of an autoimmune disease, as outlined above. Regarding the potential contribution of viral infection, genomic segments

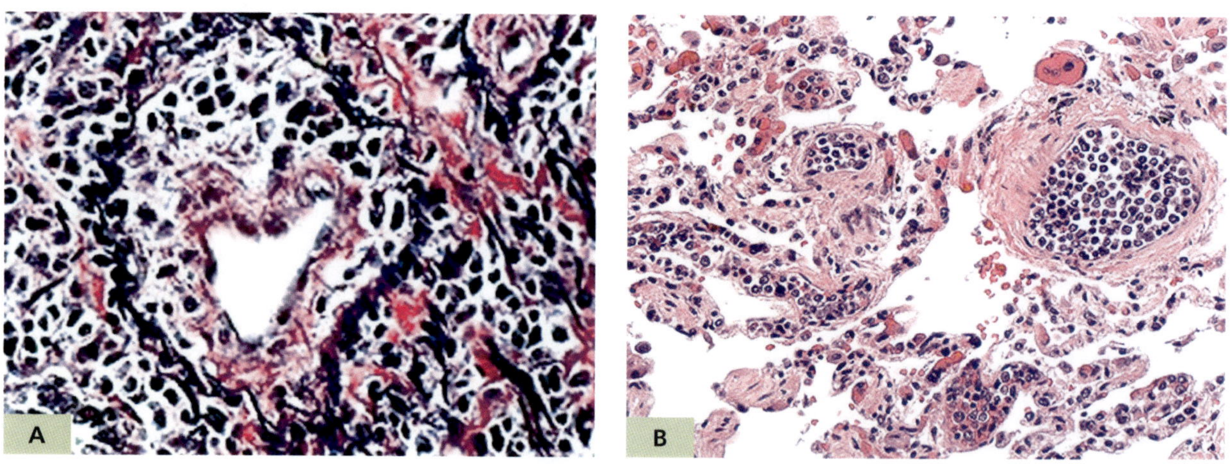

FIGURE 2.25 Marginal zone lymphoma of the lung often shows permeation of small blood vessels with undermining of the endothelium (A, Verhoeff–van Gieson elastic stain). However, that tumor type does not manifest endoluminal aggregates of large atypical lymphocytes, as seen in intravascular lymphomatosis (B). Lymphoid interstitial pneumonia manifests neither of those characteristics.

of the Epstein–Barr virus (EBV) have been identified in constituent lymphocytes in some examples of LIP (**Figure 2.26**) (295,296); moreover, that infectious agent may exert a mitogenic effect in concert with the HIV in the context of AIDS-related LIP (297). Unfortunately from a pragmatic perspective, markers of autoimmunity and EBV infection can also be present in patients with outright lymphomas.

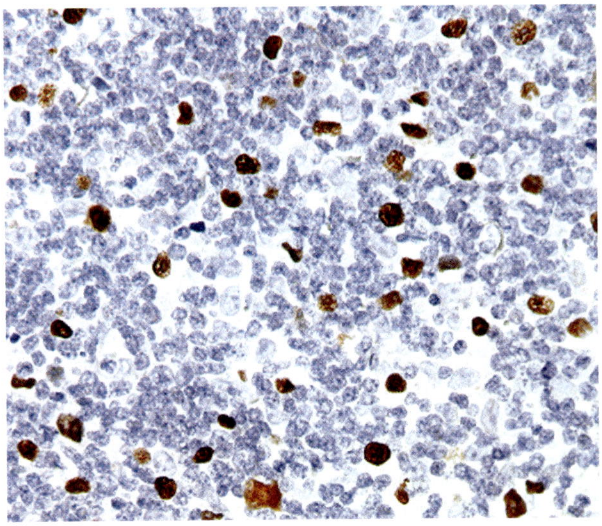

FIGURE 2.26 In some immunocompromised patients with lymphoid interstitial pneumonia, incorporated nucleic acid segments from the Epstein–Barr virus can be demonstrated in the lesional cells using in-situ hybridization.

Rarely, *Castleman's disease* (angiofollicular lymph node hyperplasia) involves only the lung parenchyma and might be confused with multinodular pulmonary lymphoid hyperplasia on cursory microscopic inspection (298). That condition will be discussed more fully later in this chapter.

Isolated examples of acute viral pneumonia are typified by exuberant interstitial lymphoid infiltrates. Nevertheless, the clinical context of that disorder—featuring a rapidly evolving course and symptoms of an infectious disease—should allow for its accurate recognition even without special pathologic studies. It is more difficult to distinguish LIP from *extrinsic allergic alveolitis* (hypersensitivity pneumonitis [HP]) histopathologically, because both of those disorders can exhibit exuberant lymphoid inflammation with small epithelioid granulomas (**Figure 2.27**). Clinical

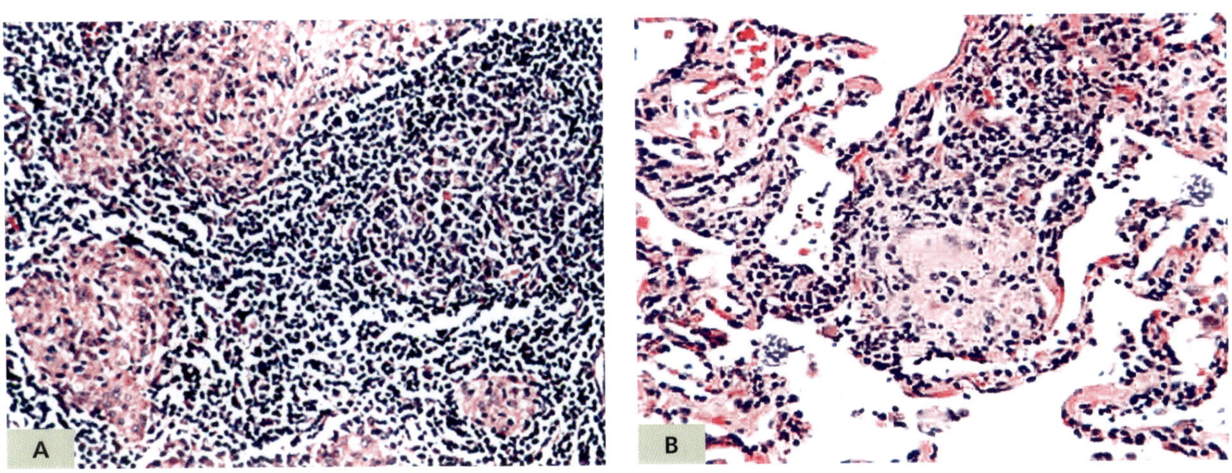

FIGURE 2.27 Occasionally, the lymphoid infiltrates in either marginal-zone lymphoma or lymphoid interstitial pneumonia may contain epithelioid microgranulomas (A). Another disorder with similar histological manifestations is represented by hypersensitivity pneumonitis (B).

information regarding hypersensitivity to certain fungi and other organic antigens is necessary to identify HP definitively. On the contrary, the microscopic presence of fibrosing bronchiolitis should shift diagnostic preference towards LIP (285).

SEVERE ALLOGRAFT REJECTION VS. POSTTRANSPLANT LYMPHOPROLIFERATIVE DISEASE

After transplantation of one or both lungs, transbronchial surveillance biopsies are commonly done to evaluate the possible presence of allograft rejection. In that setting, particularly in the first year after the transplant has been done, one may have interpretative difficulty if a dense, predominantly perivascular lymphoid infiltrate is seen in the allograft (299–301). Specifically, the differential diagnosis of that finding centers on severe cellular rejection vs. *posttransplant lymphoproliferative disease* (PTLD). Both of those conditions may manifest with a cytologically atypical but heterogeneous population of lymphoid cells that expand the perivascular interstitium and permeate outward into the surrounding lung parenchyma **(Figure 2.28)**. Each also produces clinical dysfunction, with variable dyspnea and hypoxemia.

The most helpful methods for making the cited diagnostic distinction are the use of immunohistology and genotypic evaluations of lymphoid clonality. If the infiltrate comprises a majority of CD20+ lymphoid cells (≥75%), with or without immunoreactivity for Epstein–Barr virus latent membrane protein (EBV-LMP) **(Figure 2.29)**, a diagnosis of PTLD is indicated (299,302). Positive results for EBV RNA (EBER) in the lymphoid cells using in-situ hybridization

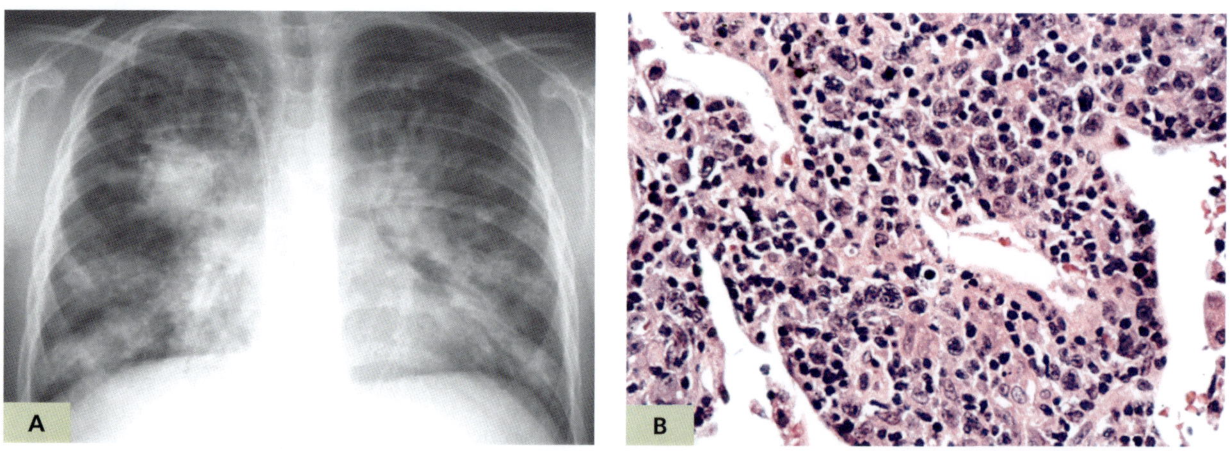

FIGURE 2.28 Following allogeneic lung transplantation, one may see dense lymphoid infiltrates in the grafted lungs (A) as a reflection of severe cellular rejection (B), or as a consequence of posttransplant lymphoproliferative disease (PTLD). *(Continued)*

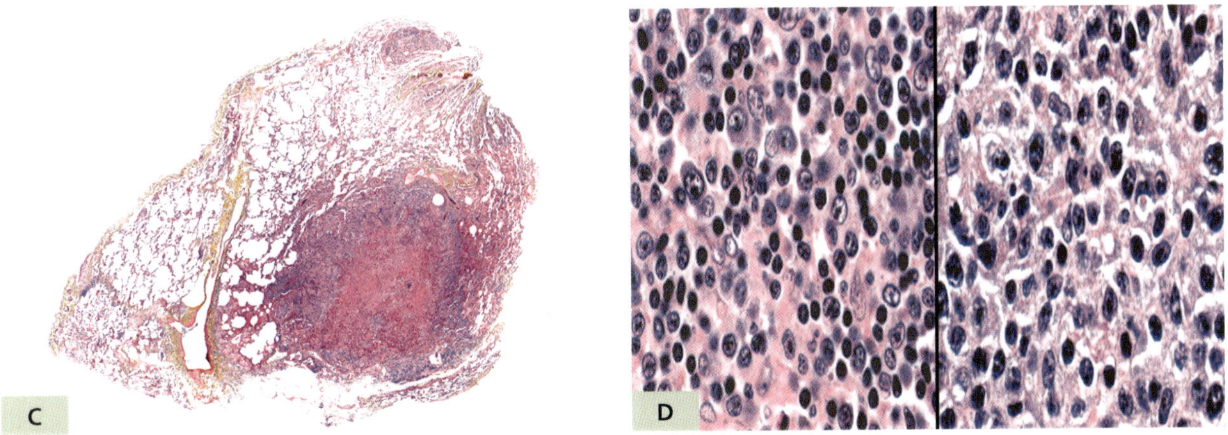

FIGURE 2.28 *(Continued)* As a general rule, rejection is a diffuse process, whereas PTLD produces one or only a few intrapulmonary lesions (C). Lymphoid infiltrates in PTLD may be either polymorphous (D, left) or monomorphic (D, right).

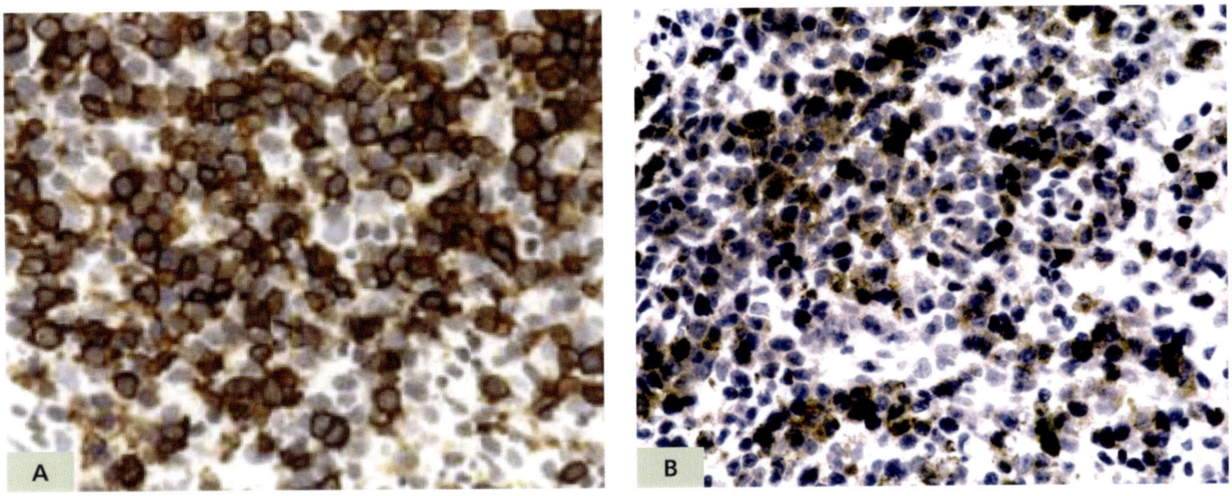

FIGURE 2.29 Immunoexpression of CD20 (A) and Epstein–Barr virus-related latent membrane protein (B) is common in posttransplant lymphoproliferative disease but is not expected in allograft rejection.

are similarly dispositive (303). In contrast, severe cellular allograft rejection features a mixed population of T and B cells, with the proportion of CD20+ cells not exceeding 25% (304), and uniform negativity for EBV-LMP and EBERS (299).

This distinction is a crucial one. Immunosuppressive therapy must be augmented for rejection and diminished in cases of PTLD. Antineoplastic therapy for the latter of those conditions may also be necessary.

ROSAI–DORFMAN DISEASE (SINUS HISTIOCYTOSIS WITH MASSIVE LYMPHADENOPATHY)

A unique pseudoneoplastic hematopoietic proliferation that involves lymph nodes, namely, sinus histiocytosis with massive lymphadenopathy (SHML; RDD) may also involve the lung as a primary lesion (305,306) in either sex and over a wide range of patient ages. Despite the name of this condition, lymphadenopathy does not always coexist with extranodal disease. When it affects the pulmonary parenchyma, RDD appears to have its epicenter in the hilar tissue and it tracks along lymphatics peripherally into both lung fields **(Figure 2.30)** (305,307). Accordingly, chest radiographs show an accentuation of central bronchovascular markings and bilateral interstitial prominence in CT scans. Pleural-based consolidation may also be apparent. Confluence of the infiltrates may yield mass-like densities in the lung fields as well. In likeness to LIP, clinical evidence of associated immune dysfunction is often evident in SHML, including autoantibody formation, polyarthritis, immune-complex glomerulonephritis, asthma, and juvenile diabetes mellitus. Fever, night sweats, and weight loss can be present (305). Justification for the classification of RDD as nonneoplastic in nature comes from molecular data that indicate its polyclonal composition (305). Nevertheless, this condition may occasionally coexist with solid malignancies—including carcinomas of the lung (308,309). That association likely arises, at least in part, because of dysfunctional immunological surveillance in SHML.

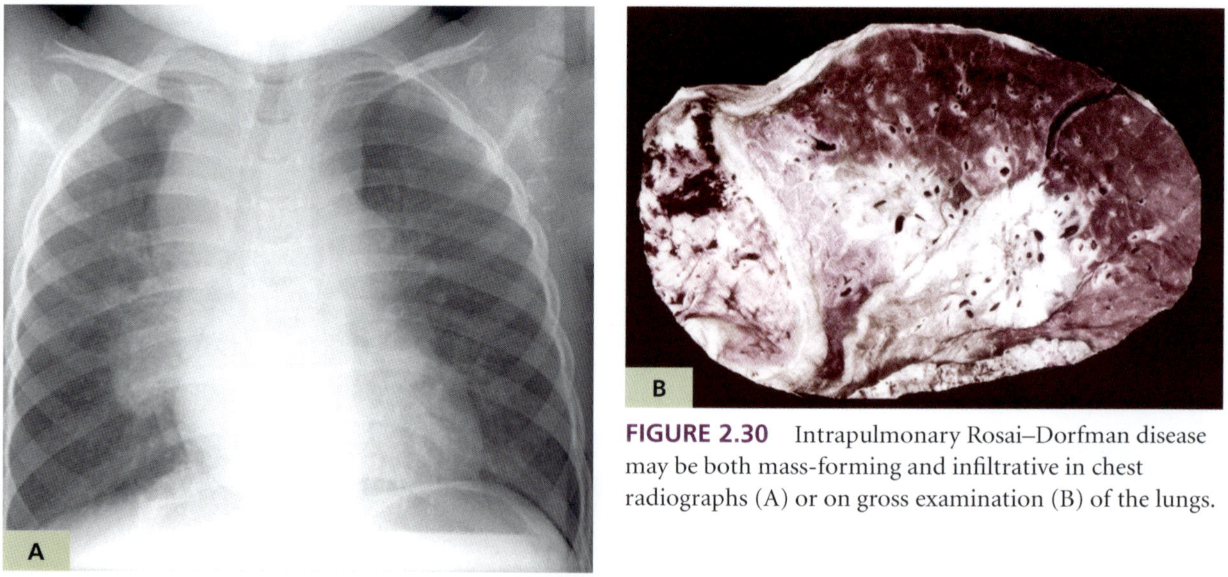

FIGURE 2.30 Intrapulmonary Rosai–Dorfman disease may be both mass-forming and infiltrative in chest radiographs (A) or on gross examination (B) of the lungs.

Pathologic specimens of the lung or lymph nodes in RDD demonstrate comparable morphologic findings. Dilated lymphatic spaces in the pulmonary parenchyma contain large pale histiocytes with abundant amphophilic cytoplasm, surrounded by lymphoid infiltrates that are punctuated by germinal centers and fibrous septa (**Figure 2.31**). The large histiocytes demonstrate a peculiar tendency to engulf intact, mature lymphocytes, representing a phenomenon known as "lymphemperipolesis." The overall image of foci of SHML in extranodal sites is therefore reminiscent of abnormal lymph nodes (305). The immunophenotype of the lesional histiocytes is singular in that it features prominent reactivity for S100 protein (**Figure 2.32**) and CD45 in the absence of CD1a. Labeling for CD68, lysozyme, MAC387, and alpha-1-antichymotrypsin may also be observed (306).

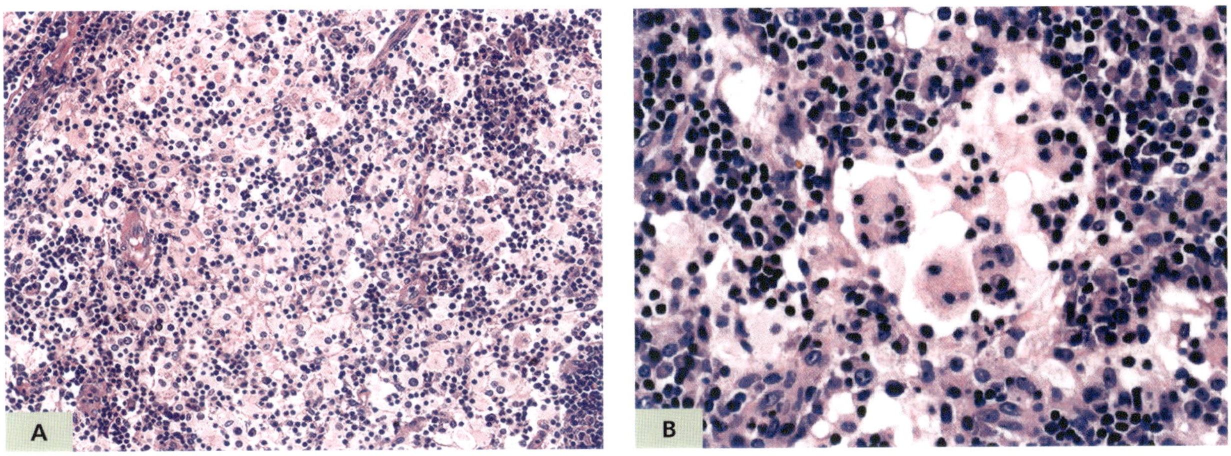

FIGURE 2.31 Rosai–Dorfman disease is typified by infiltrates of large histiocytes with abundant amphophilic cytoplasm, admixed with numerous lymphocytes (A). The histiocytes often contain intact lymphoid elements, representing so-called lymphemperipolesis (B).

FIGURE 2.32 The large histiocytes in Rosai–Dorfman disease are uniformly reactive for S100 protein.

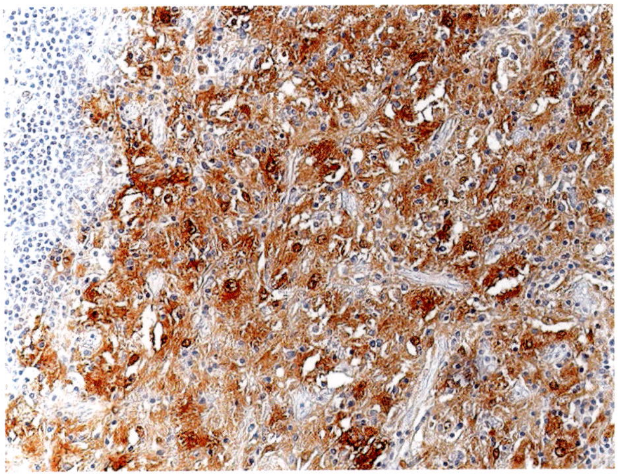

Differential diagnoses in cases of SHML potentially include *metastatic carcinoma*, *metastatic melanoma*, *Erdheim–Chester disease*, *large cell lymphoma*, and *Hodgkin's disease* (305,306). The large tumor cells in the nonhistiocytic conditions in that list differ from those in RDD immunohistologically, by their reactivity for keratin (in carcinoma), MART-1/melan-A (in melanoma), CD3 or CD20 (in non-Hodgkin's lymphoma), and CD30 (in Hodgkin's lymphoma) **(Figure 2.33)**. Practically speaking, with the exception of Erdheim–Chester disease—which is immunohistochemically similar to SHML and also com-

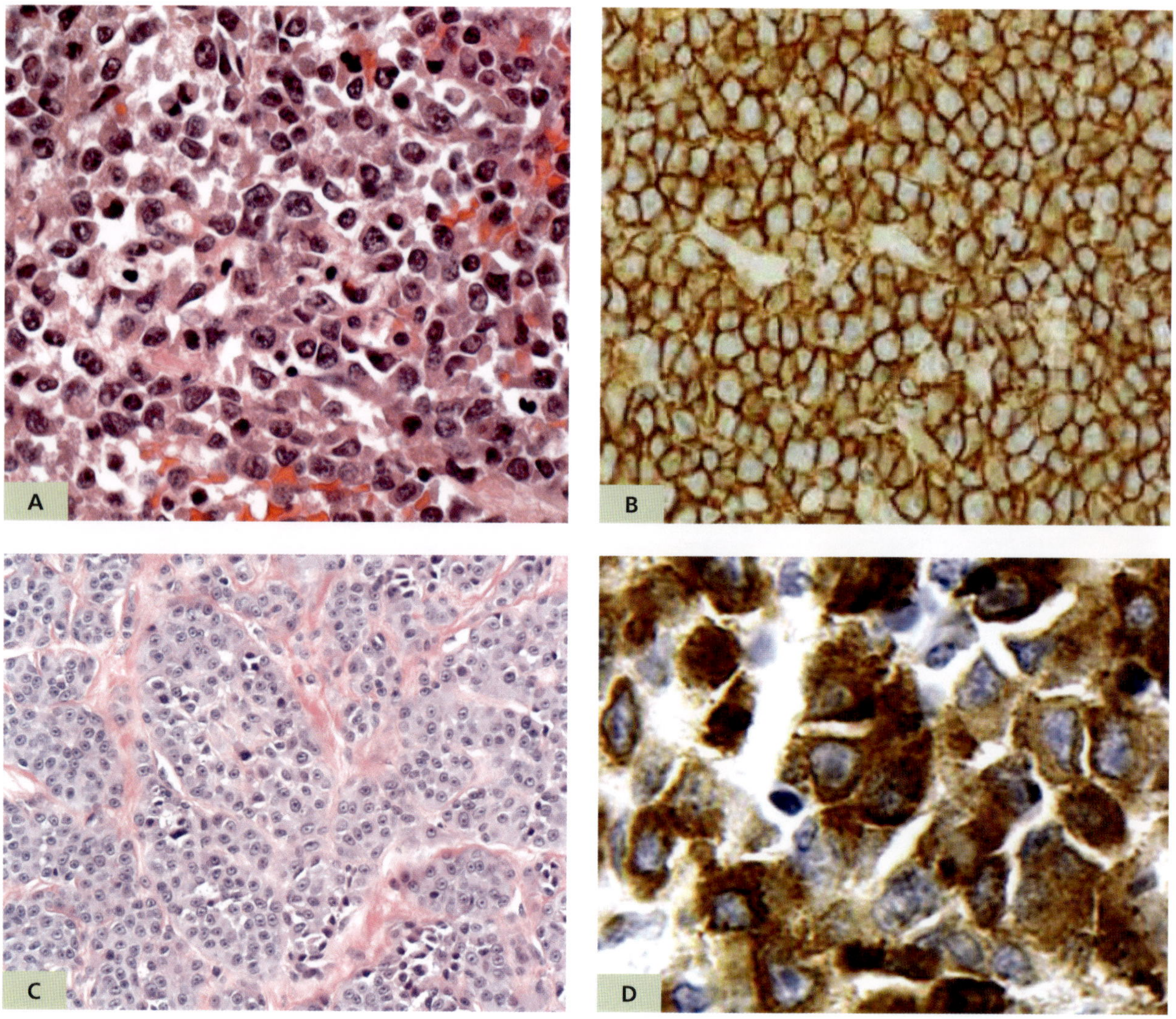

FIGURE 2.33 Differential diagnostic considerations in cases of intrapulmonary Rosai–Dorfman disease include several other pathologic entities that potentially comprise admixtures of lymphocytes and large polygonal cells. Examples are B-cell lymphomas (A & B, stained for CD20); metastatic melanoma (C & D, stained for MART-1). *(Continued)*

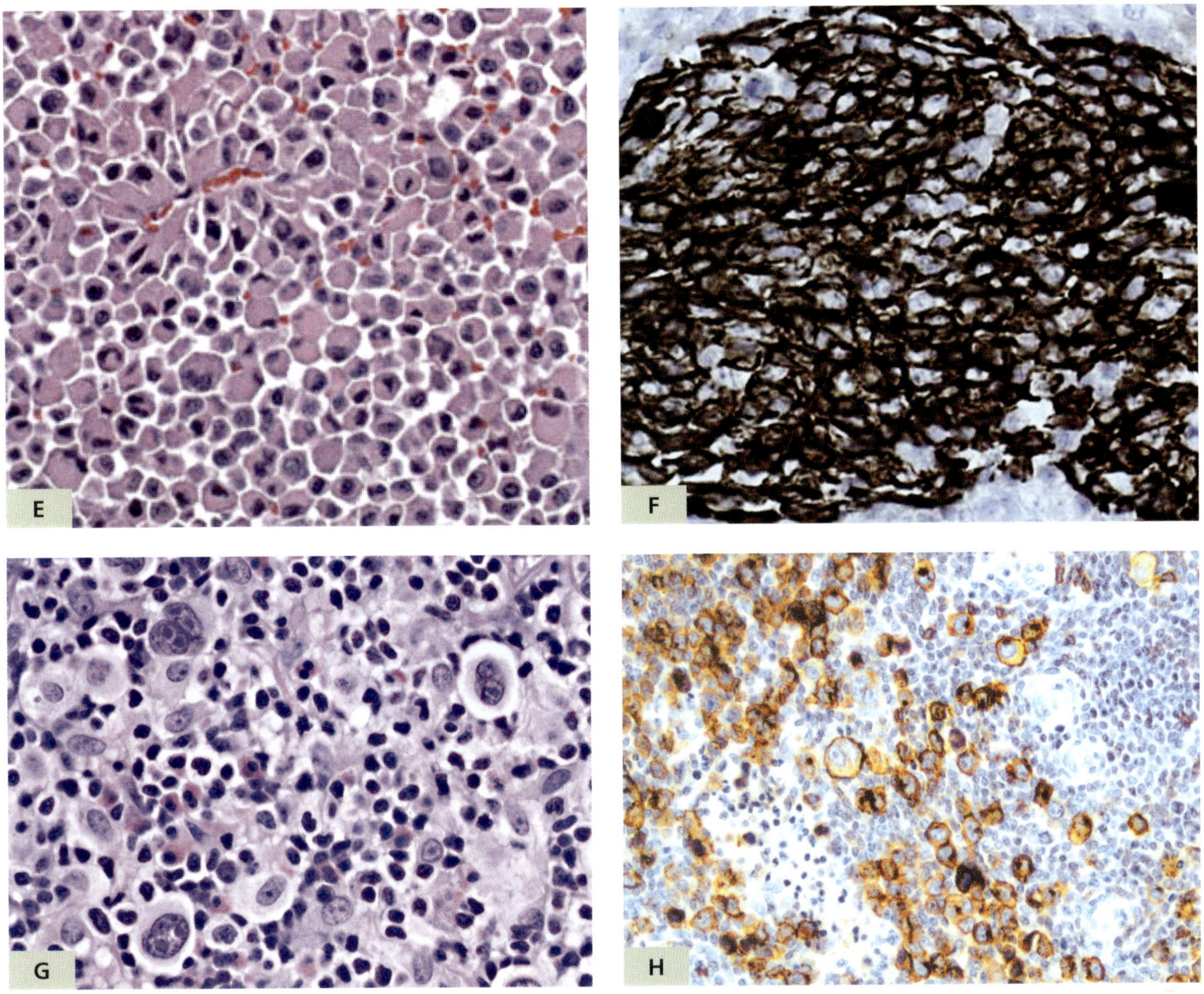

FIGURE 2.33 *(Continued)* Large-cell undifferentiated lung carcinoma (E & F, stained for pankeratin); and "syncytial" Hodgkin's lymphoma (G & H, stained for CD30).

posed of bland histiocytes—all of the other conditions also show much more cytologic atypicality than that seen in SHML. Thus, special diagnostic studies are usually not required to make the cited distinctions.

The clinical course of RDD is unpredictable. In a comprehensive summary by Foucar et al. (305), it was noted that patients with more than one site of extranodal disease and obvious immune dysfunction often had significant morbidity and possible mortality from this condition. Conversely, spontaneous remissions are also well-documented. Treatment is individualized, with antineoplastic-type interventions being reserved for those patients with serious organ dysfunction.

INTRAPULMONARY CASTLEMAN'S DISEASE

Castleman's disease (CaD) is a peculiar lymphoproliferative disorder that was first described by Dr. Benjamin Castleman and colleagues in 1956 (310). It may rarely present in the lung with single or multiple intraparenchymal nodules, imitating a malignant process (310–320).

Two main clinical forms of CaD are recognized—solitary and multicentric. The first of them is represented by a single mass, which may be completely asymptomatic (**Figure 2.34**). On the other hand, multicentric CaD manifests itself with widespread lymphadenopathy, and hepatosplenomegaly can also be present. "B" symptoms such as fatigue, night sweats, fever, and anorexia are common in multicentric CaD, and such problems are thought to be caused by lesional production of interleukin 6. Despite these similarities to the disease profiles of malignant lymphomas, both types of CaD are non-clonal (321,322,323).

The histopathologic image of solitary CaD characteristically features the presence of numerous germinal center-like structures with hyalinized vascular cores; the follicular units are surrounded by concentric arrays of lymphocytes, and plasma cells are relatively inapparent. Capillary proliferation is evident in the tissue between the germinal centers. This form of the disorder is accordingly

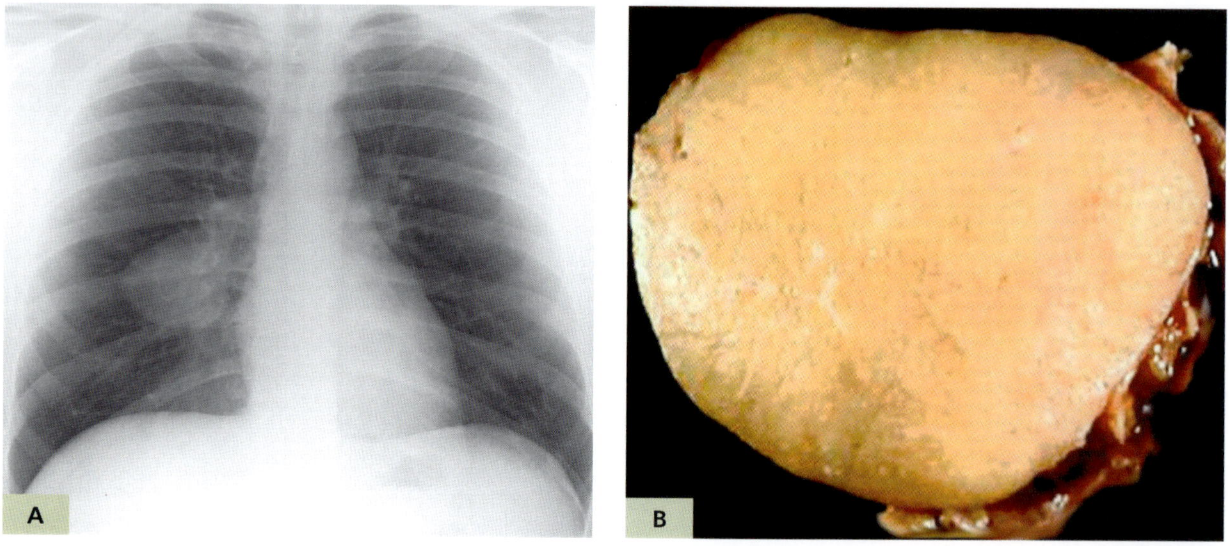

FIGURE 2.34 A & B: Rarely, Castleman's disease (angiofollicular lymphoid hyperplasia) may present as a single intrapulmonary mass. Differential diagnostic considerations in such cases include lymphoma or thymoma in the lung.

known as "hyaline-vascular" CaD **(Figure 2.35)** (324,325). Multicentric CaD demonstrates more numerous hyperplastic lymphoid follicles with larger mantle zones, as compared with the hyaline vascular form. Confluent plasma cell infiltrates are also present in interfollicular areas of the lesion, and account for the designation of "plasmacellular CaD" **(Figure 2.36)** (326,327). Some lesions in the plasmacellular CaD group also exhibit features of the hyaline-vascular variant (321). Solitary CaD is causally idiopathic, but multicentric CaD is associated with infection by HHV6 and HHV8, with or without coinfection by HIV (313).

Localized-solitary CaD is cured by surgical excision in the vast majority of cases. However, multicentric CaD may persist in several organ sites for a prolonged period of time and ultimately require antineoplastic treatment for adequate control (323). It can also be associated with Kaposi's sarcoma (328) and the "POEMS" syndrome (polyneuropathy; organomegaly; endocrine dysfunction; monoclonal protein in serum or urine; and skin lesions [glomeruloid hemangiomas]) (329).

In the lung, the differential diagnosis of CaD includes *follicular non-Hodgkin's lymphoma* (NHL) and *"micronodular" intrapulmonary ("Castlemanoid") thymoma*. The first of those possibilities lacks the hyaline-vascular cores

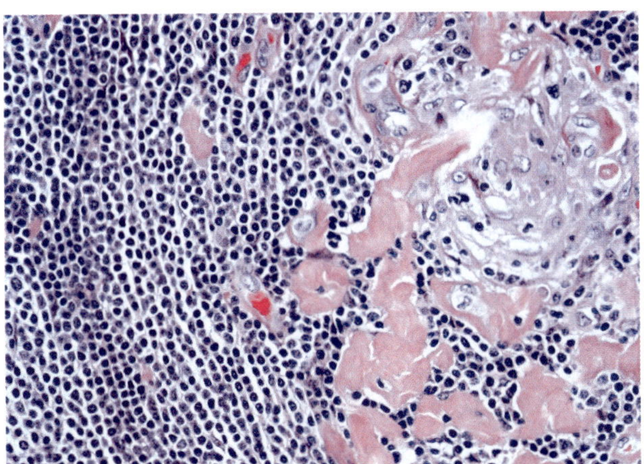

FIGURE 2.35 The "hyaline-vascular" form of Castleman's disease shows a deposition of eosinophilic and hyalinized basement membrane material amidst a lymphoid population that is organized into germinal center-like structures (GCLSs) multifocally. Other lymphocytes surround the GCLSs concentrically, resembling an onion-skin.

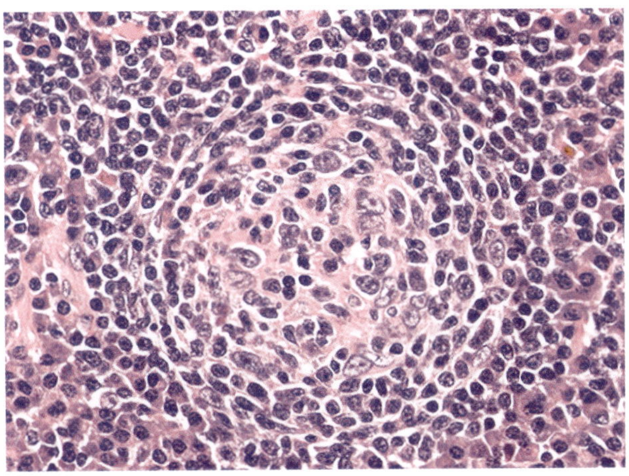

FIGURE 2.36 Plasmacellular Castleman's disease (PCD) is dominated by plasma cells and plasmacytoid lymphocytes, and lacks the eosinophilic deposits seen in the hyaline-vascular variant. PCD is more likely to be multifocal and can be associated with systemic lymphoproliferative diseases.

and plasma-cell infiltrates of CaD; it also shows immunoreactivity for *bcl*-6 protein and CD10 in constituent lymphocytes **(Figure 2.37)** (312,317,330). The latter marker is absent in CaD. Micronodular thymoma bears a striking microscopic resemblance to CaD, except that aggregates of thymic epithelium are present within the former lesion; these cell groups can be delineated with

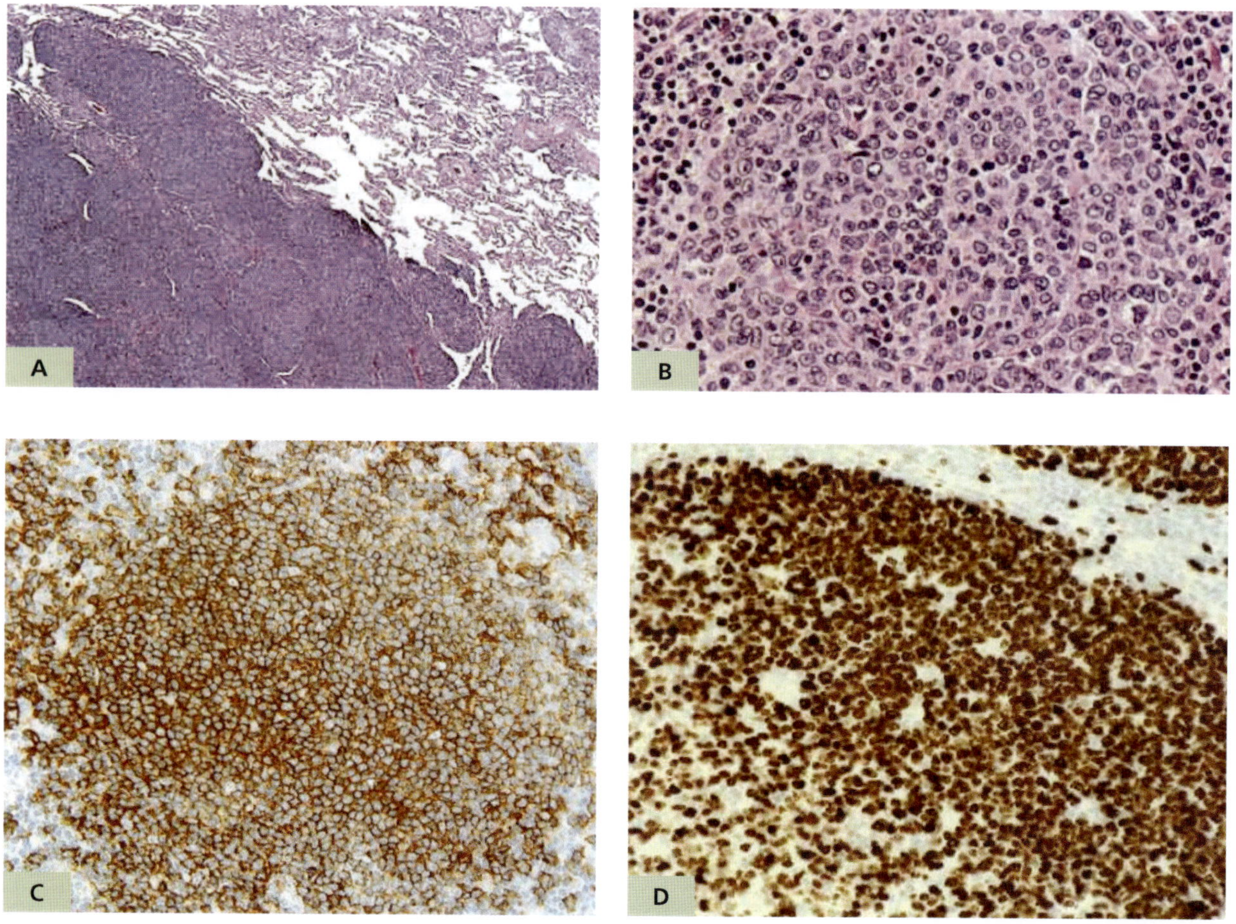

FIGURE 2.37 Castleman's disease may be confused with follicular non-Hodgkin's lymphoma (FNHL), in the lungs and elsewhere. However, FNHL shows only vague organization of lymphoid elements in its follicular foci (A & B), with an absence of hyaline-vascular deposits and scant if any plasma cells. CD10 (C) and *bcl*-6 protein (D) are evident immunohistologically in FNHL, but not in Castleman's disease.

keratin immunostains **(Figure 2.38)** (331–333). CaD contains no epithelial elements.

Interestingly, micronodular thymoma may be associated with concurrent NHL in regional lymph nodes in some instances (333). Indeed, we have encountered 2 such cases.

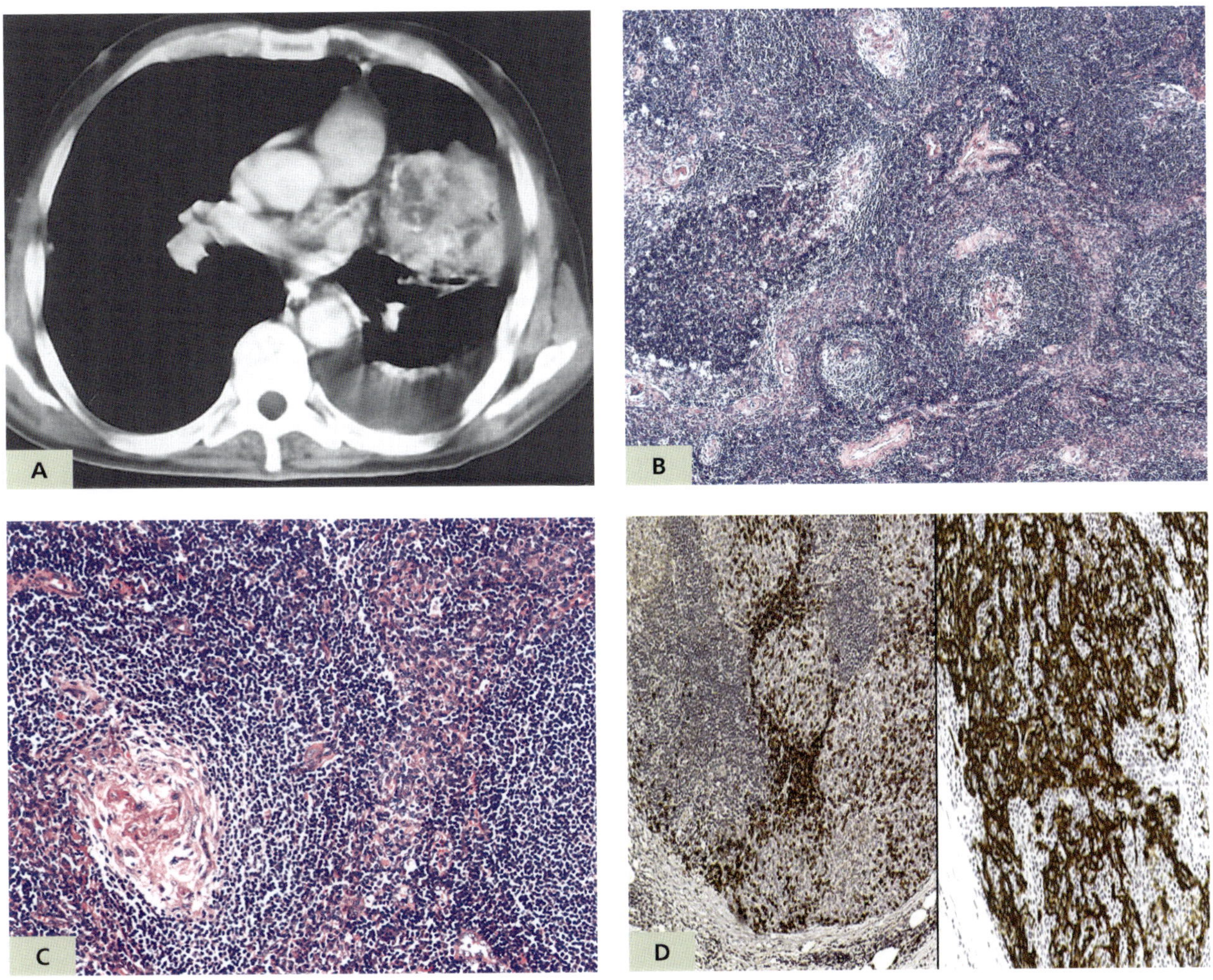

FIGURE 2.38 Another neoplasm that can be closely simulated by Castleman's disease is represented by "micronodular" intrapulmonary thymoma (MIT) (A). MIT also contains follicular units (B & C), and, unlike other forms of thymoma, they are constituted by a substantial number of B-lymphocytes (D, left). A definitive identification of MIT can be achieved with immunostains for pankeratin (D, right).

OTHER TUMEFACTIVE HEMATOPOIETIC LESIONS OF THE LUNG

In patients who have preexisting disorders of myelopoiesis—such as idiopathic myelofibrosis, constitutive hemoglobinopathies, severe hemolytic anemias, or Gaucher's disease (334–339)—myeloid tissue which has been nascent since infancy can potentially reappear in extramedullary sites with the lung and pleura being included. If the proliferation of such elements is sufficient, it may produce discrete masses in visceral structures or serosal surfaces, often imitating neoplasms macroscopically (338).

Fine-needle aspiration **(Figure 2.39)** or needle biopsy of extramedullary hematopoiesis (EMH) demonstrates a variable mixture of erythroblasts, myeloid precursors, and megakaryocytes (337). These cell lines are usually recognizable as such by conventional morphological study; however, should confirmation of their identity be desired, the Leder (chloroacetate esterase) stain and immunostains for glycophorin-A, myeloperoxidase, factor VIII-related antigen and CD61 can be used **(Figure 2.40)**.

The clinical course of patients with pulmonary EMH depends on management of the underlying hematologic disorders. If normal medullary hematopoiesis can be improved or restored, the condition often regresses

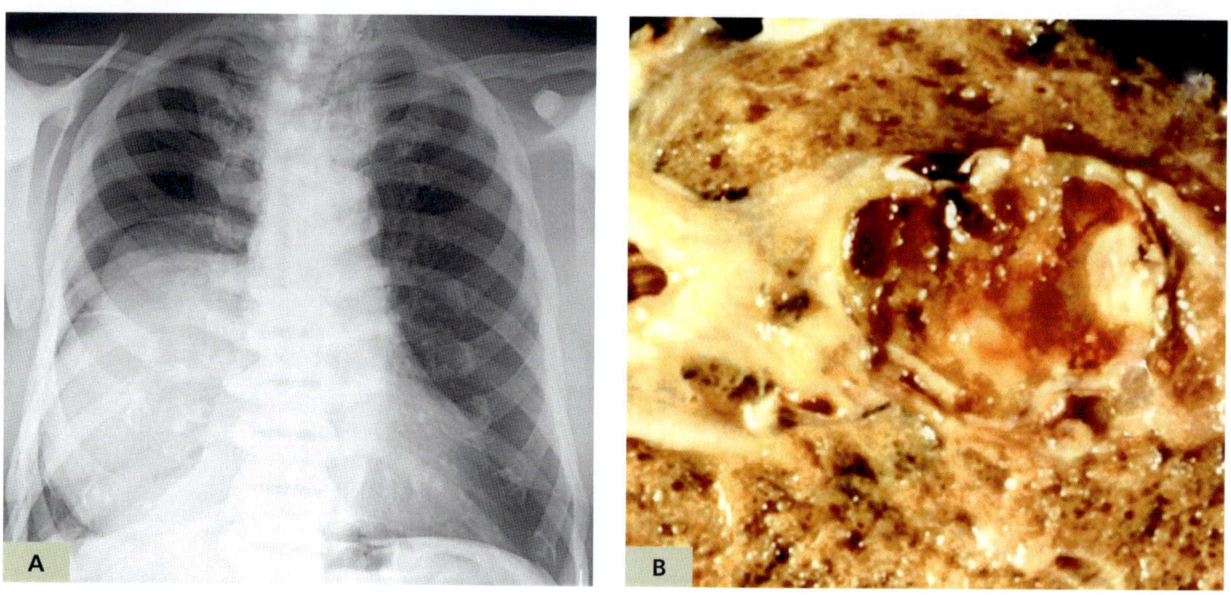

FIGURE 2.39 A & B: Especially in patients with bone marrow dyscrasias and severe chronic anemia, tumefactive extramedullary hematopoiesis can appear as a pulmonary mass.

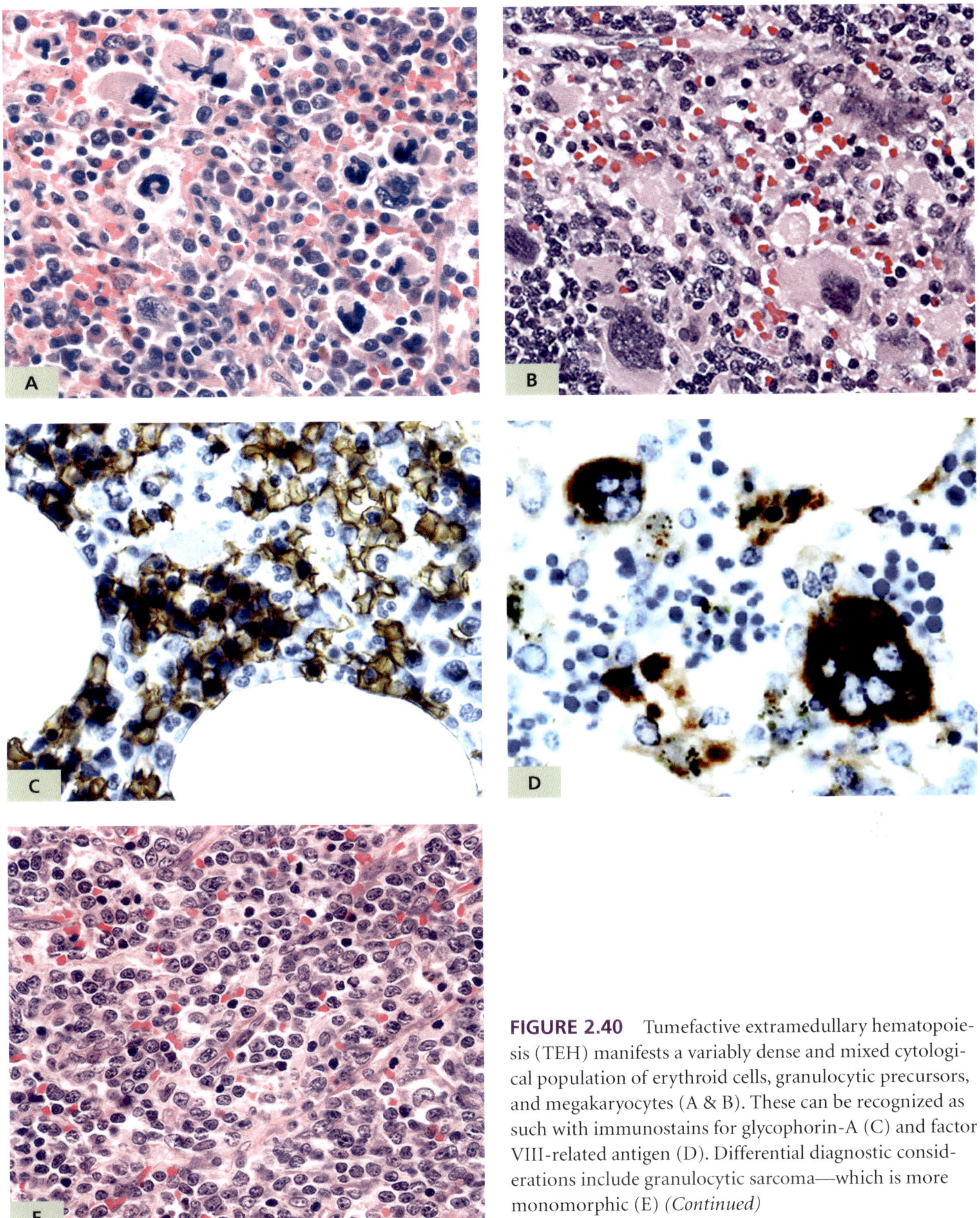

FIGURE 2.40 Tumefactive extramedullary hematopoiesis (TEH) manifests a variably dense and mixed cytological population of erythroid cells, granulocytic precursors, and megakaryocytes (A & B). These can be recognized as such with immunostains for glycophorin-A (C) and factor VIII-related antigen (D). Differential diagnostic considerations include granulocytic sarcoma—which is more monomorphic (E) *(Continued)*

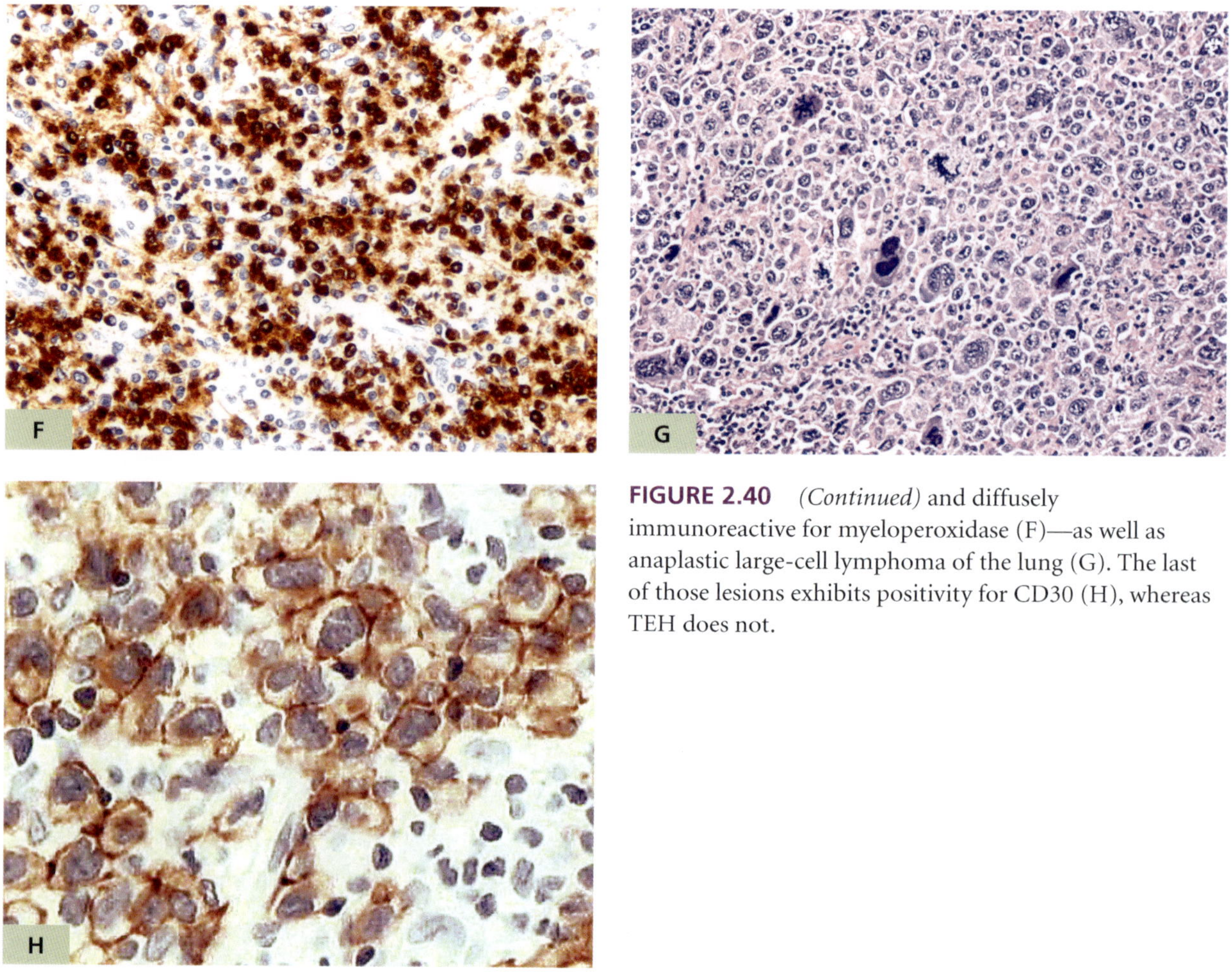

FIGURE 2.40 *(Continued)* and diffusely immunoreactive for myeloperoxidase (F)—as well as anaplastic large-cell lymphoma of the lung (G). The last of those lesions exhibits positivity for CD30 (H), whereas TEH does not.

spontaneously. In cases where tumefactive EMH is symptomatic, local-ablative therapy can be considered. However, the lesions in question may be a major source of circulating blood elements, and so this intervention should be used with caution.

Occasionally, infiltrates of EMH may be dominated by one or another hematopoietic cell line. In that eventuality, a resemblance to granulocytic sarcoma (tumefactive acute myelogenous leukemia), Hodgkin's disease, or non-Hodgkin's lymphoma may be encountered. The latter two conditions are rather easily dismissed from consideration by immunostains for B- and T-cell markers as well as CD30, all of which are absent in EMH (340). On the other hand, studies for cellular clonality may be necessary to separate granulocytic sarcoma from "lineage-lopsided" EMH.

PSEUDONEOPLASTIC CHANGES AS CONSEQUENCES OF LUNG INJURY

PROBLEMS IN RESPIRATORY CYTOLOGY AND INTERPRETATION OF SMALL LUNG BIOPSIES

Exfoliative cytology of the respiratory tract has been used as a clinical tool in the diagnosis of pulmonary neoplasms for over 65 years (341). However, inherent pitfalls in that method have been recognized and well documented, and some concern the potential for misinterpretation of reparative or inflammatory conditions in the lung as neoplastic disorders. The incidence of that eventuality should be no greater than 0.25% of all cytologic specimens, according to established guidelines (342). To a lesser extent, the same problem accompanies the interpretation of small transbronchial biopsy specimens of the lung parenchyma.

Several possible explanations exist for erroneous cytologic diagnoses of malignancy in the context of benign diseases. The pathologist or the screening technologist may simply misinterpret reparative processes or inflammatory epithelial atypia as carcinoma **(Figure 2.41)**, but this should be a rare event (343,344). Another potential source of error is the shedding of malignant cells from the oropharynx or nasopharynx into a "respiratory" cytology specimen (345,346). Both scenarios are problematic only if there are abnormalities on

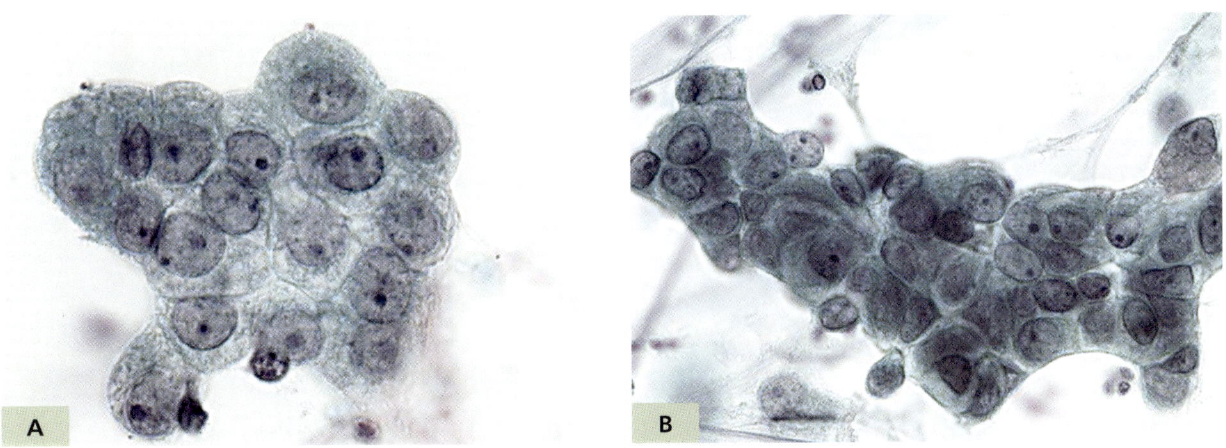

FIGURE 2.41 In several predefined clinical settings, including drug toxicity, pulmonary infections, and lung infarcts, respiratory cytology specimens may be alarmingly atypical (A–D). *(Continued)*

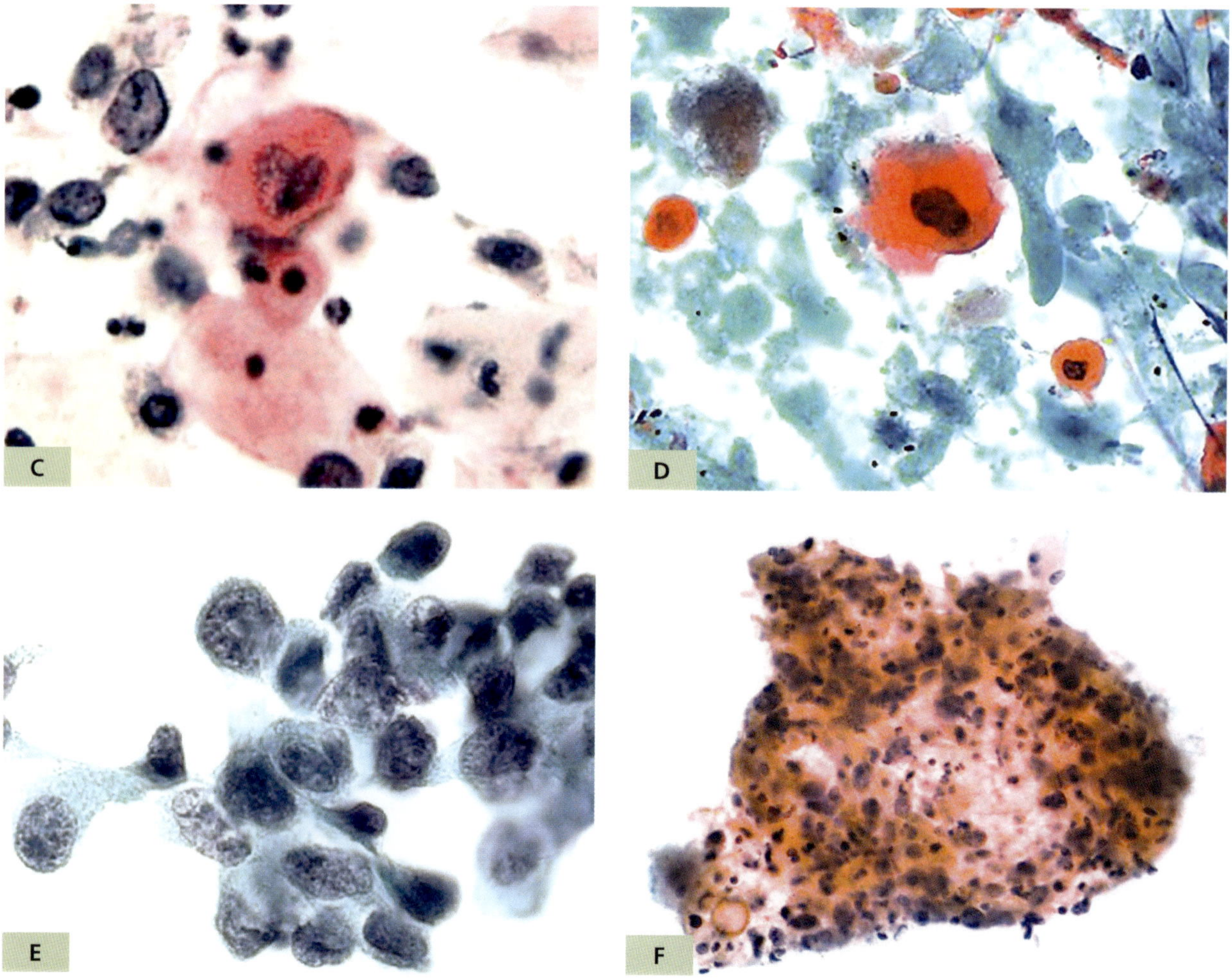

FIGURE 2.41 *(Continued)* They can simulate the appearances of adenocarcinoma (E) or squamous cell carcinoma (F).

chest radiographs that might lead to diagnostic consideration of a true neoplasm. Therefore, knowledge of the radiologic findings is an essential piece of information for cytopathologists and surgical pathologists in this setting.

Along the same lines, some radiographic "mass" lesions are capable of inciting benign but atypical epithelial proliferations in the surrounding lung parenchyma, such that exfoliated cells in those cases may be mistaken as carcinomatous in nature. These disorders include symptomatically occult pulmonary infarcts, granulomatous agglomerations, and foci of bronchiectasis with surrounding pneumonia, which are often associated with atypical squamous metaplasia of the bronchial epithelium **(Figure 2.42)** (347–352). Consequently, a misdiagnosis of *squamous carcinoma* in cytologic specimens or small tissue samples is the usual error in those circumstances.

Another group of diseases may produce morphological changes that simulate *adenocarcinoma of the lung*. It includes radiation pneumonitis, postchemotherapy atypia in alveolar lining cells, bronchiectasis, pulmonary infarction, viral pneumonias of various types, pulmonary vasculitides, inhalation of toxic chemicals, noninfectious interstitial pneumonitides, pneumothoraces, and diffuse alveolar damage **(Figure 2.43)** (353–360). Again, these conditions are

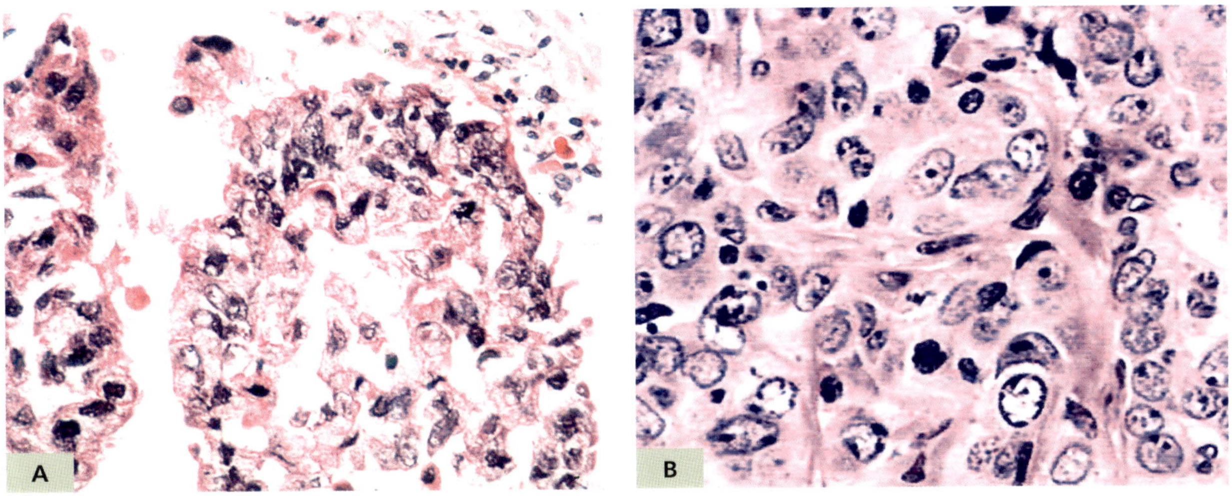

FIGURE 2.42 A & B: Atypical squamous metaplasia in tubular airway epithelium is a likely source of pseudomalignant respiratory cytology specimens.

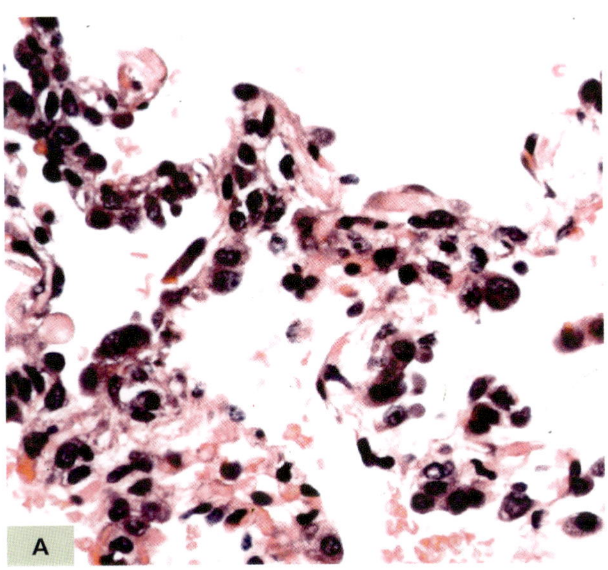

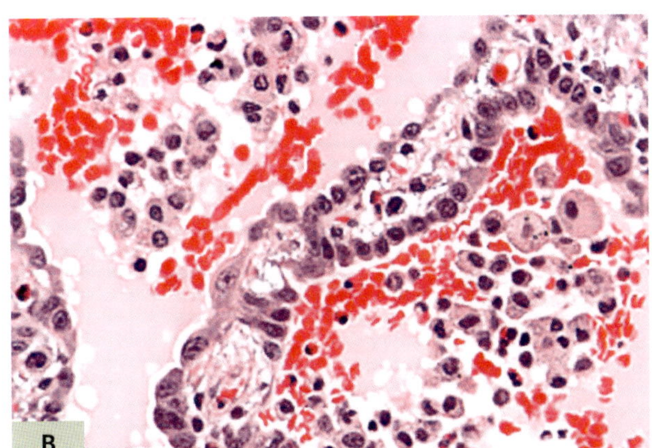

FIGURE 2.43 Damage to alveolar epithelium after cytotoxic chemotherapy (A), after pneumothoraces (B), *(Continued)*

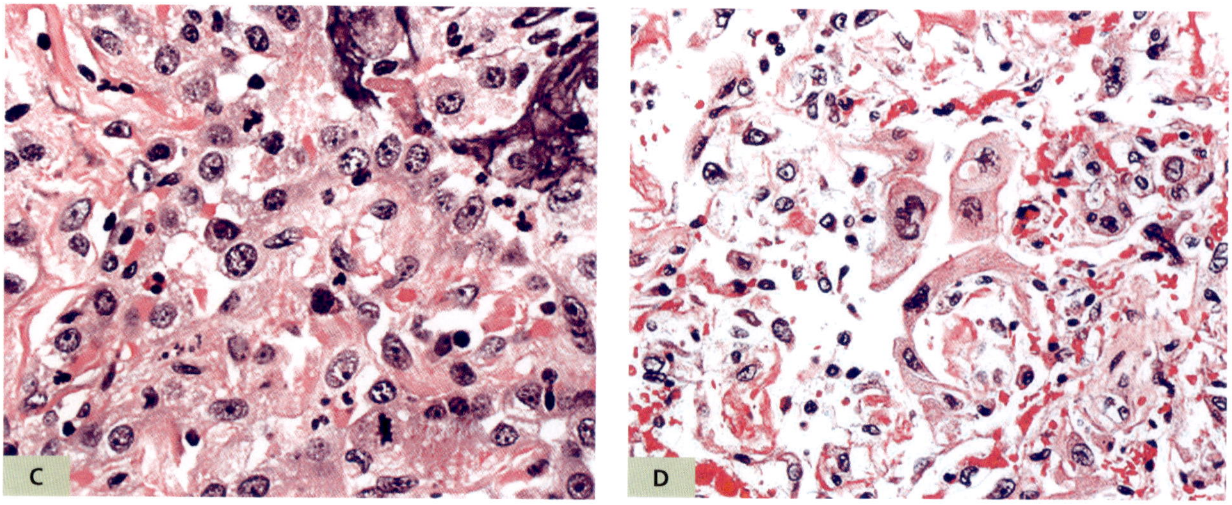

FIGURE 2.43 *(Continued)* in viral pneumonias (C), and in diffuse alveolar damage (D) can produce atypical respiratory cytology specimens.

most vexing to the cytopathologist when a localized radiographic abnormality exists in the lungs. Unfortunately, because of the broad roentgenographic spectrum attached to bronchioalveolar adenocarcinoma—including an image like that of uncomplicated pneumonia (361)—scrutiny of chest X-ray films is a less potent safeguard in this specific context. As summarized by Stanley et al. (362), pseudomalignant glandular pulmonary metaplasias may be recognized by their greater cellular heterogeneity than that seen in true adenocarcinomas, lower nuclear-to-cytoplasmic ratios than those of malignant tumors, "scalloping" of cell borders in metaplastic aggregates, and focal intercellular "windows" in pseudoneoplastic gland-like proliferations.

It is also pertinent to emphasize that special techniques—such as immunostaining for tumor-associated glycoprotein-72—are not capable of making the distinction in question and may even contribute further to misdiagnosis (363). In fact, there are no absolutely effective methods whereby mistaken cytologic or biopsy diagnoses of pulmonary malignancy can be avoided in selected cases. Pathologists and clinicians must be fully aware of that fact, while at the same time striving to maximize diagnostic accuracy by all possible means.

TRAUMATIC NEUROMA AND NECROTIZING SIALOMETAPLASIA OF THE BRONCHUS

A discrete injury-related tumefactive lesion of the bronchial mucosa was first described by Miura et al. (1364)—that of traumatic neuroma (TN). Rossi and colleagues added an additional report on that entity (1365). TN may occur

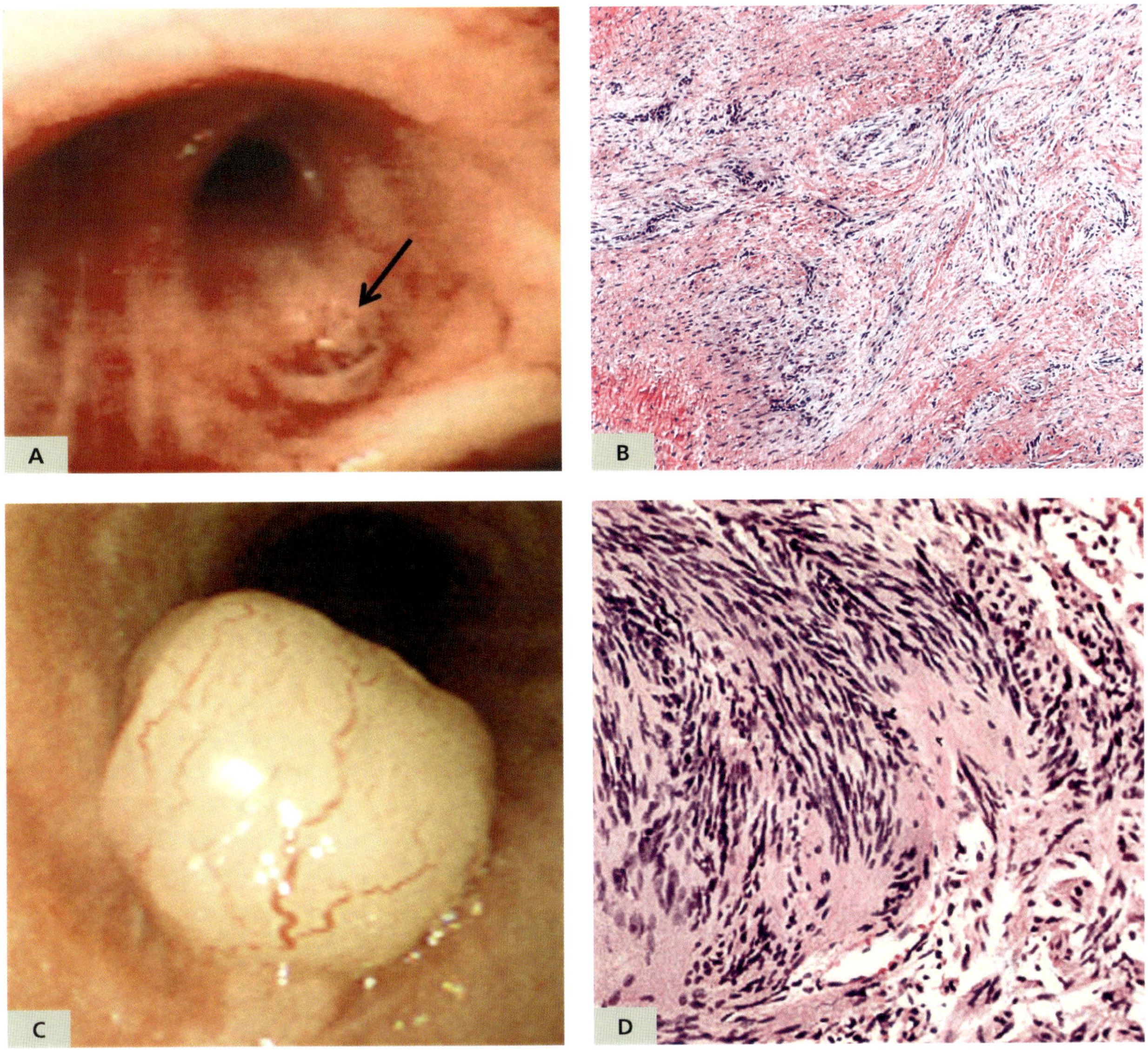

FIGURE 2.44 Traumatic neuromas can be seen in the bronchial mucosa (A, arrow) after prior injury to the airway. Microscopically, it is represented by the submucosal proliferation of regenerating and morphologically-bland neural fascicles (B). Differential diagnosis principally concerns intrabronchial neurilemmoma, which is a larger and more discrete lesion (C) with a biphasic histological appearance (D).

either spontaneously (e.g., after aspiration of food) or as a result of instrumentation-induced injury of the airway. Histologically, it shows a disorganized proliferation of mucoal nerve bundles, set in a collagenous or fibromyxoid stroma (**Figure 2.44**). The resulting image may be confused with that of *neurofibroma*. A mechanistically related process is that of necrotizing sialometaplasia, caused

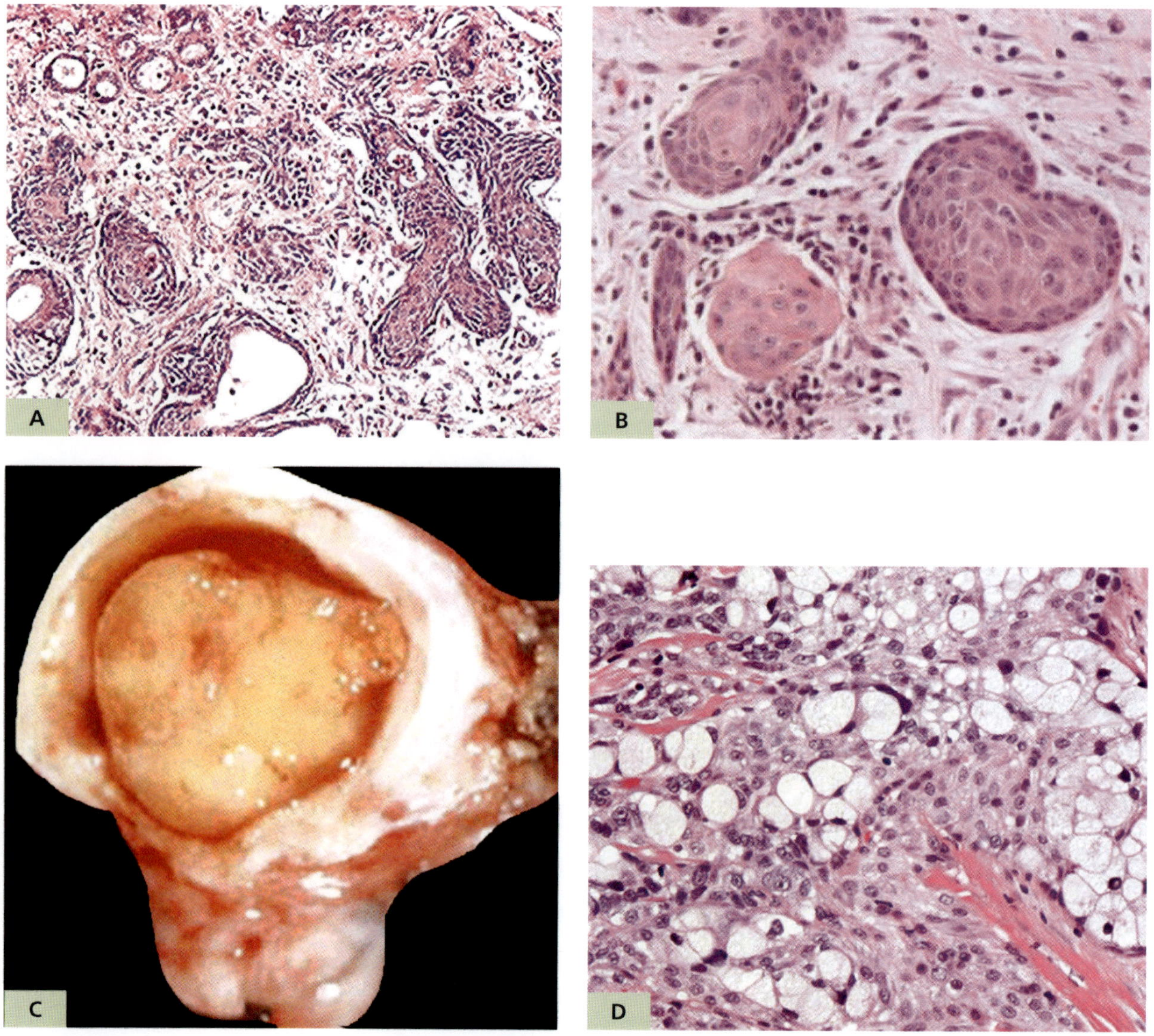

FIGURE 2.45 Another consequence of traumatic bronchial injury may be the process of submucosal sialometaplasia (SSM). In that lesion, salivary gland-type bronchial glands undergo squamous metaplasia and assume a distorted architectural relationship to one another (A & B). In the absence of clinical information, endobronchial biopsies of SSM might be mistaken for mucoepidermoid carcinoma. However, the latter neoplasm is typically a large luminal mass (C) unlike the flat, sometimes-ulcerated nature of SSM. Moreover, mucoepidermoid carcinoma comprises obviously atypical epithelial cells that are both squamoid and glandular in nature (D).

by inflammatory damage to, and pseudomalignant metaplasia of, the bronchial glands **(Figure 2.45)** (366). Confusion with *bronchial-gland adenocarcinoma* is therefore a possibility.

PERIBRONCHIOLAR METAPLASIA ("LAMBERTOSIS")

Peribronchiolar metaplasia (PBM; also known as "Lambertosis") is a reactive condition wherein metaplastic bronchiolar epithelium extensively colonizes the adjacent alveolar spaces **(Figure 2.46)** (367,368). Occasionally, the process may be so marked as to imitate the morphologic appearance of adenocarcinoma. When PBM is seen in the setting of emphysema in cigarette smokers, that worry is heightened even further. Nevertheless, the metaplastic elements in PBM are more columnar than those of bronchioloalveolar carcinoma, with less cellular atypicality than one sees in ordinary pulmonary adenocarcinomas. Focal retention of ciliation in the cells of PBM further supports its reactive benign nature, because cilia are essentially never observed in lung cancers.

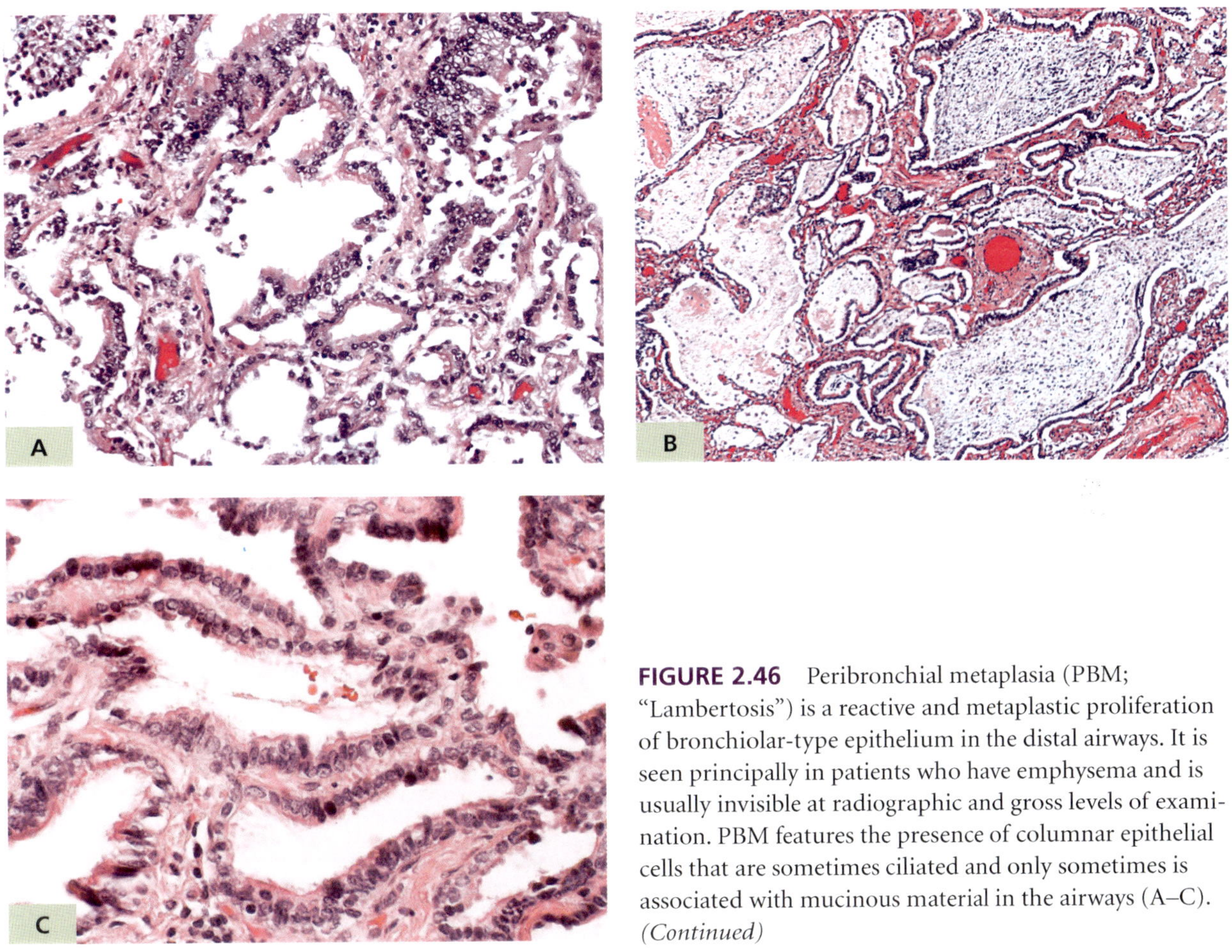

FIGURE 2.46 Peribronchial metaplasia (PBM; "Lambertosis") is a reactive and metaplastic proliferation of bronchiolar-type epithelium in the distal airways. It is seen principally in patients who have emphysema and is usually invisible at radiographic and gross levels of examination. PBM features the presence of columnar epithelial cells that are sometimes ciliated and only sometimes is associated with mucinous material in the airways (A–C). *(Continued)*

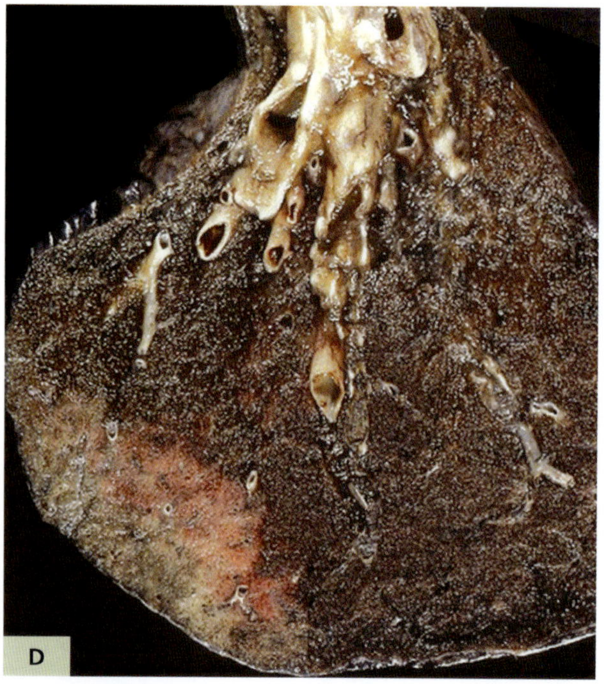

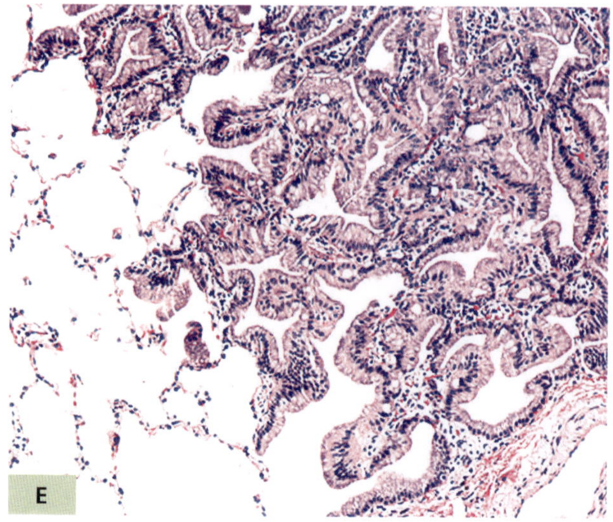

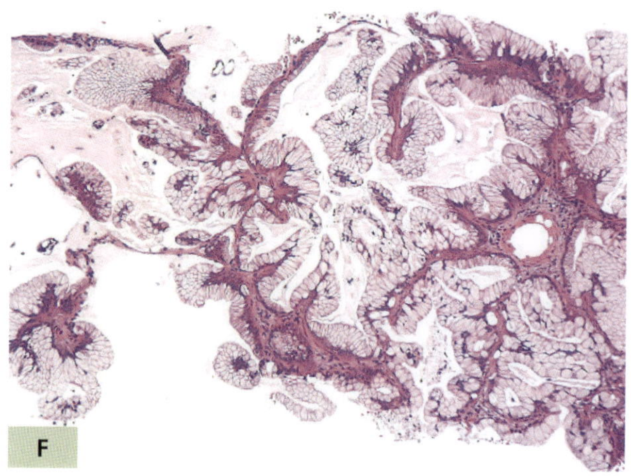

FIGURE 2.46 *(Continued)* In contrast, bronchioloalveolar carcinomas (BACs), with which PBM can be confused, comprise a mass-forming, monomorphic, and lepidic proliferation of atypical epithelium (D & E), often with intranuclear cytoplasmic invaginations. Mucinous BACs contain cytoplasmic and intracellular as well as extracellular mucin (F).

MALAKOPLAKIA OF THE LUNG

In immunocompromised patients who have AIDS or miliary tuberculosis, one may encounter malakoplakia—a peculiar proliferation of histiocytes in the bronchi and pulmonary parenchyma (369–373). It is thought to be an idiosyncratic reaction to infectious agents, most often represented by *Rhodococcus equi* or several species of mycobacteria.

Histologically, malakoplakia comprises sheets of eosinophilic polygonal cells with interspersed acute and chronic inflammation. The lesional cells

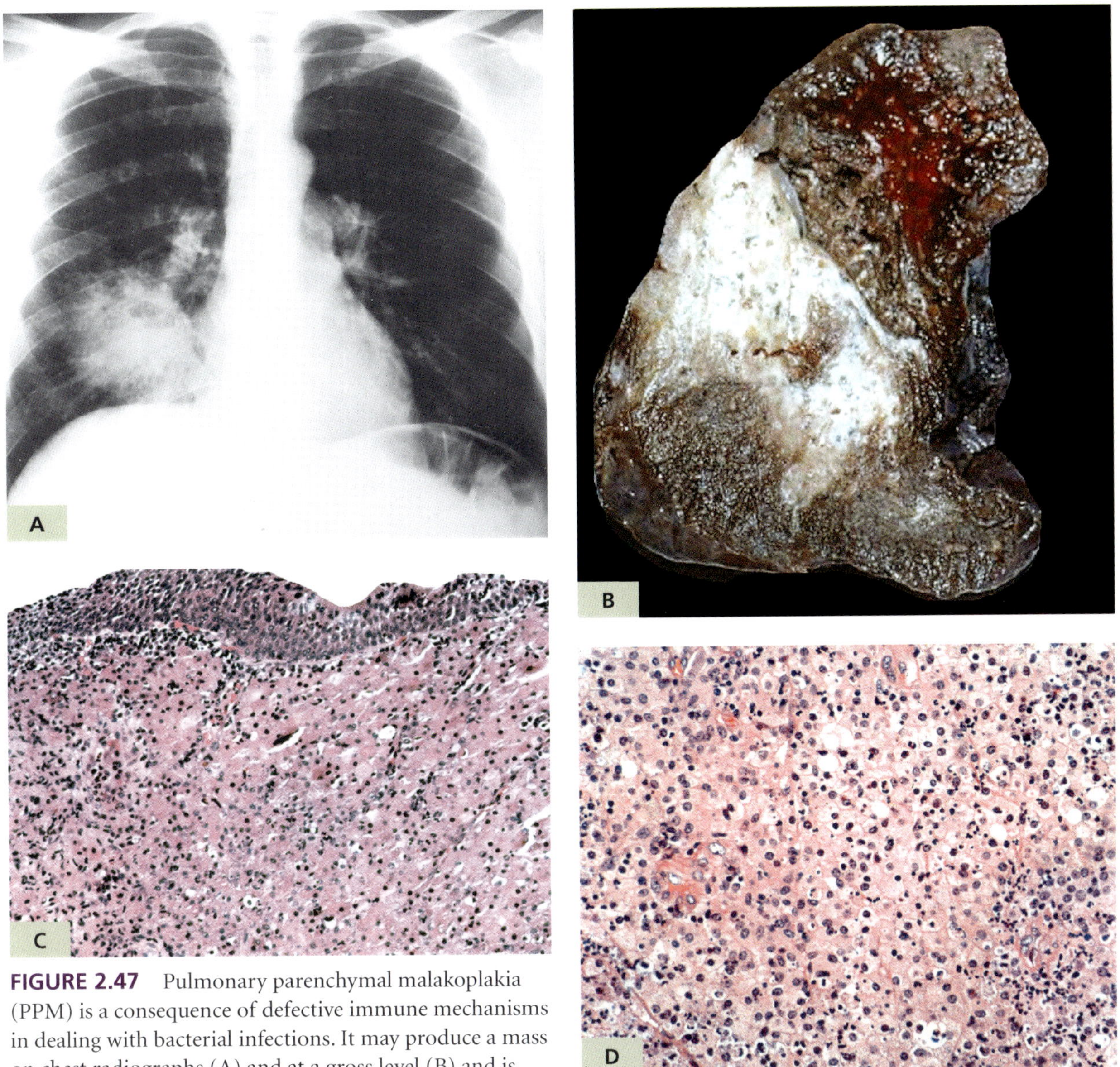

FIGURE 2.47 Pulmonary parenchymal malakoplakia (PPM) is a consequence of defective immune mechanisms in dealing with bacterial infections. It may produce a mass on chest radiographs (A) and at a gross level (B) and is composed of sheets of histiocytes that manifest modest nuclear atypia and are admixed with other inflammatory cells (C & D).

may demonstrate modest nuclear atypia (**Figure 2.47**). A subpopulation of them contains cytoplasmic inclusions, called "Michaelis–Gutmann bodies" (MGBs) which are diagnostic of malakoplakia. They can be highlighted with histochemical stains, including Perls' method and the von Kossa technique **(Figure 2.48)** (369).

The differential diagnosis of pulmonary malakoplakia primarily concerns two neoplastic entities; namely, *large-cell non-Hodgkin's lymphoma* and *granular cell tumor*. Neither of the latter lesions contains MGBs; moreover, they both lack immunoreactivity for CD163 (as seen in malakoplakia). Granular cell tumor can be labeled for S100 protein and alpha-inhibin **(Figure 2.49)** (374), but both of those markers are absent in malakoplakia.

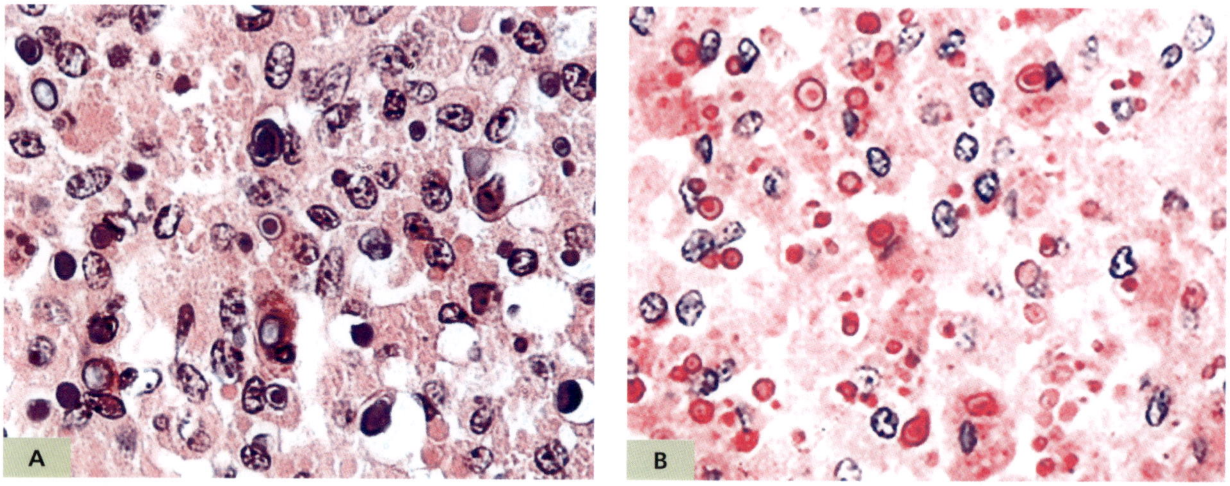

FIGURE 2.48 A singular feature of pulmonary malakoplakia is the presence of concentrically ringed inclusions in the cytoplasm of constituent histiocytes (A). These are known as Michaelis–Gutmann bodies and can be highlighted with the alizarin-red stain (B) as well as Perls' method and the von Kossa technique.

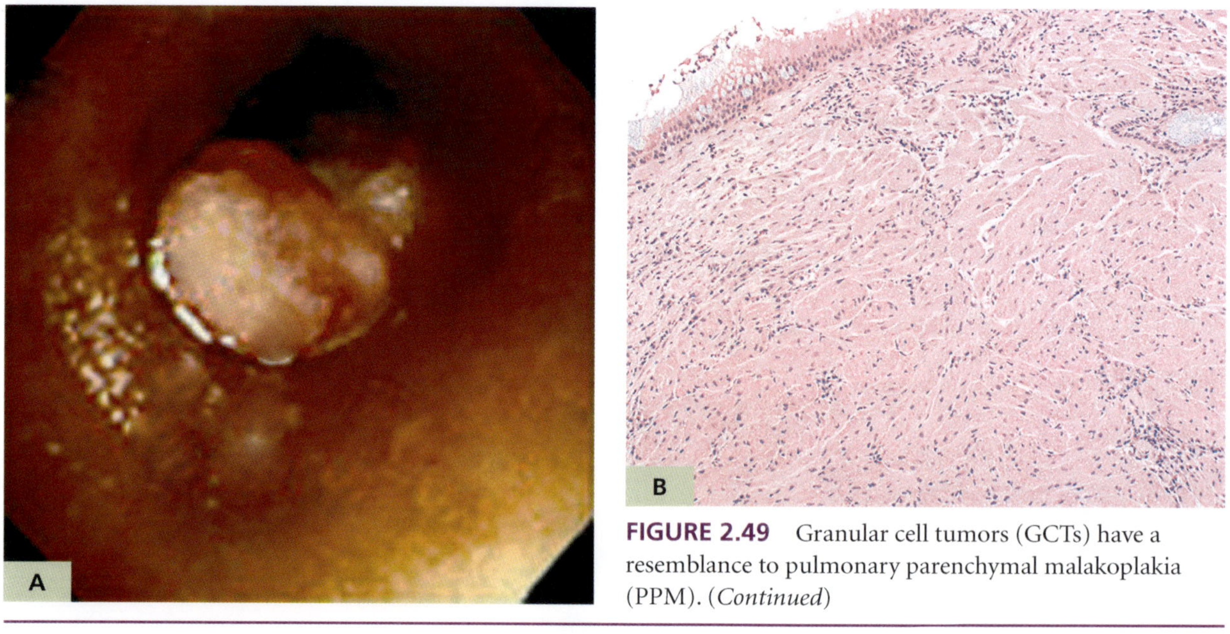

FIGURE 2.49 Granular cell tumors (GCTs) have a resemblance to pulmonary parenchymal malakoplakia (PPM). (*Continued*)

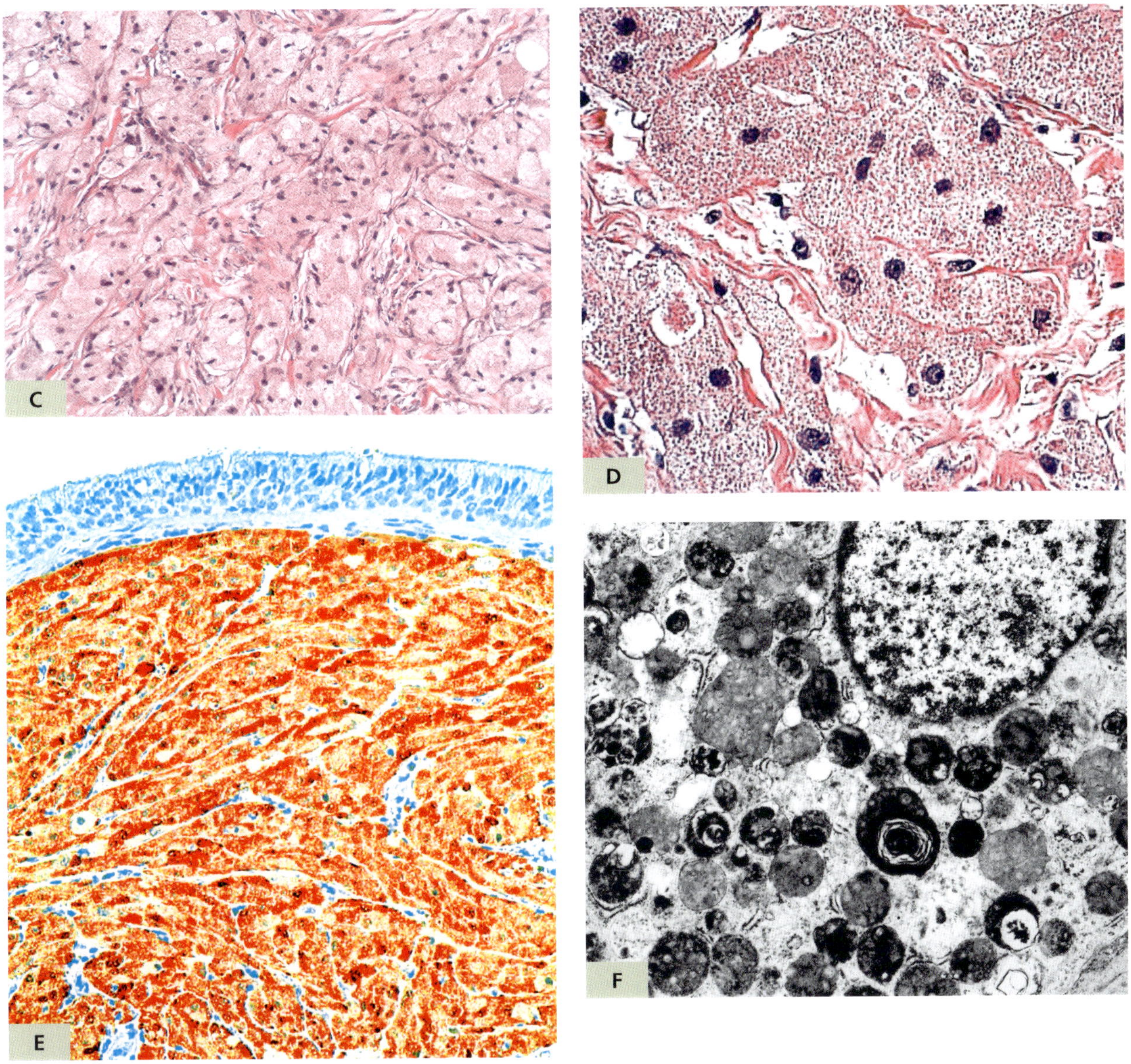

FIGURE 2.49 (*Continued*) However, GCT is usually a central lesion in large airways (A), in contrast to the more peripheral location of PPM. Furthermore, GCT comprises polygonal eosinophilic cells with uniform cytoplasmic granulation, and a lack of Michaelis–Gutmann bodies (B–D). Immunoreactivity for alpha-inhibin is seen in GCT (E), and ultrastructural studies demonstrate numerous cytoplasmic phagolysosomes (F). Neither one of those findings is apparent in malakoplakia.

3 Pleural Lesions

- REACTIVE MESOTHELIAL PROLIFERATIONS
- SMALL LYMPHOCYTIC EFFUSIONS/ LYMPHOCYTIC PLEURITIDES
- HYALINE PLEURAL PLAQUES
- DIFFUSE PLEURAL FIBROSIS (CHRONIC FIBROSING PLEURITIS; FIBROUS PLEURISY)
- OTHER PLEURAL PSEUDONEOPLASMS

Pseudoneoplastic processes in the pleura are also represented by a limited number of lesions. Perhaps the most common of them is principally a cytopathologic entity, namely, mesothelial hyperplasia, as seen in pleural effusion specimens **(Figure 3.1)**. Cytopathological mimics of malignancy encompass such a wide variety of entities that they cannot be addressed completely in this text; for a complete discussion the reader may consult more comprehensive treatises on cytology (375–377).

Nonetheless, several distinct pseudoneoplastic pleural lesions can be misinterpreted as tumors in surgical pathology. Moreover, because several of those

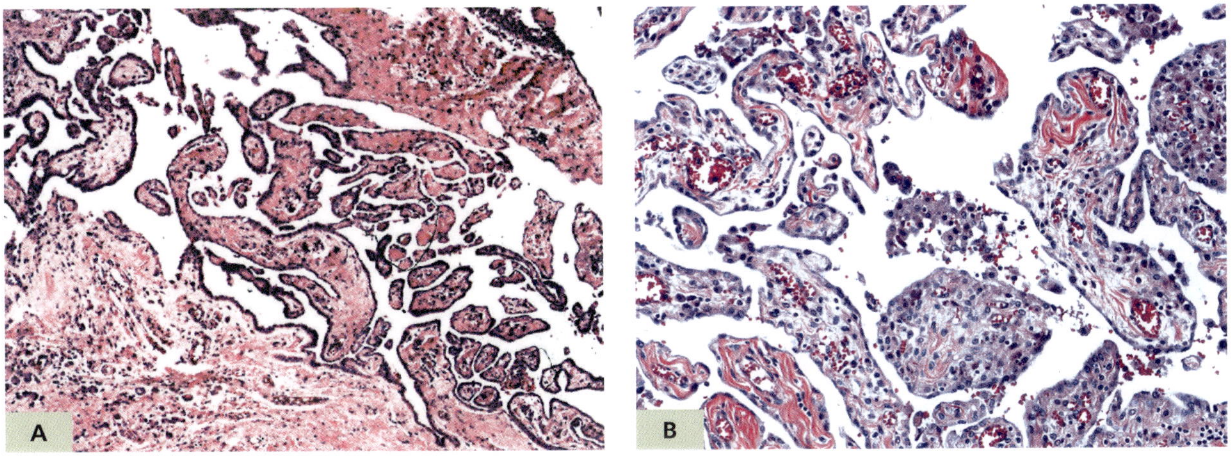

FIGURE 3.1 A & B: Mesothelial hyperplasia of the pleura may produce markedly papilliform structures that raise concern over possible diagnoses of mesothelioma or metastatic adenocarcinoma.

entities can be associated with asbestos exposure, they may be part of legal actions in which the pathologist becomes involved.

REACTIVE MESOTHELIAL PROLIFERATIONS

The correct microscopic classification of mesothelial lesions can be challenging (378,379). The principal problem here centers on the distinction of reactive proliferations from *mesothelioma* or *metastatic carcinoma*.

In the past, reactive mesothelial cell proliferations were often dispatched with the descriptive but vague label of "atypical mesothelial cells present" in regard to cytologic specimens (380). Because that terminology implies a possible connection to malignancy, or, at least, premalignancy, we do not advocate its continued use. Instead, it is better to simply indicate that "activated" but benign mesothelial cells are hyperplastic or reactive (381). Such proliferations can be seen in association with a variety of underlying conditions, including cirrhosis, anemia, viral infections, collagen vascular diseases, radiation pleuritis, responses to pleural metastases, and chronic pleural infections (382). Needless to say, an adequate clinical history is, therefore, an absolute necessity when evaluating pleural fluid specimens or pleural biopsies (383).

Features that favor a malignancy in pleural cytology specimens or small biopsies include the presence of papillae or other complex architectural structures, notable nuclear atypia (**Figure 3.2**), necrosis, and pathologically shaped mitotic figures (383). Inflammation in mesothelioma is generally scant, or it is seen primarily in areas of the lesion that are farthest away from the pleural surface.

As summarized by Bedrossian and coworkers, contrasting criteria exist for reactive or hyperplastic mesothelial lesions (384). These benign processes are characterized by only superficial entrapment of cellular nests in the stroma; an intense inflammatory infiltrate that is heaviest near the mesothelial surface; marked vascular proliferation with only scant spindle cells; the lack of overtly aberrant cytologic features; and an absence of atypical mitoses.

Despite the almost-universal reference to "cytologic atypia" in the literature on mesotheliomas, our experience with pleural biopsies suggests that this finding is often unimpressive in some mesothelial malignancies. On the other hand, it can be paradoxically striking in reactive mesothelium (**Figure 3.3**) (385). The cytologic criteria for mesothelioma include elevated nucleocytoplasmic ratios, irregularity of the nuclear membranes, and coarse, irregularly clumped chromatin. Studies by Marchevsky et al. (386), Kwee and colleagues (387), and Oberholzer and coworkers (388) all have suggested that nuclear morphometry—including such details as mean nuclear profile diameter, nuclear/cytoplasmic area, and "nuclear texture"—can discriminate benign from malignant mesothelial cell populations. In contrast, however, other authors have disagreed with that conclusion (389), and the general unweildiness of performing morphometric studies in daily practice is another detriment.

Selected attributes of mesothelial cells are common to both benign and malignant proliferations in cytologic specimens. These include cytoplasmic vacuolization, binucleation or multinucleation, and a brush-border pattern over the entire free surface of the cells **(Figure 3.4)**, corresponding to the

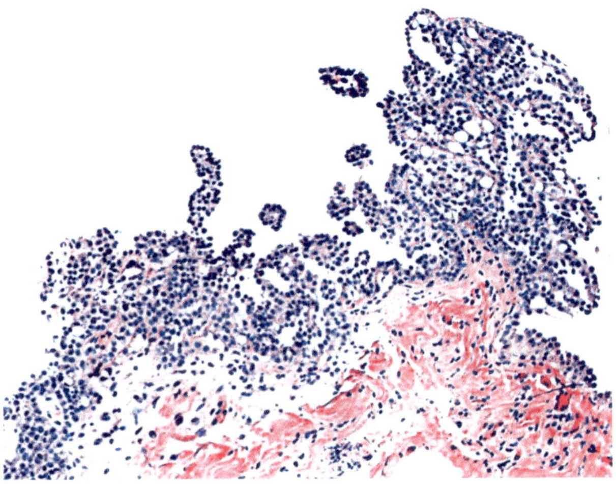

FIGURE 3.2 Architectural complexity in some examples of mesothelial hyperplasia is extreme.

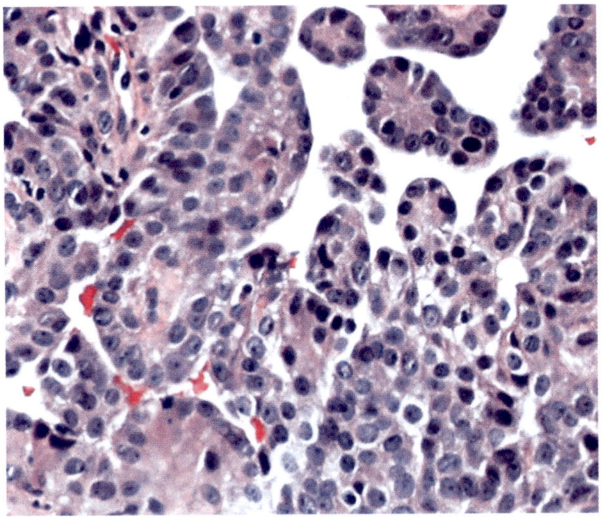

FIGURE 3.3 Moderate nuclear atypia is evident in what proved to be a case of mesothelial hyperplasia.

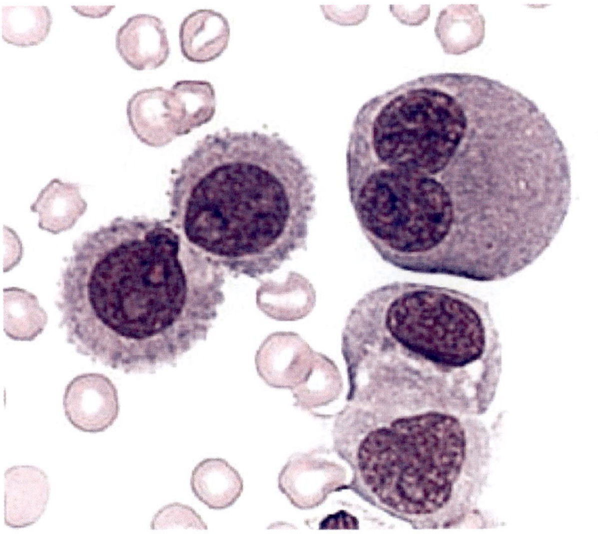

FIGURE 3.4 Effusion cytology specimens from pleural mesothelial proliferations feature the presence of "fuzzy" cell borders that reflect the presence of long microvilli.

ultrastructural finding of elongated microvilli **(Figure 3.5)** (390). In general, reactive cells tend to exfoliate singly or in small clusters (375). Large formations, including morular structures with "knobby" cellular outlines or papillary structures **(Figure 3.6)**, should raise suspicion for a diagnosis of mesothelioma. The same comment applies to the presence of dense hypercellularity in an effusion specimen (391).

Incidentally, one must understand that the foregoing discussion applies principally to the epithelial or biphasic varieties of malignant mesothelioma.

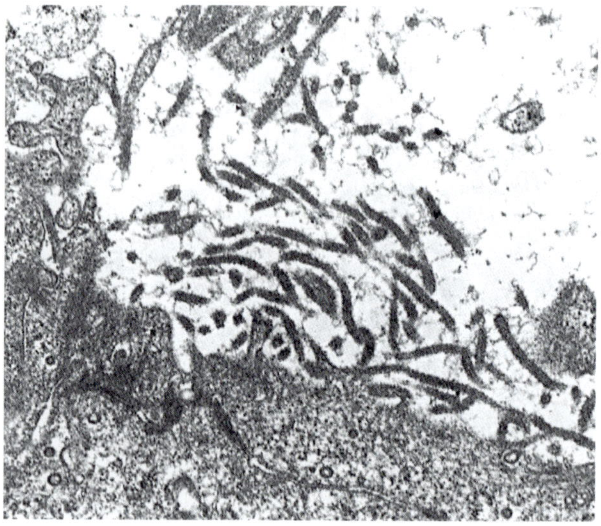

FIGURE 3.5 Electron microscopic studies of mesothelial lesions demonstrate long, branching microvilli on the cellular surfaces, with length-to-diameter ratios that usually exceed 10.

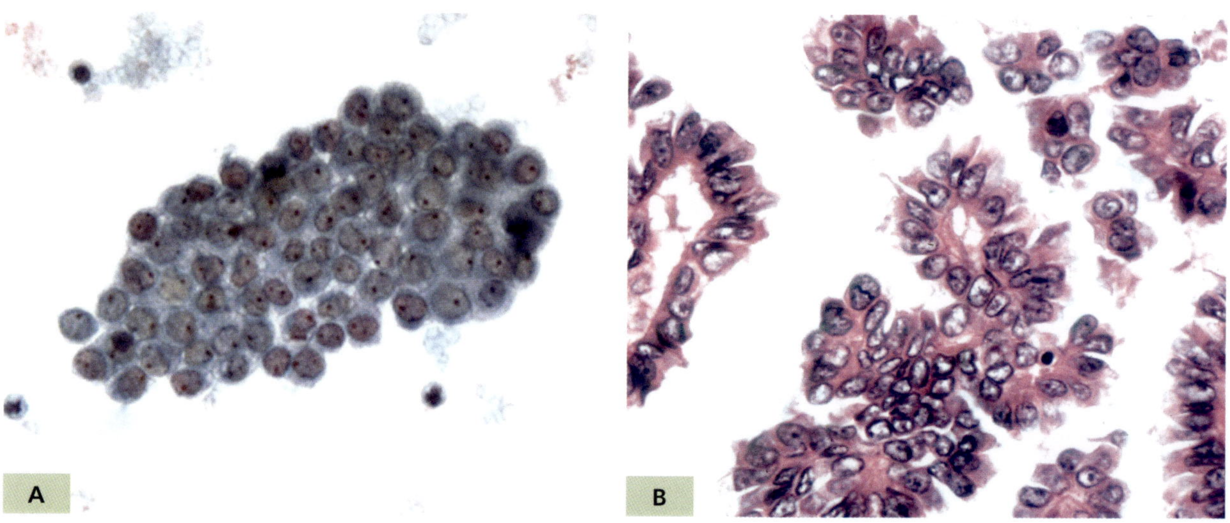

FIGURE 3.6 Tubulopapillary malignant mesotheliomas may be deceptively-bland cytologically, in effusion specimens or pleural biopsies (A & B). *(Continued)*

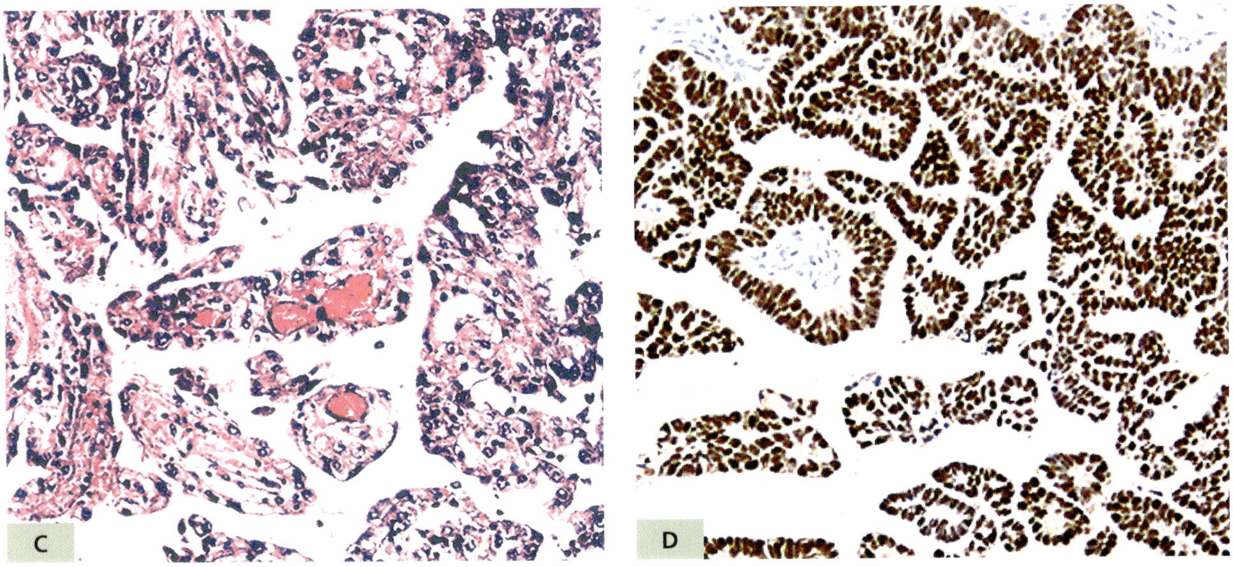

FIGURE 3.6 *(Continued)* Moreover, selected metastatic adenocarcinomas—such as papillary renal cell carcinoma (C & D, stained for PAX-2) can be confused with mesothelial hyperplasia as well.

That is so because *sarcomatoid* neoplasms rarely shed ***any*** malignant cells into body cavities. If effusions are present in those cases, they often contain only inflammatory cells and reactive but cytologically benign mesothelia (392).

The concept of "mesothelioma *in situ*" has been introduced for flat, noninvasive, microscopic mesothelial proliferations (393). Nonetheless, reliable pathological criteria for the prospective distinction of reactive proliferations from such putatively early lesions in small biopsies or cytologic specimens are still lacking.

In our opinion, immunohistochemical studies have limited value in making the distinction between reactive and malignant mesothelia. Both of those cell populations express a comparable spectrum of keratin types (394). Suggestions have been made that purely epithelioid mesotheliomas are reactive for a dense band of plasmalemmal epithelial membrane antigen (EMA) **(Figure 3.7)** and cytoplasmic vimentin, whereas benign mesothelial cells are negative for both markers (395). However, our own experience has not tended to validate these assertions. Hasteh et al. (396) likewise concluded

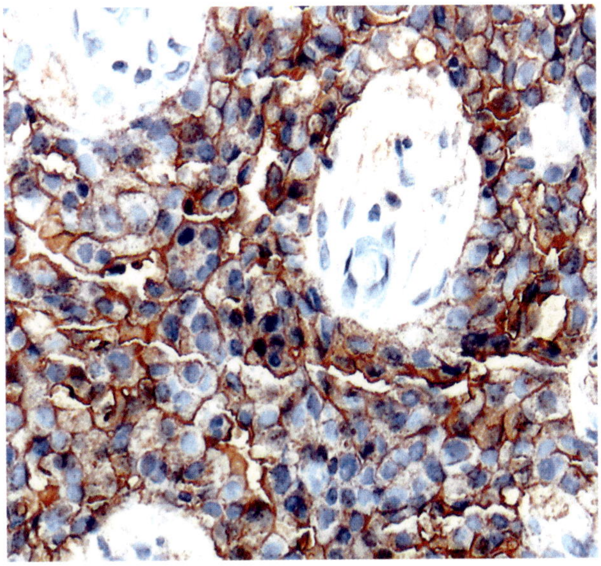

FIGURE 3.7 Dense cell-membrane-based immunoreactivity for epithelial membrane antigen has been said by some observers to favor a diagnosis of mesothelioma over one of mesothelial hyperplasia.

that immunoreactivity for GLUT-1 also favors a diagnosis of mesothelioma, but systematic validations of that proposition—especially as focused on cytologically indeterminate proliferations—have yet to be published.

Both benign and malignant mesothelia are nonreactive for carcinoembryonic antigen (CEA), CA72.4 antigen (the target of the B72.3 antibody), BG8, MOC-31, and CD15. Thus, that panel of reactants is helpful in distinguishing adenocarcinoma from mesothelioma, but it cannot separate benign from malignant mesothelial proliferations (397).

Interest has also grown with respect to immunostains for gene products that might suggest malignancy. Markers of cellular proliferation, such as proliferating cell nuclear antigen and Ki-67, have been advocated in this context (398), and mutant p53 protein has also received considerable attention (399–402). Some authors have found that p53 immunostaining is often present in mesothelioma **(Figure 3.8)** but is rarely seen in benign or reactive mesothelial proliferations (399–401). Although it may provide some interpretative assistance, sole diagnostic reliance on immunohistology for mutant p53 protein is unwise. That analyte must always be integrated with histologic and cytologic findings, as well as other clinicopathologic details (402).

In view of the generally dismal outcome in mesothelioma cases and the continuing absence of effective therapy for that tumor, diagnostic caution is generally appropriate in this context. It is much less satisfactory to label a reactive proliferation as mesothelioma than it would be to "undercall" an abnormal, but less than completely diagnostic specimen. With the passage of time, morphologically-ambiguous cases will declare themselves as mesothelioma if that is what they truly represent.

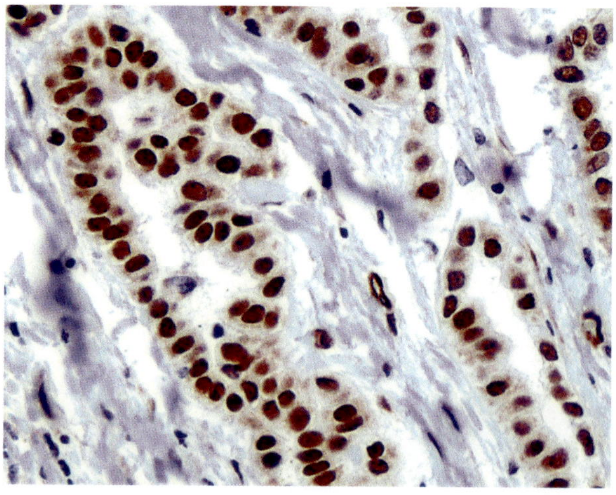

FIGURE 3.8 Nuclear positivity for putatively mutant p53 protein is another finding that has been used to distinguish mesotheliomas—which area said to be positive—from mesothelial hyperplasias.

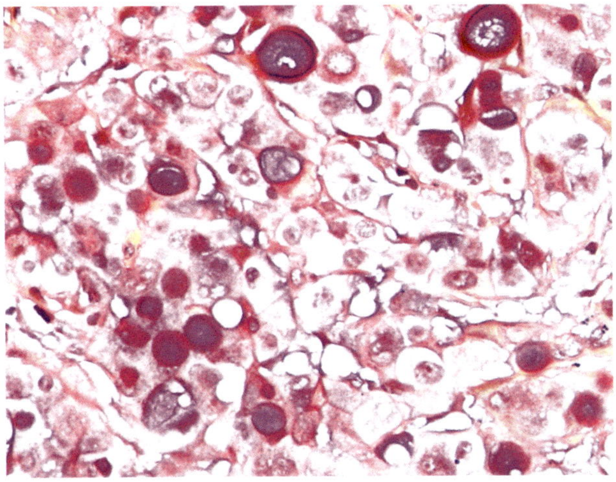

FIGURE 3.9 Histochemical positivity with the digested periodic acid-Schiff method for epithelial mucin eliminates the diagnostic possibilities of mesothelial hyperplasia and mesothelioma and supports an interpretation of metastatic adenocarcinoma in the pleura.

In regard to the distinction of reactive mesothelial cells from metastatic carcinoma, more clear-cut criteria exist (384). The cytologic attributes of benign mesothelial cells include relative cellular monomorphism (375). In contrast, carcinomatous effusions often feature a dimorphic cellular population (375). Periodic acid–Schiff stains, done after diastase digestion, will identify epithelial-type mucin in a substantial number of metastatic adenocarcinomas **(Figure 3.9)** but not in mesothelial proliferations (390,403). On the other hand, some intracytoplasmic vacuoles in mesothelial cells contain hyaluronic acid that is stainable with Alcian blue or colloidal iron methods at pH 2.5; it is digestible with hyaluronidase (403).

As documented above, a selected panel of immunostains can detect the great majority of metastatic carcinomas in the serosae, but it will not label reactive or malignant mesothelial cells (375–377,380,381,384, 390,403–408). Stains for oncogene products, including c-*erb*-B2, mutant p53, and H-ras proteins (409), may also be useful in selected instances in this specific context. Useful "pro-mesothelial" markers include calretinin, WT-1 gene product, and podoplanin.

SMALL LYMPHOCYTIC EFFUSIONS/LYMPHOCYTIC PLEURITIDES

Another common problem pertaining to pseudoneoplastic pleural lesions concerns lymphocyte-rich effusions. This conundrum almost never involves a question of large-cell or high-grade lymphoma but rather revolves around the differential diagnosis of small, relatively mature lymphocytic proliferations (e.g., *small lymphocytic lymphoma* [SLL], *mantle-cell lymphoma*, or *chronic lymphocytic leukemia* versus benign lymphoid infiltrates). A short list of benign conditions that can produce lymphocyte-rich pleural effusions includes tuberculosis, laceration of the intrathoracic lymphatic vessels, and autoimmune serositides as seen in rheumatoid arthritis or lupus erythematosus **(Figure 3.10)** (377).

The cytologic features of benign and malignant small lymphocytic lesions can be remarkably similar; both may comprise compact, round, uniform lymphocytes **(Figure 3.11)**, admixed with a few mesothelial cells. Although pleural effusions are rare as a presenting manifestation of SLL, they may be seen in a substantial number of cases as that disease progresses. Adjunctive pathologic techniques may be useful in excluding benign infiltrates. The great majority of cases of SLL are B-lymphocytic in nature (375,377). Thus, immunostains showing a predominance of cells expressing CD20, CD79a, or *PAX5*, and in situ hybridization studies for monotypic light chain immunoglobulins (LCIs) are potentially definitive diagnostically. Conjoint expression of CD20 (a pan-B-cell marker) and CD43 (a pan-T-cell marker) may also be helpful. In contrast, one expects reactive lymphoid infiltrates of the serosae to be composed mainly of T-cells (410,411). Polymerase chain reaction-based techniques for immunoglobulin

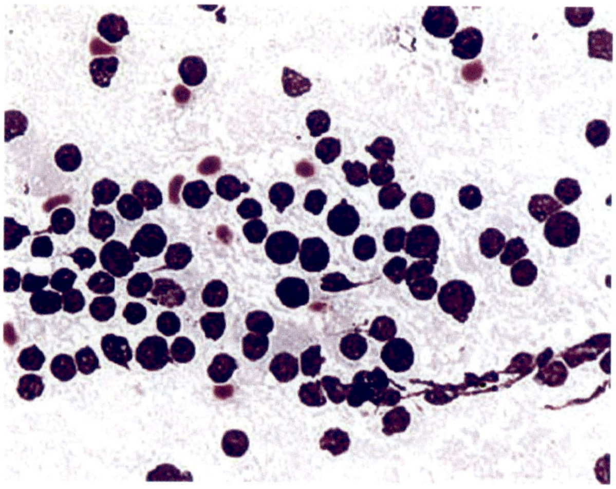

FIGURE 3.10 An abundance of mature lymphocytes in pleural effusion cytology specimens is associated with a sizable differential diagnosis. It includes pleuritis caused by collagen vascular diseases or mycobacterial infections, as well as trauma to intrathoracic lymphatic vessels, chronic lymphocytic leukemia, and small lymphocytic lymphoma.

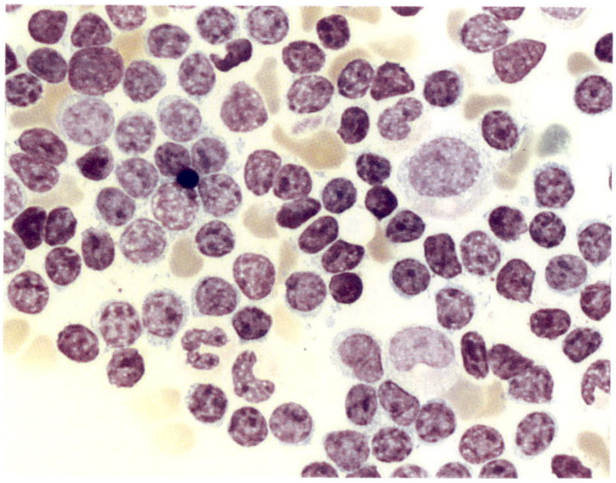

FIGURE 3.11 In cases of lymphocytic effusions that feature mature lymphoid cells, it is usually impossible to distinguish benign from malignant infiltrates based on morphology alone.

heavy chain gene rearrangements can be applied successfully to cytologic material or small biopsies, to document lymphoid monoclonality (411).

In a pragmatic sense, it is important to remember that malignant effusions typically reaccumulate over a short time. If immunostains and other data are insufficient for a firm diagnosis of any given cytological specimen, more pleural fluid can be readily obtained if the lesion is truly lymphomatous. Morphological reanalysis, together with flow cytometry, is certainly more cost-effective than reflexive application of other adjunctive pathologic procedures to every lymphocytic effusion specimen.

HYALINE PLEURAL PLAQUES

Hyaline pleural plaques (HPPs) constitute important lesions, because of their association with occupational dust exposures and the necessity of distinguishing them from true neoplasms of the pleura. HPPs were first described several decades ago in association with asbestos exposure (412–431).

A review of autopsy studies by Schwartz (430) revealed a widely variable incidence of pleural plaques in routine necropsies, with an average of 12.2%. Virtually all analyses have failed to demonstrate the presence of asbestos fibers in the plaques themselves, but instead have demonstrated those minerals in subjacent pulmonary parenchyma. Warnock and coworkers (429) opined that all types of asbestos were potentially linked to the development of HPPs, although most were associated with amosite and crocidolite fibers. Additional studies by Churg (414,415) and others (418,419,422,429) have likewise found a predominance of intrapulmonary amphibole fibers in association with HPPs. The number of fibers is above that seen in age- and sex-matched control individuals without past asbestos exposure, but it is far smaller than the asbestos burden of individuals with documented asbestosis (422,429).

The foregoing comments apply principally to individuals with ***bilateral, parietal*** pleural plaques **(Figure 3.12)**. In contrast, one-sided plaques or visceral pleural hyalizing fibrosis may occur whenever chronic pleural irritation has existed from any cause. Other conditions that can produce ***unilateral*** HPPs include tuberculosis, bacterial empyema, chronic or recurrent pleural hemorrhage, and trauma to the chest wall (419,426,427).

Plaques are most often detected in individuals in the seventh and eighth decades of life (414,426). Those associated with asbestos exposure develop after a latent period of approximately 20 years from the time of initial dust inhalation

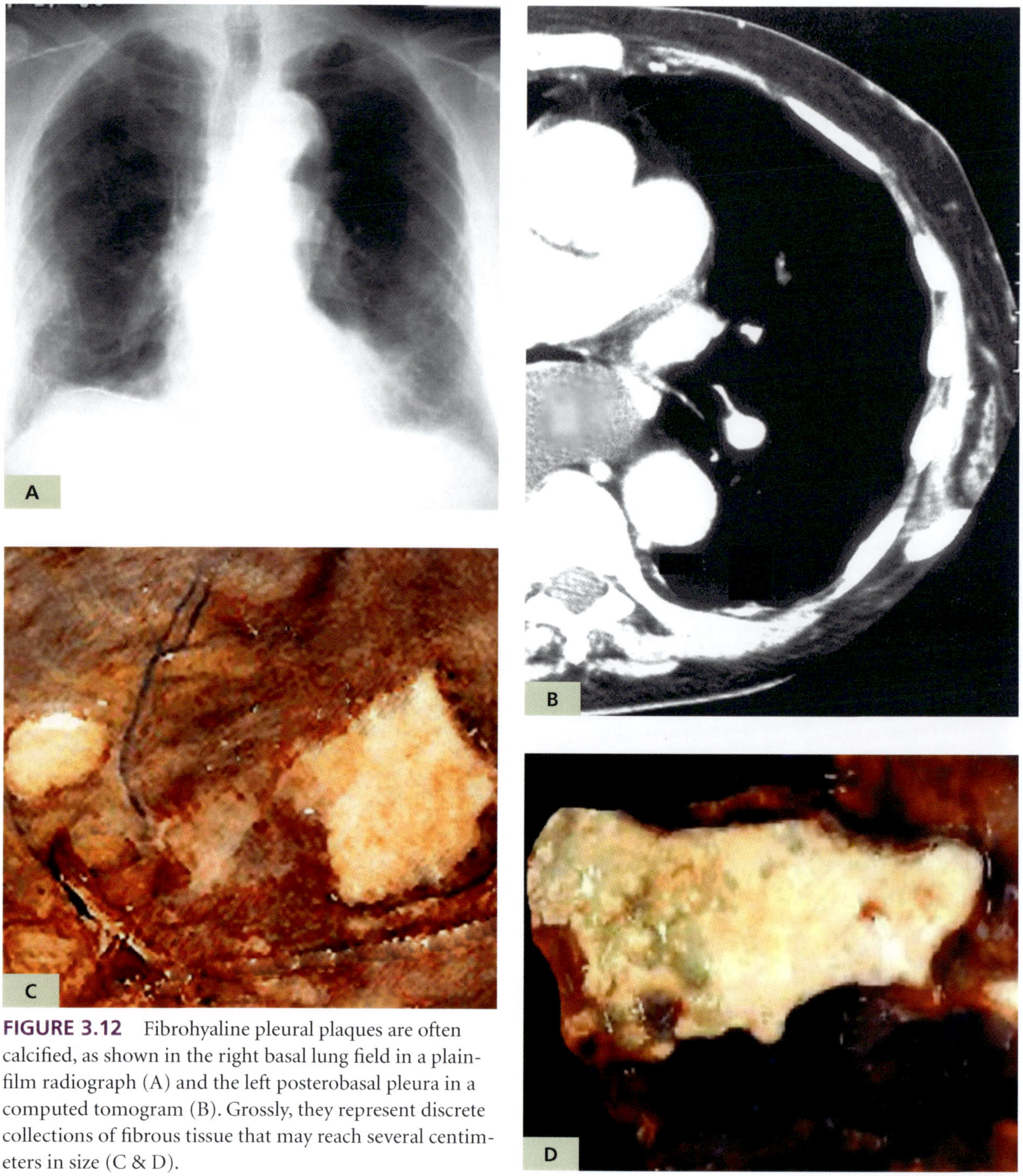

FIGURE 3.12 Fibrohyaline pleural plaques are often calcified, as shown in the right basal lung field in a plain-film radiograph (A) and the left posterobasal pleura in a computed tomogram (B). Grossly, they represent discrete collections of fibrous tissue that may reach several centimeters in size (C & D).

(414–429). HPPs most often develop in the lower thorax and principally involve the basal parietal pleural surfaces. They may show an orientation that is parallel to the ribs (420). Less often, one sees involvement of the visceral pleura, and, rarely, HPPs can occur in the pericardium as well (417,428). Affected individuals have no symptoms that can be related directly to the plaques themselves. Pulmonary function abnormalities in such patients are caused by associated chronic obstructive pulmonary disease or other disorders of the lung parenchyma (414,415). Plain-film chest radiographs have limited sensitivity for the detection of HPPs, unless they are calcified (420,422). The use of computed tomography has greatly improved the visualization of these lesions (431).

Histologically, HPPs comprise dense and hypocellular aggregates of collagen, often with a lamellated "basket-weave" pattern **(Figure 3.13)**. Foci of associated chronic inflammation may be seen, and calcification is multifocal and amorphous. The proposed mechanism for formation of HPPs is that of recurrent organizing pleuritis.

The most important differential diagnostic consideration in cases of HPP is that of *desmoplastic mesothelioma* (DM). Both lesions can be constituted by relatively bland spindle cells that are separated by dense bands of collagen (432). Nonetheless, DM only extraordinarily presents as a solitary and localized mass, and one expects to see greater cellularity in that tumor as compared

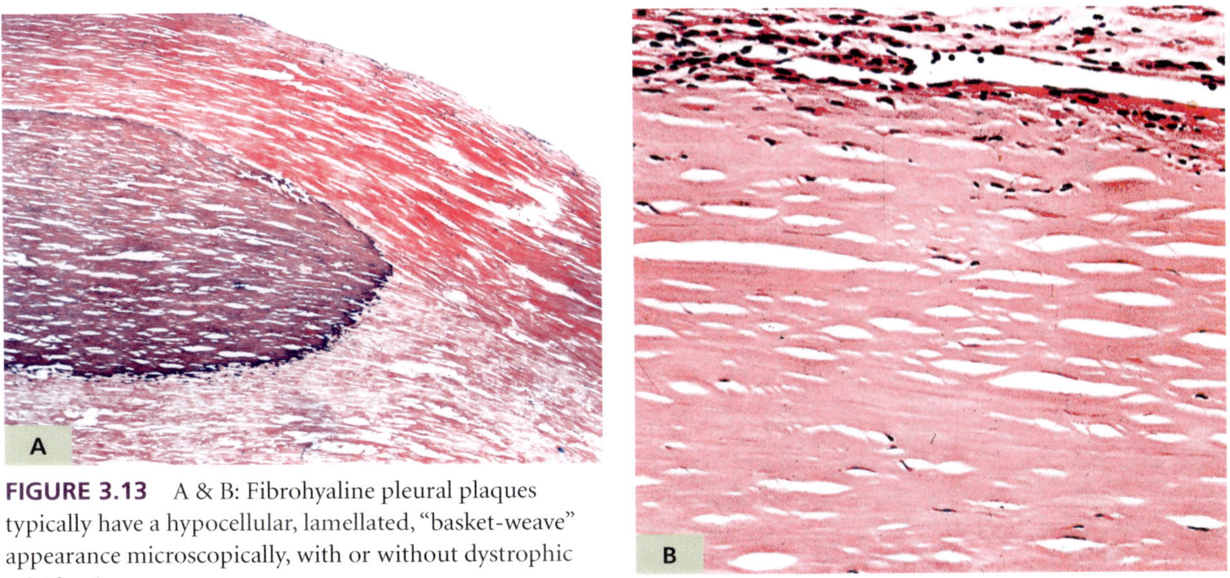

FIGURE 3.13 A & B: Fibrohyaline pleural plaques typically have a hypocellular, lamellated, "basket-weave" appearance microscopically, with or without dystrophic calcification.

with HPP. Intralesional calcification is distinctly unusual in DM as well (432). The cells of DM also exhibit a greater degree of nuclear pleomorphism and hyperchromasia (**Figure 3.14**). Involvement of the visceral pleura and diffuse effacement of the pleural space are preferential features of DM and argue

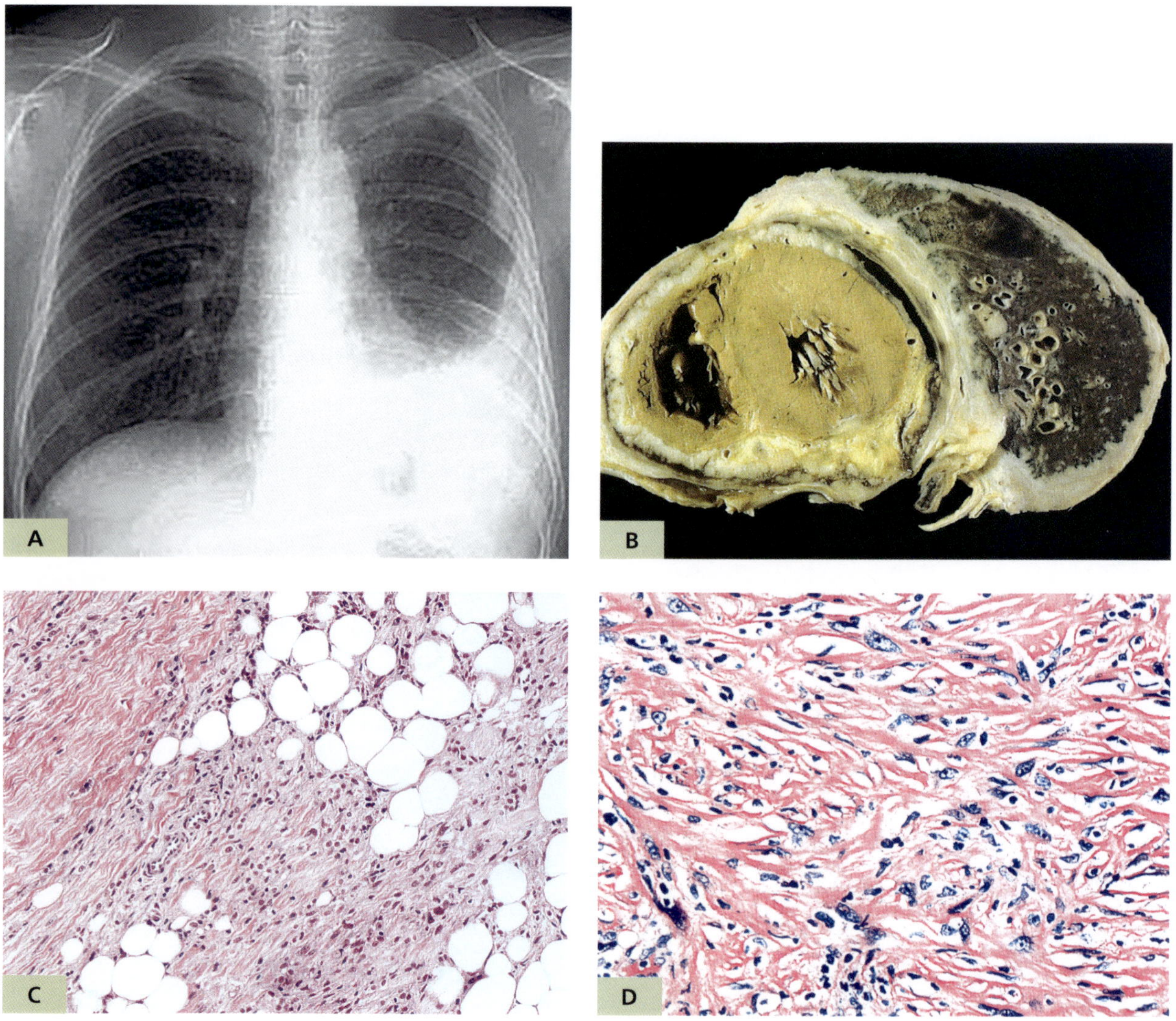

FIGURE 3.14 Desmoplastic mesotheliomas (DMs) are diffuse lesions that often cause pleural effusions (A), in contrast to fibrohyaline plaques. DMs may encase both the lungs and the heart (B), and they show obvious invasion of the subpleural adipose tissue (C). These features are important in differential diagnosis, because the histologic appearance of DM may be only marginally different from that of a fibrohyaline plaque in limited biopsies (D).

strongly against an interpretation of HPP (433), which is typically spheroid and well-circumscribed.

Immunohistological studies have limited use in this context. Both HPP and DM are diffusely immunoreactive for keratin and vimentin (390,434–436). DM may also show immunoreactivity for such myogenic determinants as actin, desmin, and h-caldesmon, but those markers are seen in a minority of cases. Activated submesothelial fibroblasts may also show keratin-positivity (394), as seen in organizing pleuritis. Markers that are often used to separate *epithelioid* mesothelioma from metastatic carcinoma have no value in the analysis of spindle cell lesions of the pleura, because they are essentially never seen in that tumor group (437). Electron microscopy is also unhelpful in this setting because the cells of both DM and HPP resemble fibroblasts or myofibroblasts ultrastructurally (438).

Sclerotic solitary fibrous tumors (SSFTs) of the pleura may also contain keloidal collagen as seen in HPPs. In comparison, however, SSFTs are more cellular overall and often exhibit a variety of histologic growth patterns **(Figure 3.15)**. These include storiform, hemangiopericytoma-like, and "patternless" configurations (439). Solitary fibrous tumors have no causal relationship to

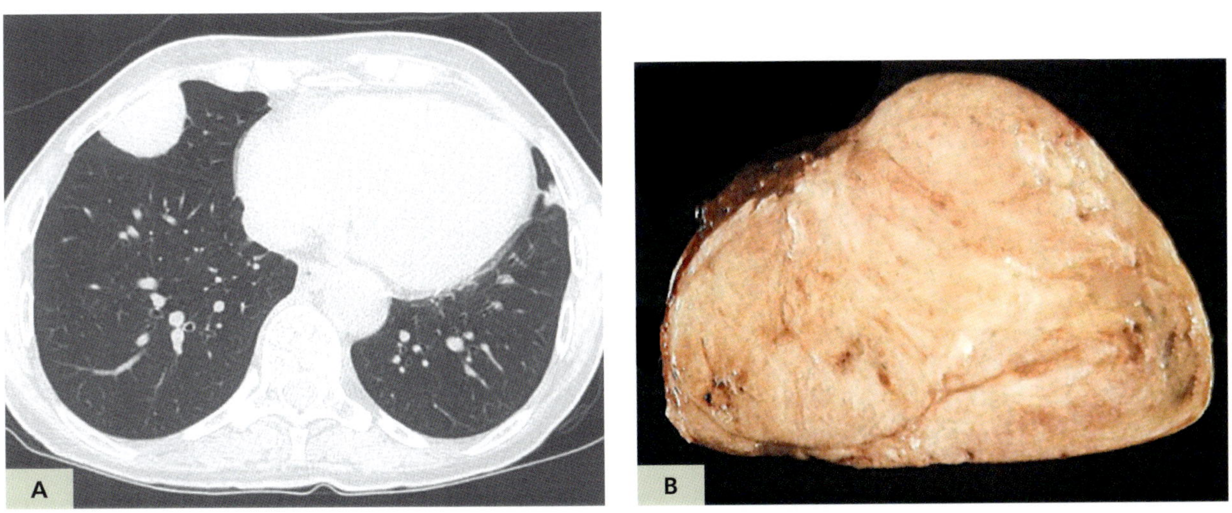

FIGURE 3.15 Solitary fibrous tumors (SFTs) of the pleura are localized nodular lesions, in similarity to pleural plaques at a radiographic level (A). However, they are "fleshier" masses grossly, with a firm, but not hard, tan-white cut surface (B). *(Continued)*

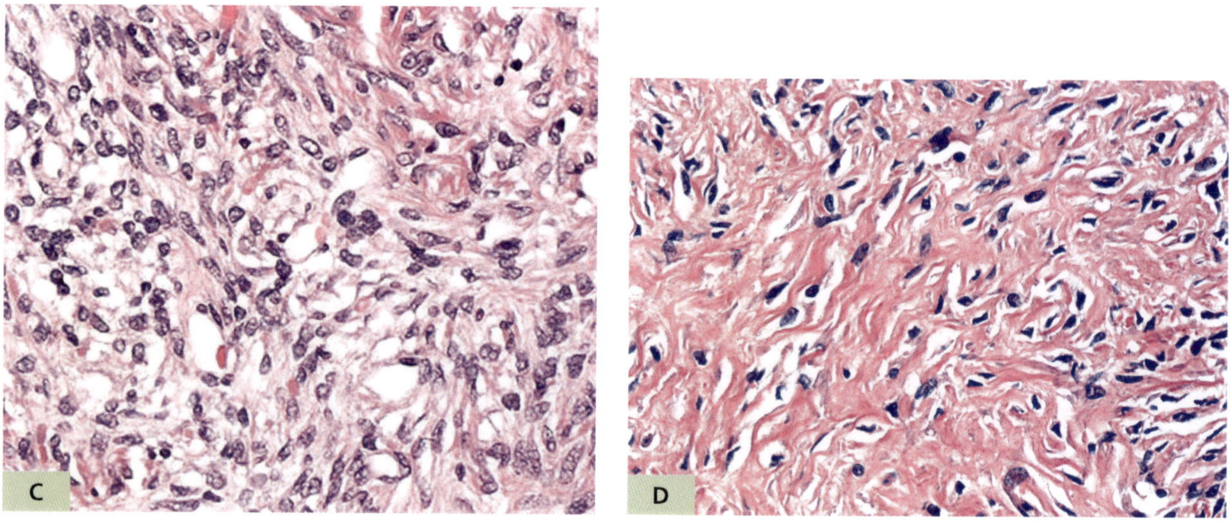

FIGURE 3.15 *(Continued)* Microscopically, SFTs may show a cellular proliferation of variably-atypical spindle cells in a collagenized stroma (C), or they may be paucicellular with stromal hyalinosis (D). The last of those images approximates that of fibrohyaline plaques.

asbestos exposure and are immunoreactive for CD34, CD99, or bcl-2 protein **(Figure 3.16)** (439,440). All of those determinants are absent in HPPs. A further differential diagnostic consideration is that of "*calcifying fibrous tumor*," another lesion that is also usually CD34-positive (441). Moreover, the calcifications in

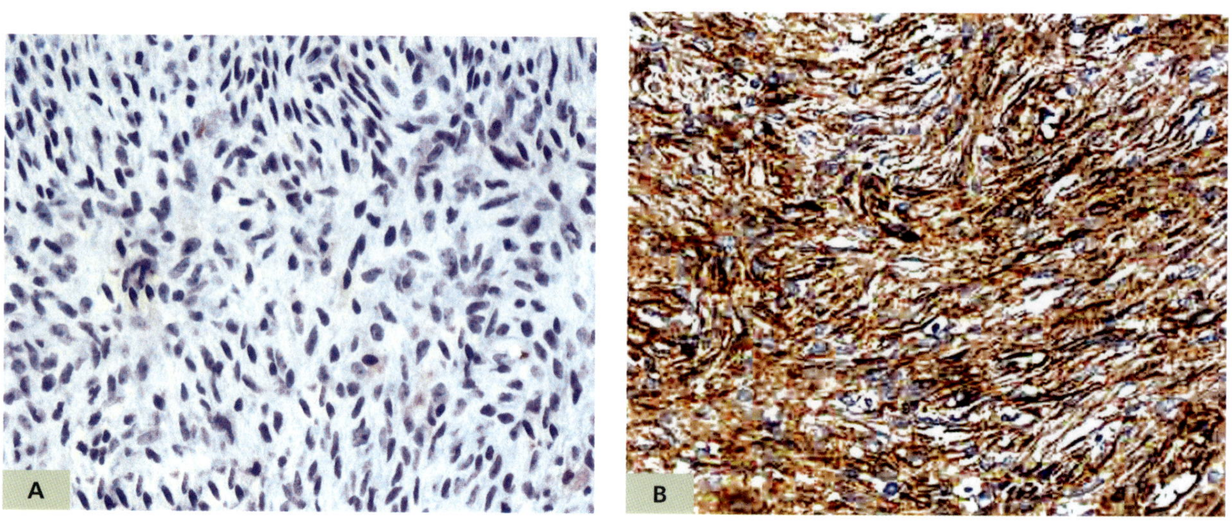

FIGURE 3.16 Immunohistochemically, solitary fibrous tumors of the pleura are non-reactive for keratin (A), and positive for CD34 (B), bcl-2 protein (C), or CD99 (D), and combinations thereof. The latter three markers are absent in pleural plaques. *(Continued)*

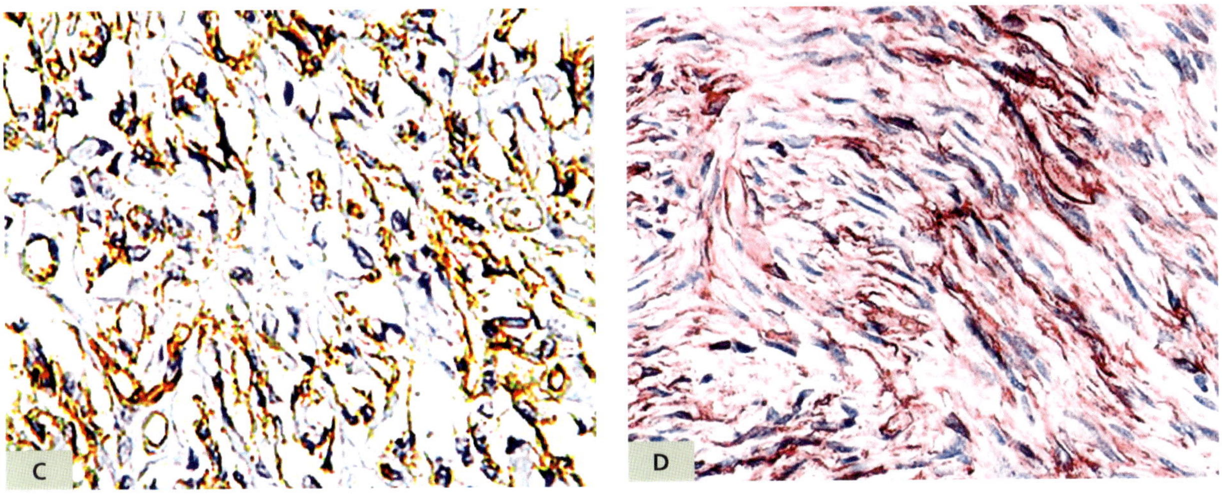

FIGURE 3.16 *(Continued)*

calcifying fibrous tumor are small and psammoma body-like **(Figure 3.17)**, differing from the broad zones of dystrophic calcium deposition in HPP.

As stated earlier, HPPs themselves produce no symptoms or organ dysfunction (415,442). Hence, there is no reason for the surgical removal of such lesions.

The concept of a relationship between asbestos-related HPPs to bronchogenic carcinomas and mesotheliomas has been addressed in many publications, which have been reviewed in other texts (443). The overwhelmingly consensual

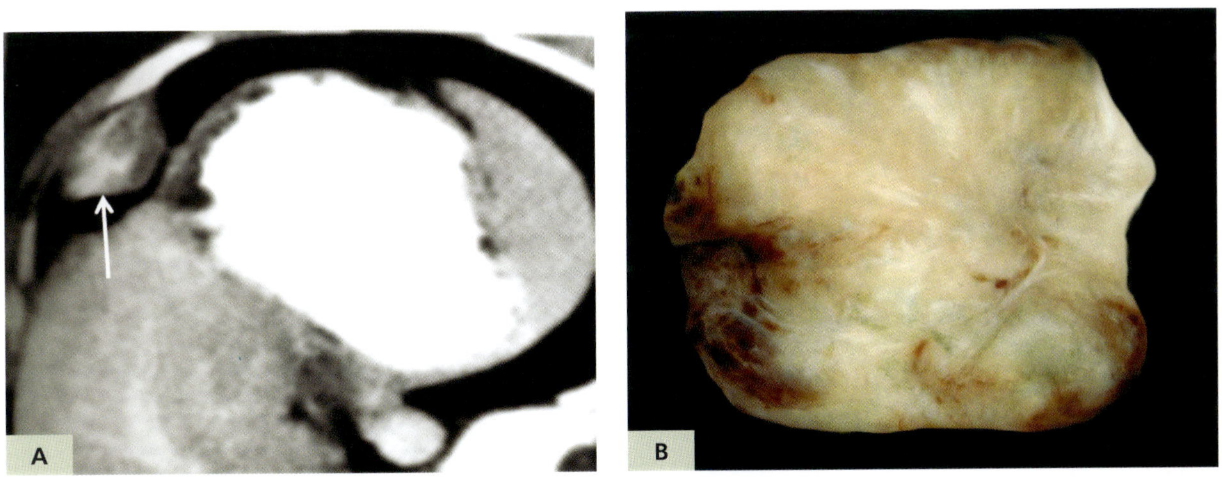

FIGURE 3.17 Another neoplasm that may be imitated by pleural plaques is represented by calcifying fibrous tumor (CFT) (A, arrow). That lesion is again fleshier than plaques are (B). *(Continued)*

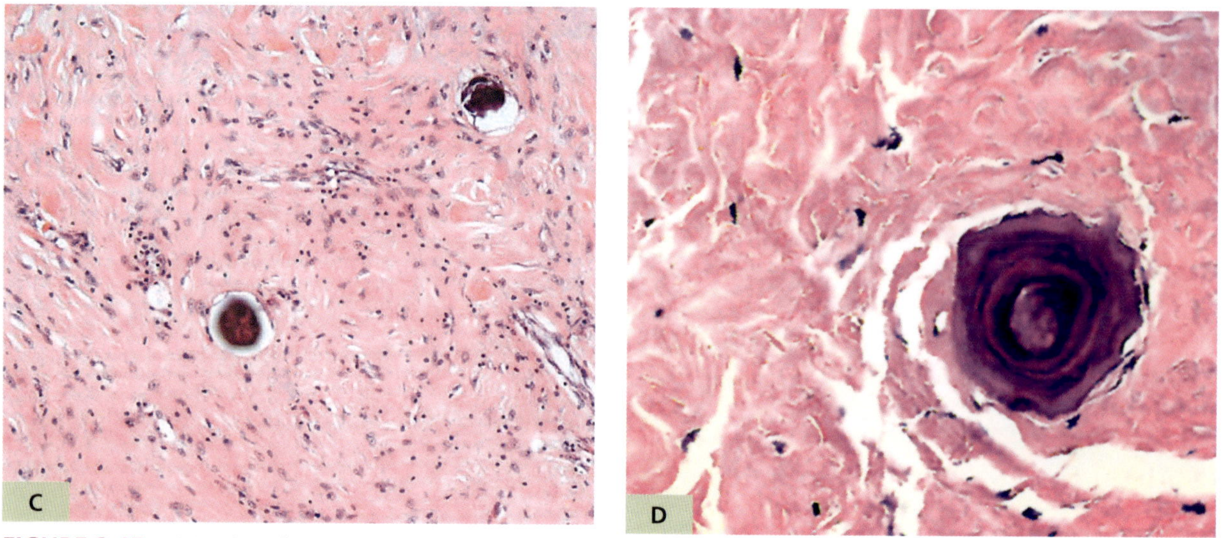

FIGURE 3.17 *(Continued)* It contains characteristic psammomatoid calcifications (C & D), which are absent in fibrohyaline plaques.

conclusion on this topic is that pleural plaques are not, in any way, precursors of true pleuropulmonary neoplasms. HPPs merely serve as markers of prior exposure to mineral dusts.

DIFFUSE PLEURAL FIBROSIS (CHRONIC FIBROSING PLEURITIS; FIBROUS PLEURISY)

Diffuse pleural fibrosis (DPF) may be associated with collagen vascular diseases, chronic infections, IgG4 disease (444), or prior asbestos exposure, although it is completely nonspecific in regard to any of those associations (445–449). Unlike pleural plaques, DPF typically involves the visceral pleura and the pulmomary apical serosa. In advanced cases, obliteration of the pleural space may occur because of fusion of the visceral and parietal pleural layers (448,449).

Histologically, one sees bland, modestly cellular fibrous tissue in DPF, generally (but not always) without the overtly lamellated appearance of hyaline plaques **(Figure 3.18)** (450,451). Hypervascularity may be observed as well, with foci of chronic inflammation including plasma cells, lymphocytes, and histiocytes. As discussed in connection with HPPs, the main differential diagnostic task in cases of DPF is the exclusion of *DM* (451,452). Morphologic nuances do exist that tend to separate the two conditions. DPF tends to exhibit a stratified internal pattern of collagen and elastic deposition, with vertically

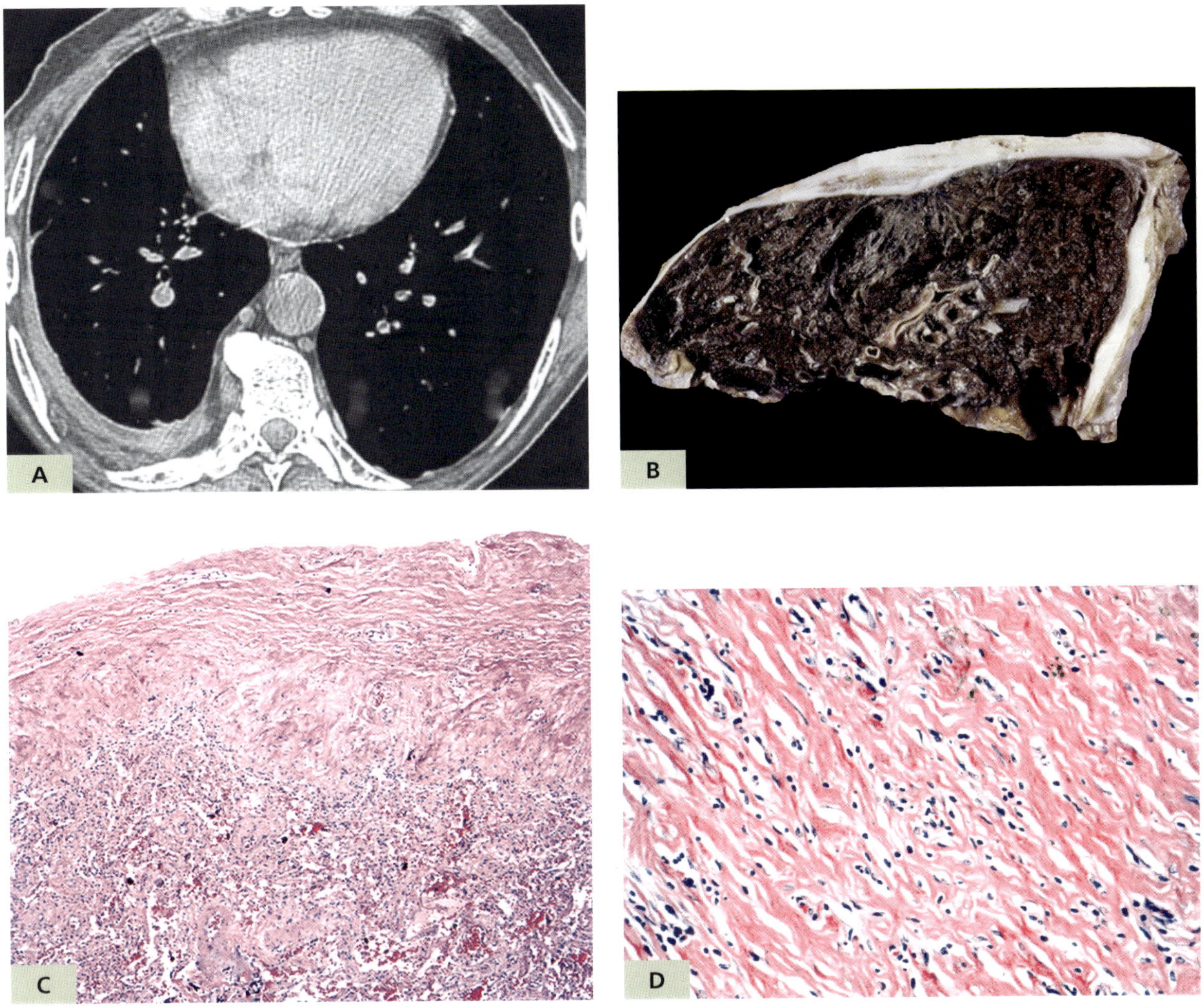

FIGURE 3.18 Diffuse pleural fibrosis (DPF) may follow episodes of sterile pleuritis, pleural empyema, or surgical procedures in the thorax. It may present with unilateral or bilateral pleural thickening (A & B), which may be striking. In contrast to desmoplastic mesotheliomas, DPF typically shows a zonation or lamellation in the deposition of fibrous tissue in the pleura (C & D), and it does not extend into the subpleural adipose tissue.

aligned stromal blood vessels and sparing of the parietal submesothelial fat **(Figure 3.19)**. DM manifests random collagenization and vascular orientation; it is a more cellular process and typically grows into the subpleural soft tissue, at least focally **(Figure 3.20)** (435,451). These findings are crucial because the clinical presentations and immunophenotypes of DPF and DM are potentially so similar (450). Both conditions have the ability to encase the lung in a dense rind of fibrosis with variable thickness **(Figure 3.21)**.

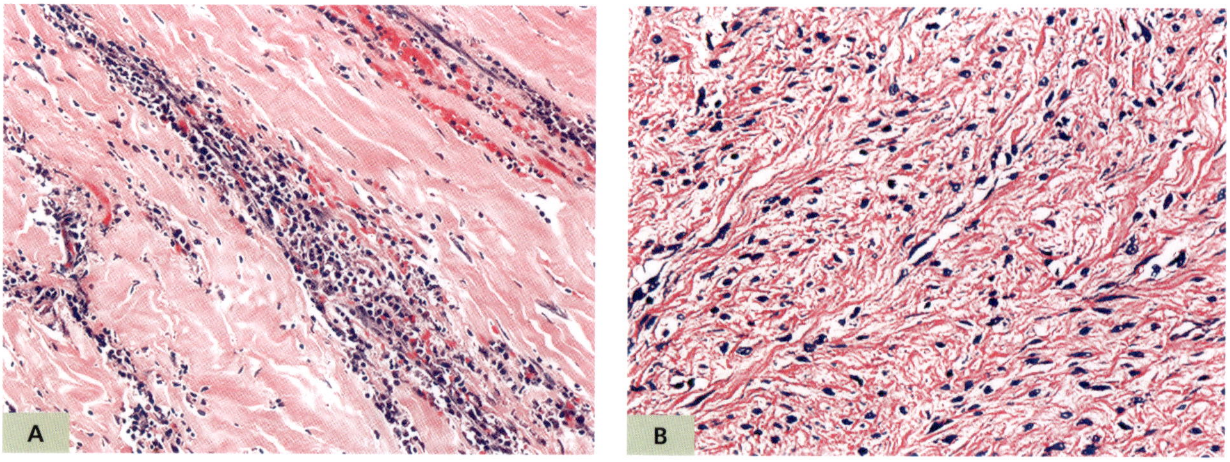

FIGURE 3.19 A & B: The lamellar and stratified nature of diffuse pleural fibrosis is well seen in these photomicrographs.

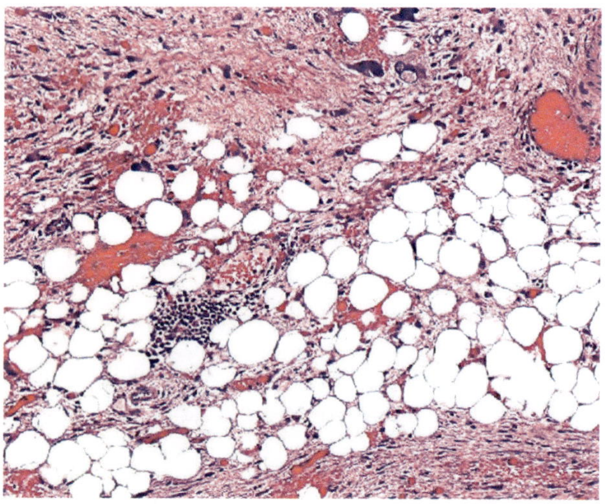

FIGURE 3.20 Extension into the subpleural adipose tissue by tumor is common in cases of desmoplastic mesothelioma.

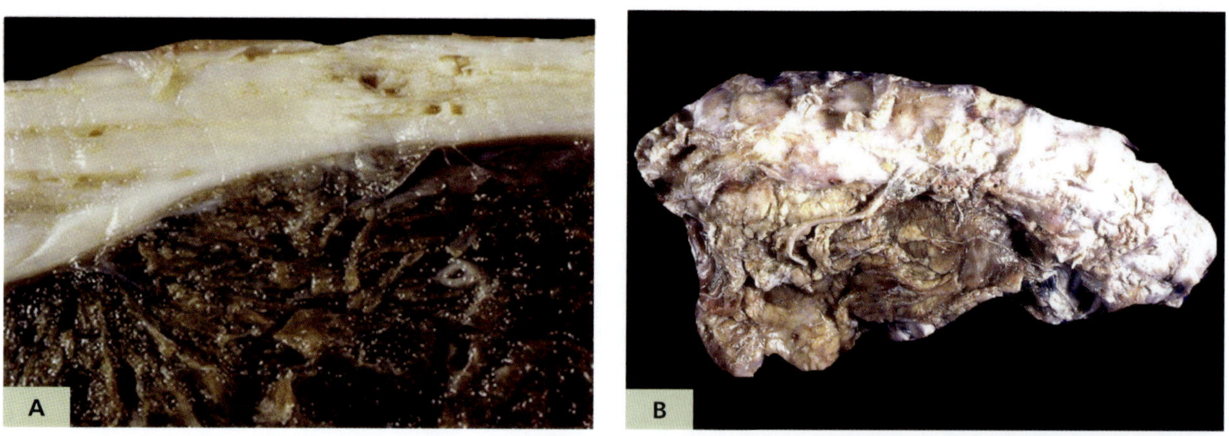

FIGURE 3.21 Diffuse pleural fibrosis (fibrous pleurisy) may create a very thick fibrous "rind" around the lung, but it maintains a sharp distinction from the pulmonary parenchyma (A). In contrast, desmoplastic mesothelioma usually infiltrates across the visceral pleura into the peripheral lung (B).

OTHER PLEURAL PSEUDONEOPLASMS

The pleural surfaces may also play host to ***extramedullary hematopoiesis*** (453–455), ***Rosai–Dorfman disease*** (456,457), ***malakoplakia*** (458), and ***Castleman's disease*** (459–461) as discussed above in reference to pulmonary lesions. Differential diagnostic considerations and clinicopathologic points of dissimilarity with true neoplasms are identical to those which have been outlined earlier in this discussion.

4 Thymic and Mediastinal Lesions

- INFLAMMATORY PSEUDOTUMORS
  - Idiopathic Fibrosing Mediastinitis
    - (Tumefactive Fibroinflammatory Lesion)
- MESOTHELIAL INCLUSIONS IN MEDIASTINAL LYMPH NODES
- MULTILOCULAR THYMIC CYSTS
- TUMEFACTIVE SARCOIDOSIS AND SARCOIDAL REACTIONS
- THYMIC HYPERPLASIA
- OTHER PSEUDONEOPLASTIC MEDIASTINAL LESIONS

Relatively few pseudoneoplastic proliferations of the mediastinum and thymus gland have been reported. These are principally represented by inflammatory pseudotumor (IPT) and tumefactive fibroinflammatory lesions (TFILs) such as fibrosing mediastinitis (FM).

INFLAMMATORY PSEUDOTUMORS

Only anecdotal reports of "plasma cell granuloma," or IPT, as described above, have been recorded in the mediastinum. Marchevsky (462) illustrated such a lesion in an adult patient of unstated age and gender, and he related that the clinical, radiologic, and macroscopic features of this mass closely simulated those of an invasive thymoma. We have seen another similar example in a 36-year-old man who presented with a 3-month history of progressive cough and who is well 15 years after subsequent thymectomy. The resected specimen demonstrated only a fascicular proliferation of bland fibroblasts, as characteristic of IPT in general, and a mixture of chronic inflammatory cells was also dispersed throughout the mass **(Figure 4.1)**. The immunohistochemical characteristics of thymic IPT were not addressed by Marchevsky (462) or in another case report by Tazzioli et al. (463). However, our case showed an absence of keratin and epithelial membrane antigen, but vimentin was instead detectable in the proliferating spindle cells. The lesional lymphocytes had

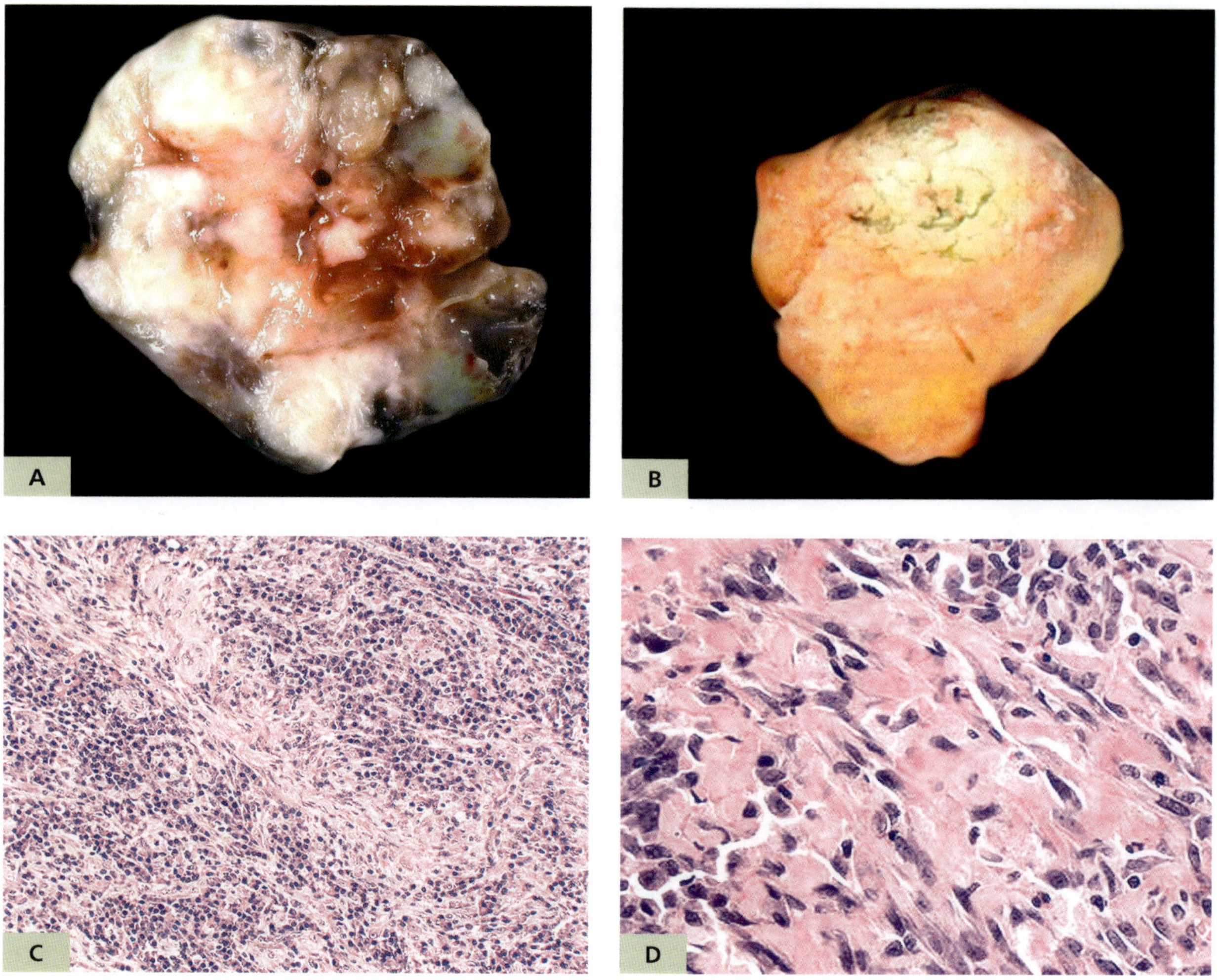

FIGURE 4.1 "True" IPT of the thymus has a fleshy appearance grossly (A & B). Microscopically, it shows an admixture of lymphocytes, plasma cells, and hyalinizing collagenous stroma (C & D).

a T-cell immunophenotype, and plasma cells in the mass were polytypic for light-chain immunoglobulins.

These features aid in excluding the primary differential diagnostic alternatives to thymic IPT, namely, *spindle-cell thymoma* and *nodular sclerosing Hodgkin's lymphoma* or *sclerosing large-cell non-Hodgkin's lymphoma* (464). Thymomas are typically definable on the basis of their conventional morphologic attributes alone (**Figure 4.2**). However, sclerosing lymphomas may show such a high density of collagenized stromal connective tissue that careful examination is necessary to detect the atypical lymphocytes in those neoplasms (465,466).

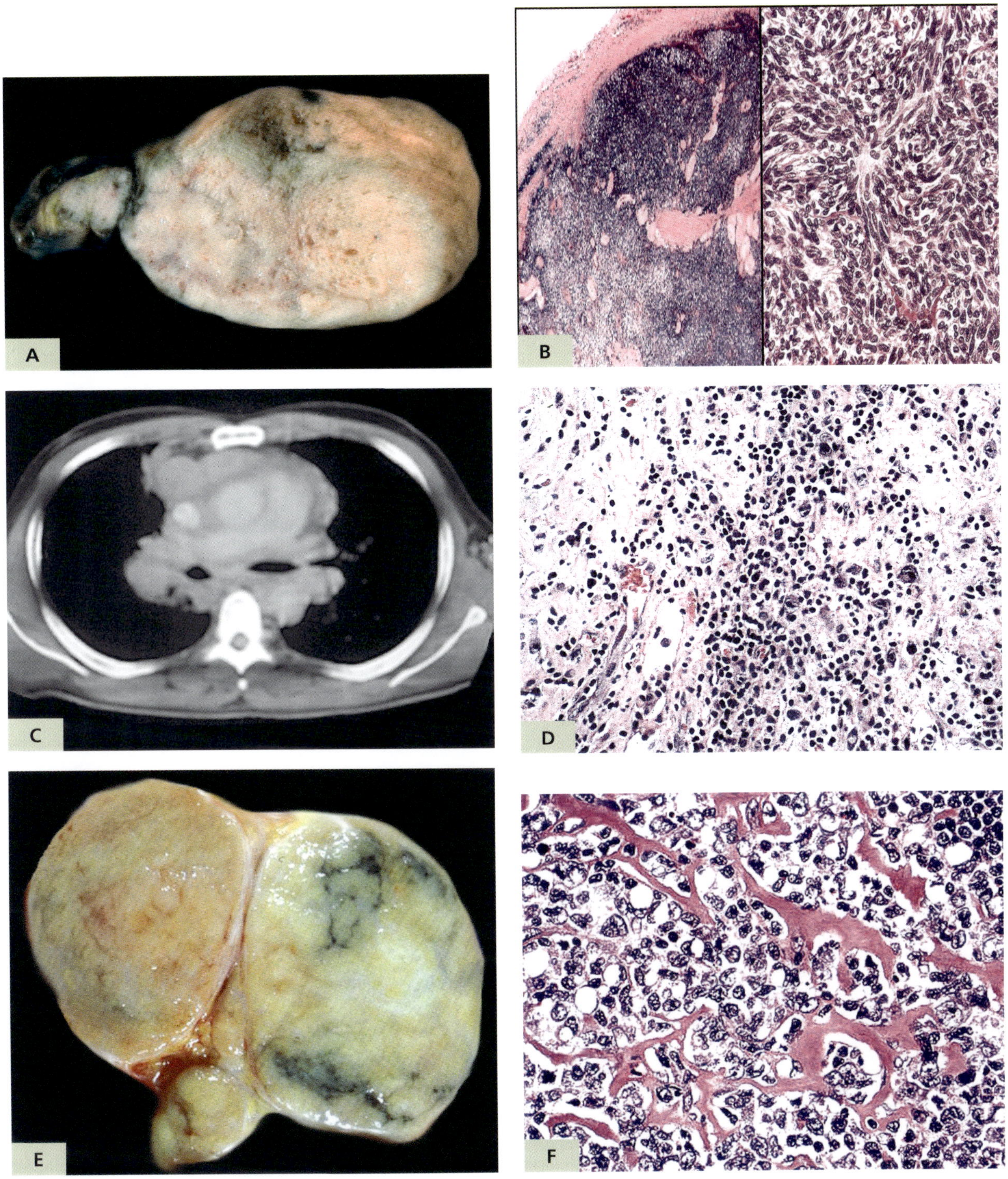

FIGURE 4.2 Differential diagnosis in cases of true inflammatory thymic pseudotumor includes spindle-cell thymoma (A & B); nodular sclerosing Hodgkin's lymphoma (C & D); and sclerosing large-cell non-Hodgkin's lymphoma (E & F).

IDIOPATHIC FIBROSING MEDIASTINITIS (TUMEFACTIVE FIBROINFLAMMATORY LESION)

Reports on FM have been made under a plethora of diagnostic synonyms, including "desmoid retraction," "lipogranuloma," "sclerosing xanthogranuloma," "isolated lipodystrophy," "IPT," and "fibrosing Weber–Christian disease." These diverse terms reflect the fact that the pathogenesis of FM has been linked by sundry authors to that of many other conditions. However, the most common cause of mediastinal fibrosis is an idiosyncratic reaction to infection of the mediastinal lymph nodes by mycobacterial or fungal organisms **(Figure 4.3)** (467–476). Hence, one is always obliged to address the possible presence of those agents in FM.

The most common clinical manifestation of FM is that of progressive dyspnea or cough. In addition, the superior vena caval syndrome—with suffusion of the soft tissues of the head and neck, and dilatation of accessory thoracic subcutaneous veins **(Figure 4.4)**—is a distinct possibility. Unlike mediastinal fibrosis associated with infection, as cited above, fever, and sweats are typically absent in idiopathic FM. Patients are generally adults over the age of 40 years, and there is no apparent predilection for either gender. In unusual cases, a mass may be felt on deep palpation of the infraclavicular fossae; however, most examples of *Idiopathic* fibrosing mediastinitis (IFM) are detected

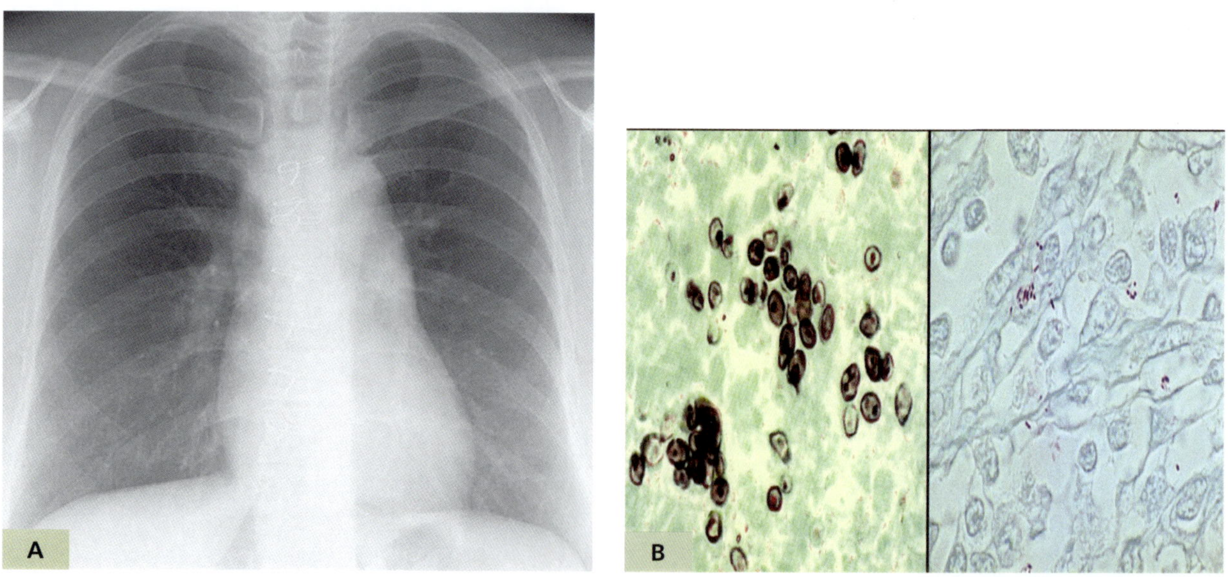

FIGURE 4.3 Patients with fibrosing mediastinitis show a widened mediastinal compartment on chest radiographs (A). In a substantial number of cases, infection of mediastinal lymph nodes with fungi—especially *Histoplasma* (B, left) or with mycobacteria (B, right) is the underlying etiological process.

only through the results of radiologic studies. These show irregular widening and density of the mediastinal soft tissue on plain films of the thorax (475). Computed tomography (CT) or magnetic resonance imaging (MRI) are more specific in delineating the presence of a mass (or multiple masses) containing variable quantities of entrapped fat and fibrous tissue **(Figure 4.5)** (476); internal calcification may also be evident.

Histologically, one observes densely hyalinized tumefactive fibrous tissue in the mediastinum with a haphazard pattern of involvement of anatomic subcompartments **(Figure 4.6)**. The fibrosis may extend into the lungs and great vessels and may markedly compromise the luminal diameter of mediastinal or hilar pulmonary vasculature. The latter finding probably secondarily explains the fat necrosis that may accompany the above-cited changes as well. Scattered throughout the mass in a regional fashion, one finds aggregates of mature lymphocytes, plasma cells, histiocytes, foam cells, and occasional eosinophils (467–477). None of these hematopoietic elements shows any cytologic atypia or monomorphism.

IFM is probably a member of the family of fibroinflammatory IgG4 diseases **(Figure 4.7)** (478). An association between FM and elevated serum IgG4 levels was reported by Zen et al. (479), but there has been no systematic evaluation of this relationship to date in a series of cases.

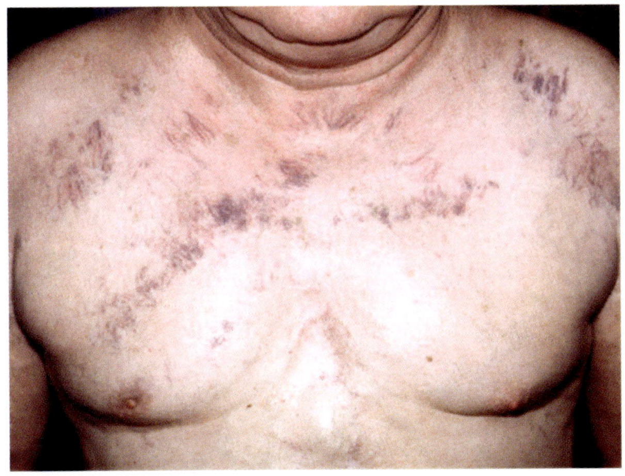

FIGURE 4.4 Fibrosing mediastinitis incites the development of numerous collateral vessels in the thorax, including the subcutis, as shown here. The superior vena cava syndrome may also be present.

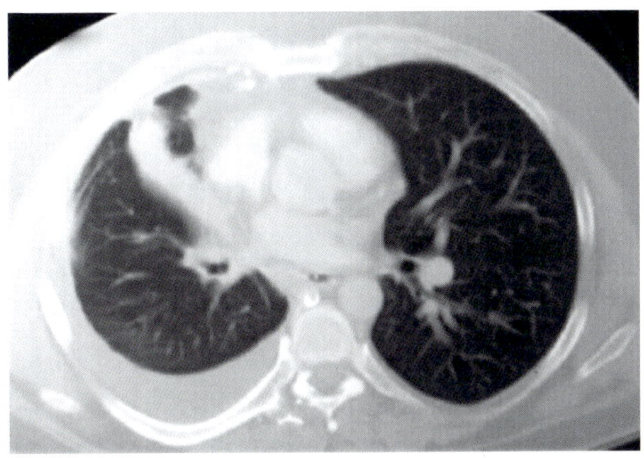

FIGURE 4.5 Computed tomograms of the thorax show entrapment of the great vessels and mediastinal fibroadipose tissue by the sclerotic mass in fibrosing mediastinitis.

Some examples of *metastatic carcinoma* or *malignant lymphoma* may involve the mediastinal soft tissue in a fashion that grossly and microscopically simulates the clinicopathologic profile of IFM (480,481). Thus, extensive sampling and careful inspection of histologic sections must be undertaken to exclude an occult malignancy in the midst of an exuberant fibrotic response.

Because of its macroscopic features, one may sometimes confuse FM with *aggressive fibromatosis* (desmoid tumor) (482,483). Nonetheless, those

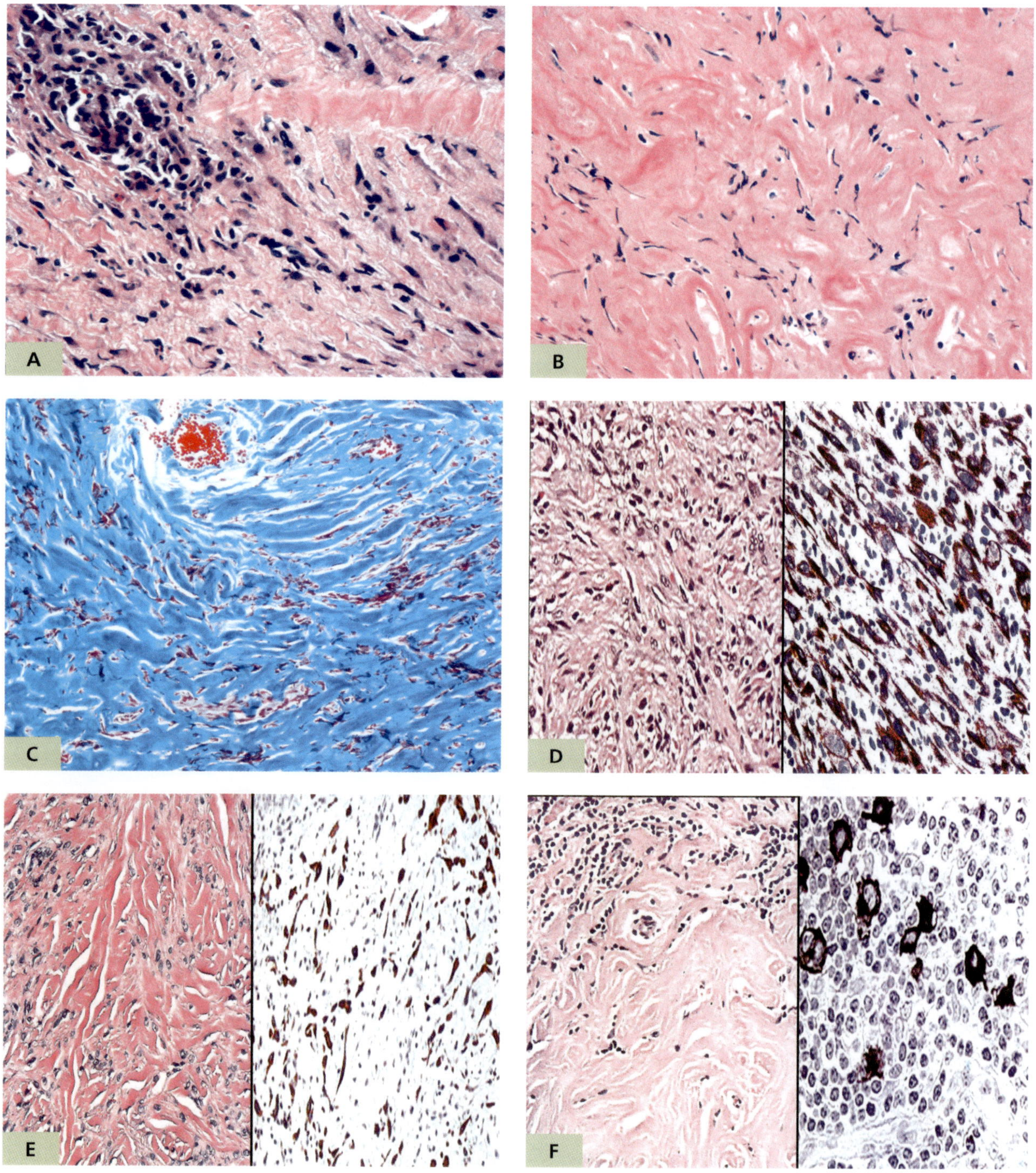

FIGURE 4.6 Fibrosing mediastinitis (FM) shows a variable amount of chronic inflammation (A) that is interspersed throughout a densely collagenous mass (B), which stains blue with the Masson trichrome method (C). Differential diagnostic considerations include desmoplastic mesothelioma (D—immunostained for pankeratin); metastatic sclerosing carcinoma (from the lung or alimentary tract) (E—immunostained for pankeratin); and "obliterative" nodular sclerosing Hodgkin's lymphoma (F—immunostained for CD30). FM expresses neither pankeratin nor CD30.

conditions are quite separate. FM is markedly hypocellular and uniformly collagenized with only regional inflammation. Fibromatosis is characterized by a distinctive fusiform and stellate-cell proliferation that is regularly punctuated by thick-walled small blood vessels (**Figure 4.8**); it is further typified by a myxoid stroma, a relative absence of lymphocytes and plasma cells, and nuclear immunolocalization of beta-catenin (**Figure 4.9**) (483,484). The latter marker is seen only in the cytoplasm of fibroblasts in FM, if it is present at all.

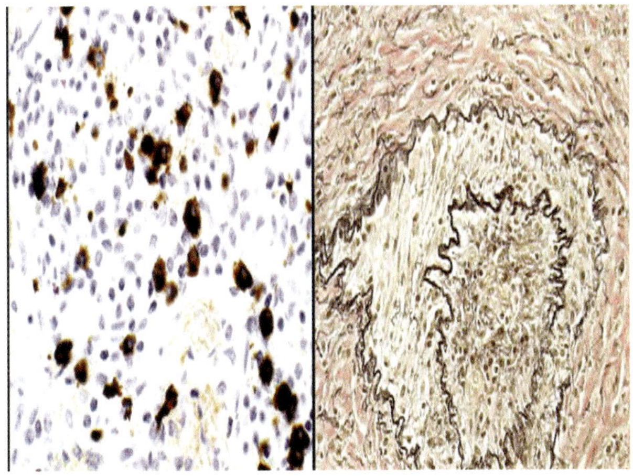

FIGURE 4.7 Idiopathic fibrosing mediastitis (i.e., unassociated with underlying infections) is likely a member of the family of IgG4-mediated autoimmune diseases. Those disorders feature an increased number of plasma cells that can be immunolabeled for IgG4, as shown here.

Following the seminal description of the concept of TFILs by Wold and Weiland (485), in reference to masses of the head and neck, other authors embraced that terminology and the paradigm attached to it (486,487). This model groups several histologically similar diseases mechanistically and suggests that they are all probably autoimmune in nature (478,481). Such disorders include not only FM but also Riedel's thyroiditis (and possibly also sclerosing lymphocytic thyroiditis), retroperitoneal fibrosis (Ormond's disease), primary sclerosing cholangitis, and "retractile mesenteritis" (488–495). It is interesting

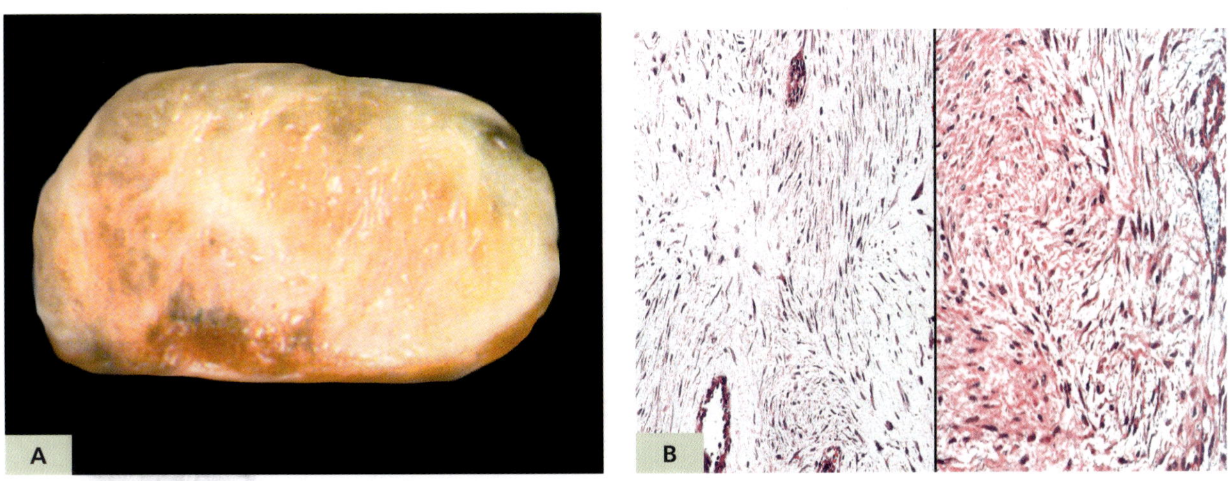

FIGURE 4.8 Another diagnostic alternative in cases of fibrosing mediastinitis (FM) is desmoid fibromatosis, a neoplastic and locally infiltrative lesion. It may have a deceptively circumscribed appearance on gross examination (A), differing from the macroscopic image of FM. In addition, desmoids are more cellular than FM is, with myxofibrous stroma and well-delineated stromal blood vessels (B).

pathobiologically that some patients have had more than one of those conditions synchronously or metachronously. To reiterate, it would appear that the presence of IgG4-bearing inflammatory cells is the common denominator in this pathologic cluster (478).

Treatment for mediastinal fibrosis is individualized and usually conservative, and it is intended principally to relieve symptoms and signs of the disorder. Only rare patients require surgical debulking of the fibrous mass, and the general outlook for FM is favorable. Some individuals with TFILs have benefited from the administration of exogenous steroids (444).

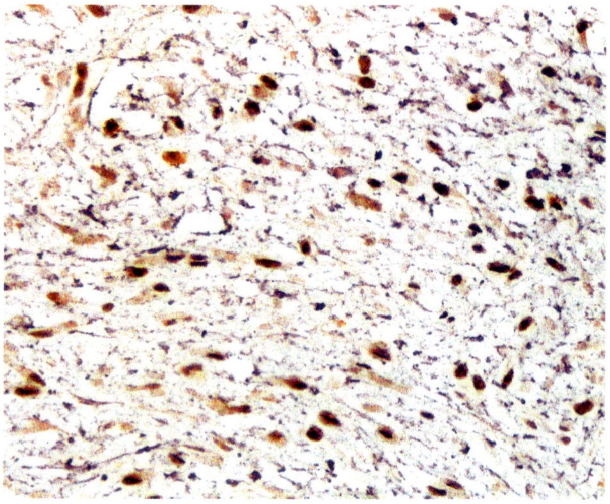

FIGURE 4.9 Nuclear immunoreactivity for beta-catenin is characteristic of desmoid fibromatosis, as shown here.

MESOTHELIAL INCLUSIONS IN MEDIASTINAL LYMPH NODES

Another mediastinal lesion that merits inclusion here is that of mesothelial cell inclusions in mediastinal lymph nodes. In the original description of this phenomenon, Rutty and Lauder (496) reported a case of a 23-year-old man with a mediastinal T-cell lymphoma. An incidental histologic finding was the subcapsular presence of small nests of bland cells in several mediastinal lymph nodes. The cells were polygonal with eosinophilic cytoplasm and bland oval nuclei. No mitoses, pleomorphism, or glandular differentiation were present. That constellation of findings dissuaded the authors from the diagnostic interpretation of a *metastatic epithelial malignancy*. The lesional cells co-expressed keratin and vimentin, and ultrastructural examination showed features of mesothelial cells including slender microvilli and desmosomes. Similar lesions have also been described by other investigators **(Figure 4.10)** (497–499).

MULTILOCULAR THYMIC CYSTS

Thymic cysts are encountered clinically mainly in patients between 20 and 50 years of age, most of whom are asymptomatic. It is now clear that congenital unilocular cysts and acquired multilocular cysts of the thymus both exist as distinct entities (500–504). In imaging studies, they are rounded and circumscribed masses in the anterior mediastinum **(Figure 4.11)**. Unilocular cysts have a water-like density on computed tomograms, but multilocular cysts demonstrate a higher attenuation. Both types may demonstrate calcification of the lesional periphery, and their maximum size extends up to 18 cm.

The epithelial component of multilocular thymic cysts (MTCs) is more generous than that of unilocular cysts, with multiple layers of squamous cells, or squamous elements admixed with cuboidal, columnar, or micropapillary

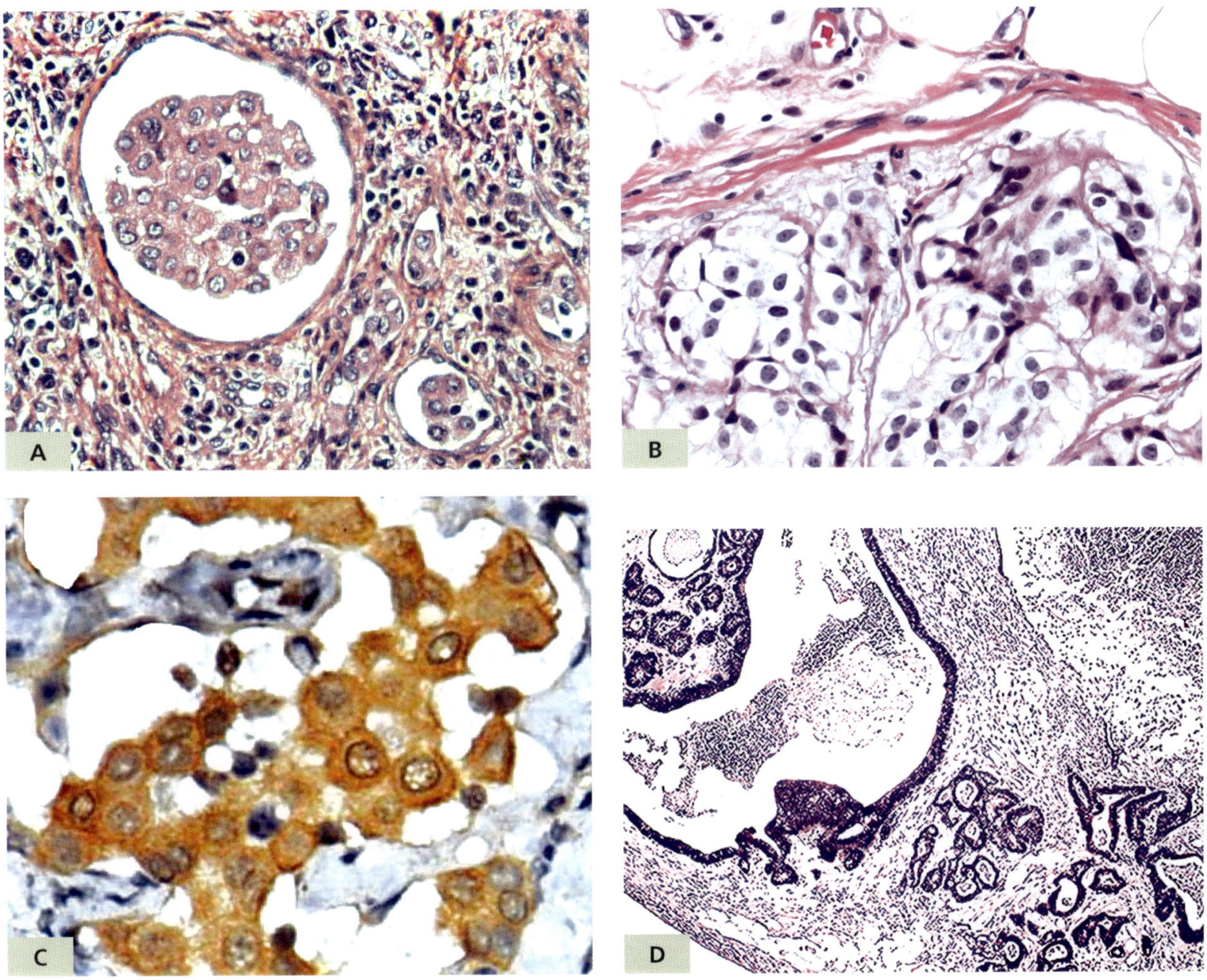

FIGURE 4.10 Benign mesothelial inclusions may rarely be encountered in intrathoracic lymph nodes; these are characteristically banal cytologically (A & B) and can be labeled immunohistologically for calretinin (C). In contrast, metastatic adenocarcinoma in thoracic nodes may be cystic (D) *(Continued)*

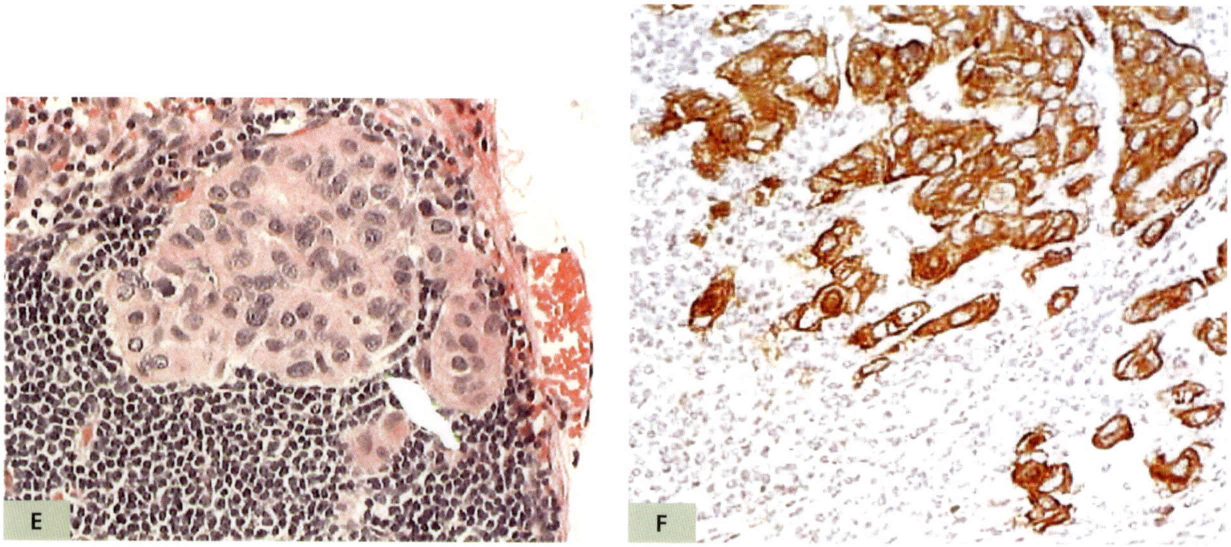

FIGURE 4.10 *(Continued)* or solid (E) and are immunoreactive for glandular markers such as MOC-31 (F).

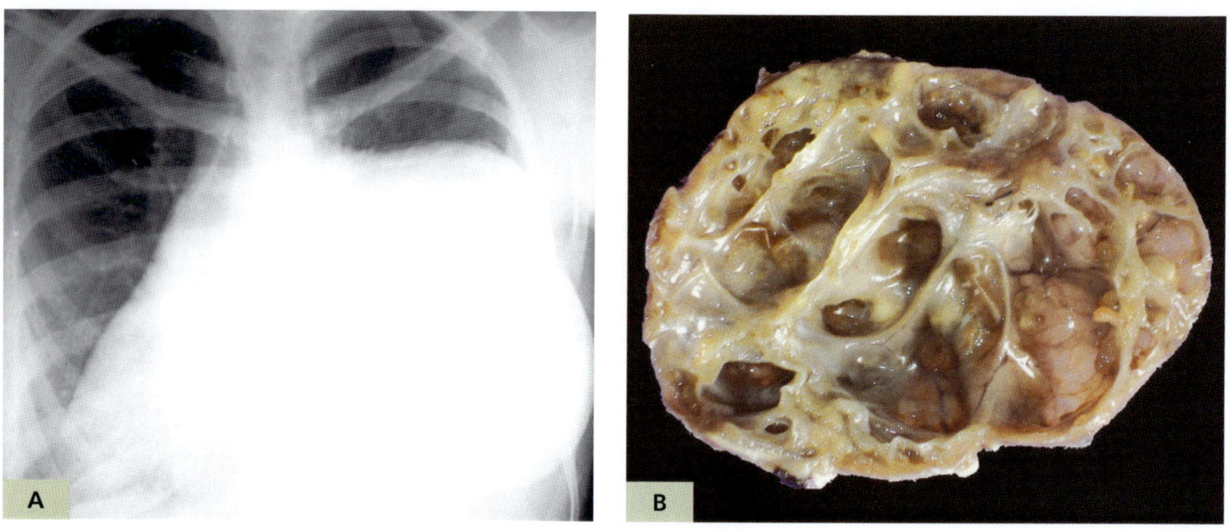

FIGURE 4.11 Chest radiographs of multilocular thymic cysts (MTCs) demonstrate a mediastinal mass of variable size that projects into one of the hemithoraces. An unusually large example is shown here (A). Grossly, MTC comprises several locular compartments that are bounded by fibrous septa (B).

glandular epithelium **(Figure 4.12)**. Small foci of parathyroid or salivary glandular epithelium can be observed rarely. In that eventuality, one may wish to employ the diagnostic terms "third pharyngeal pouch cyst" or "mixed multilocular thymic cyst" (505). Mature lymphocytes, granulation tissue, hemorrhage, and cholesterol granulomas are consistently present in the walls

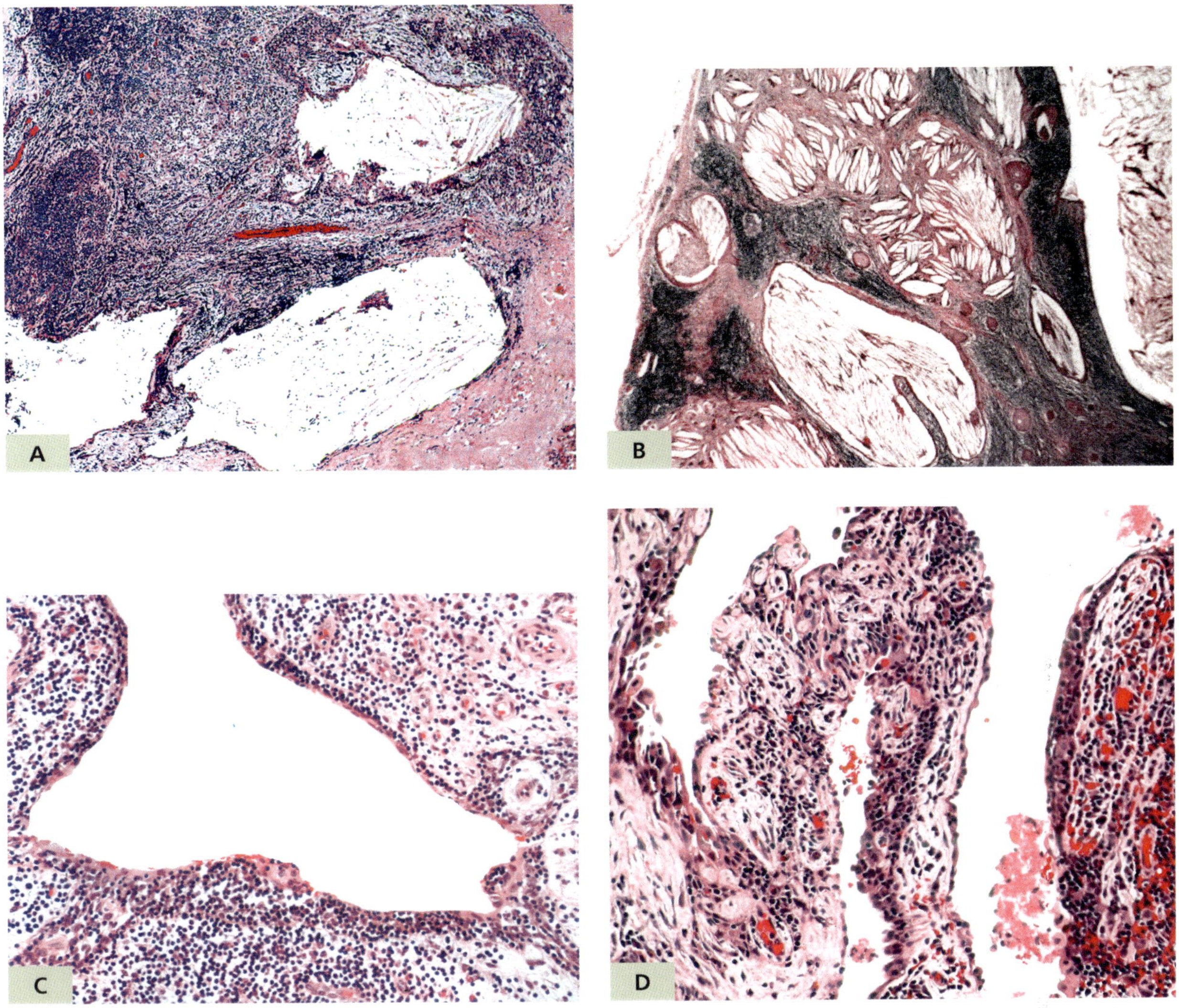

FIGURE 4.12 A–D: The compartments in multilocular thymic cyst are lined at least partially by bland squamoid epithelium, with abundant stromal lymphocytes. Spaces in the cyst often contain cholesterol clefts and amorphous material.

and cavities of MTCs. The cause of the inflammatory process that is felt to be the etiology of these lesions is currently undetermined.

A distinctive subtype of MTC is the "proliferating" variant (506). It is similarly morphologically to cysts that are seen in the skin and called "proliferating epidermoid cyst" and "proliferating trichilemmal cyst" (507). Narrow, interconnecting tongues of squamoid epithelium extend outward from the cyst lining into the surrounding connective tissue **(Figure 4.13)**. This change reflects the presence of pseudoepitheliomatous hyperplasia in

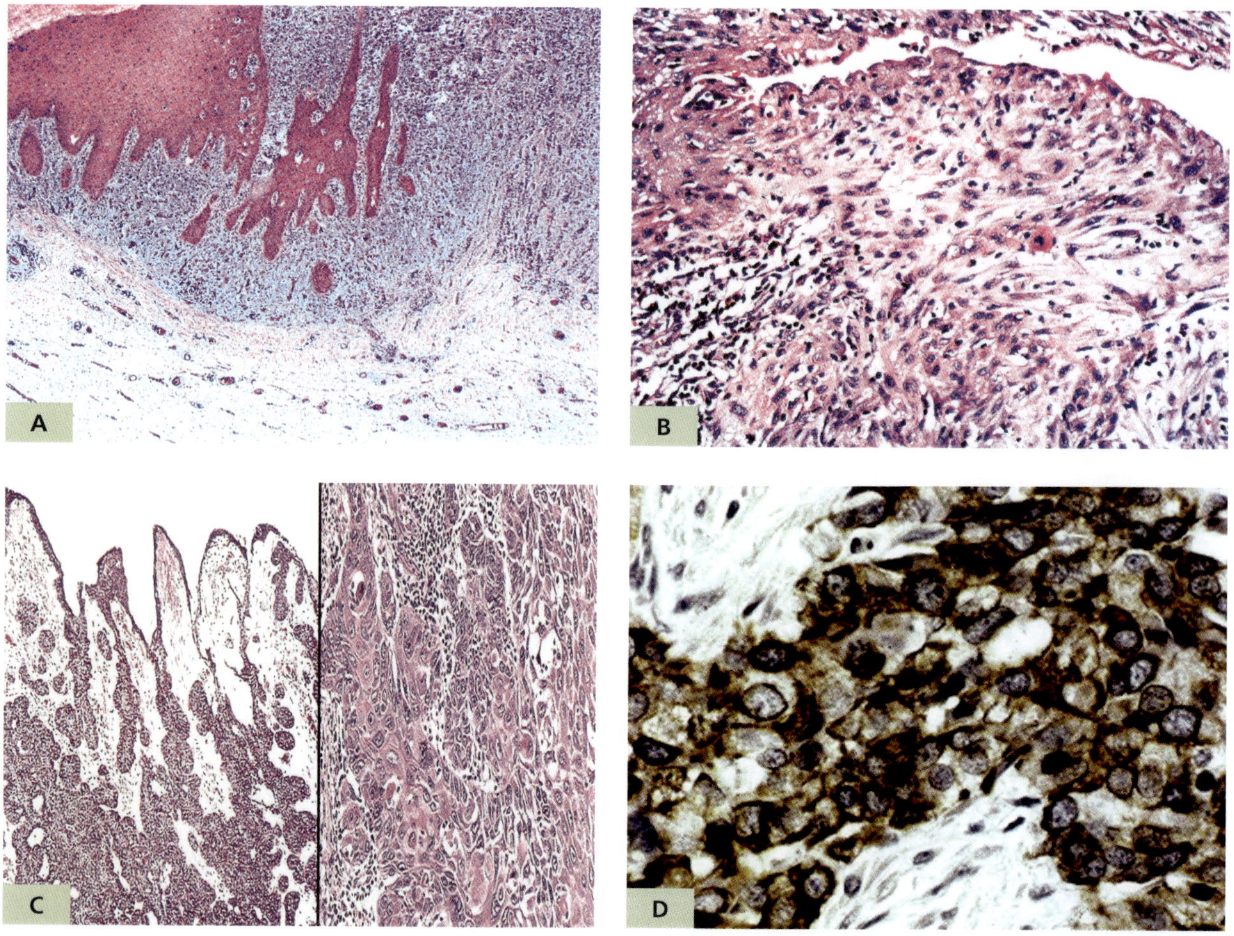

FIGURE 4.13 Proliferating multilocular thymic cysts show outward projections of squamous epithelium from the loculated linings of the cyst into the surrounding stroma (A). Modest nuclear atypia may be seen in the epithelial elements as well (B). In contrast, true thymic carcinomas that take origin in thymic cysts are overtly aberrant cytologically (C) and can often be labeled for CD5 (D). That marker is not seen in proliferating multilocular thymic cysts.

thymic cysts. The cytologic features of the proliferating epithelium are bland, and there is no true invasion of the intervening stroma. Mitoses are present but they are physiological in nature. The significance of proliferating thymic cysts is, obviously, the danger that they may be overinterpreted as *secondary carcinomas. Bona fide* malignant alteration in thymic cysts is rare (508–510), and the tumors in those cases (usually basaloid squamous carcinomas) have been obviously invasive clinically.

Another morphological variation in MTC is that of lymphoid hyperplasia, with the formation of germinal centers in a prominent stromal lymphocytic infiltrate. This eventuality should bring the possibility of acquired immunodeficiency syndrome to mind, inasmuch as it is associated with systemic infection by HIV (511–515). The presence of *lymphomas* in MTCs has not been described.

Thymus glands that are involved by *Hodgkin's disease* (HD) may also undergo cystic transformation **(Figure 4.14)**, as may others that have been traumatized by surgery or other physical injuries. The coexistence of thymic cysts with mediastinal HD was originally felt to represent the effects of therapeutic

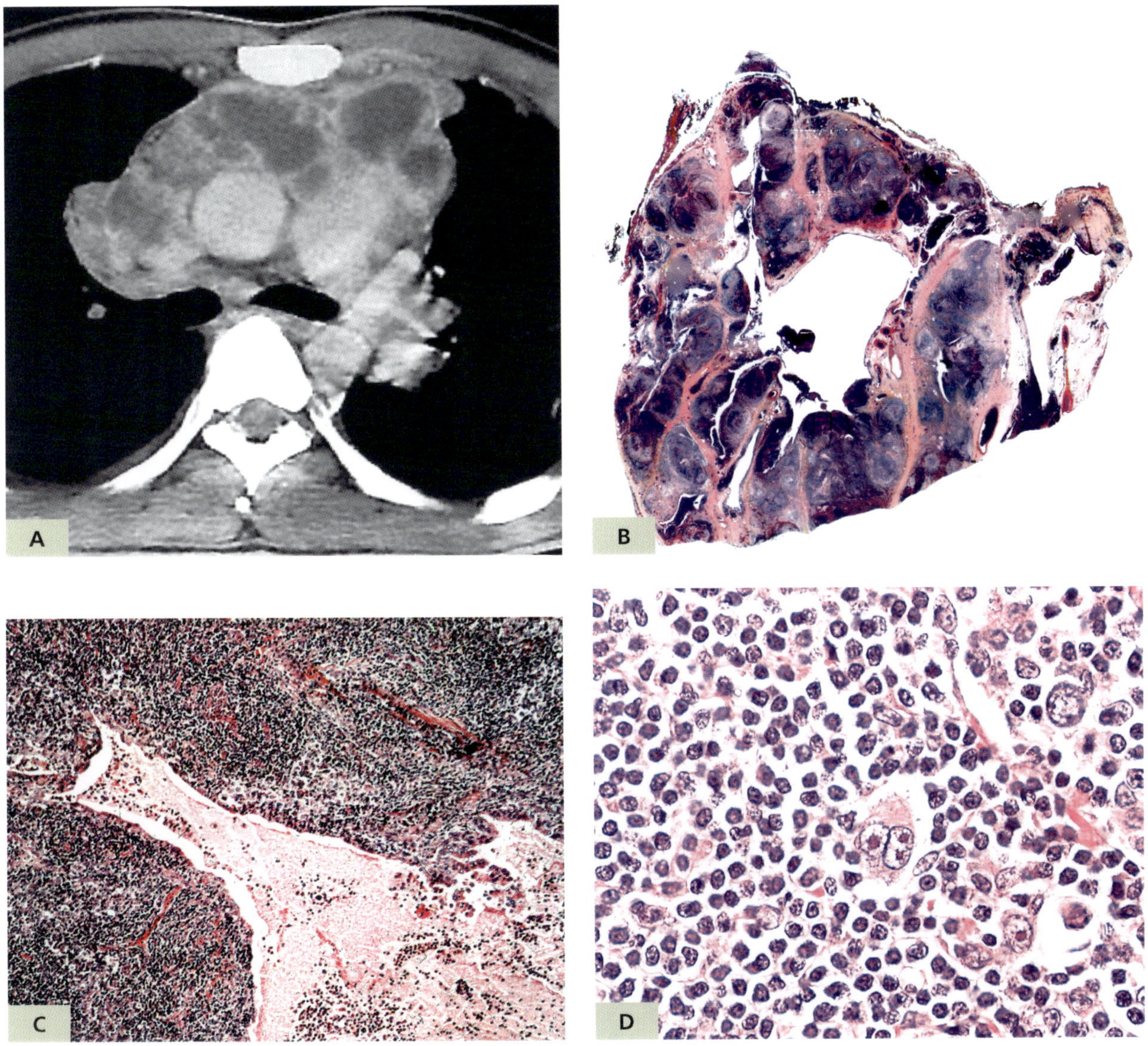

FIGURE 4.14 Internal cystic change may occur in masses of Hodgkin's lymphoma in the mediastinum (A–D), following irradiation or chemotherapy. Typically, however, at least some identifiable tumor tissue remains upon microscopic examination of those lesions (D).

irradiation or systemic chemotherapy (516–520). However, this concurrence has been observed in untreated Hodgkin's lymphoma cases as well (521).

Other mediastinal neoplasms may also undergo extensive cystification **(Figure 4.15)**. They include *thymoma*, *seminoma*, low-grade thymic *neuroendocrine carcinoma* ("thymic carcinoid"), and rare examples of *metastatic carcinoma* (522–526). In particular reference to cystic thymoma, hemorrhage and cellular debris can occupy nearly all of the lesional substance, and extensive sampling may be necessary to visualize the residual tumor.

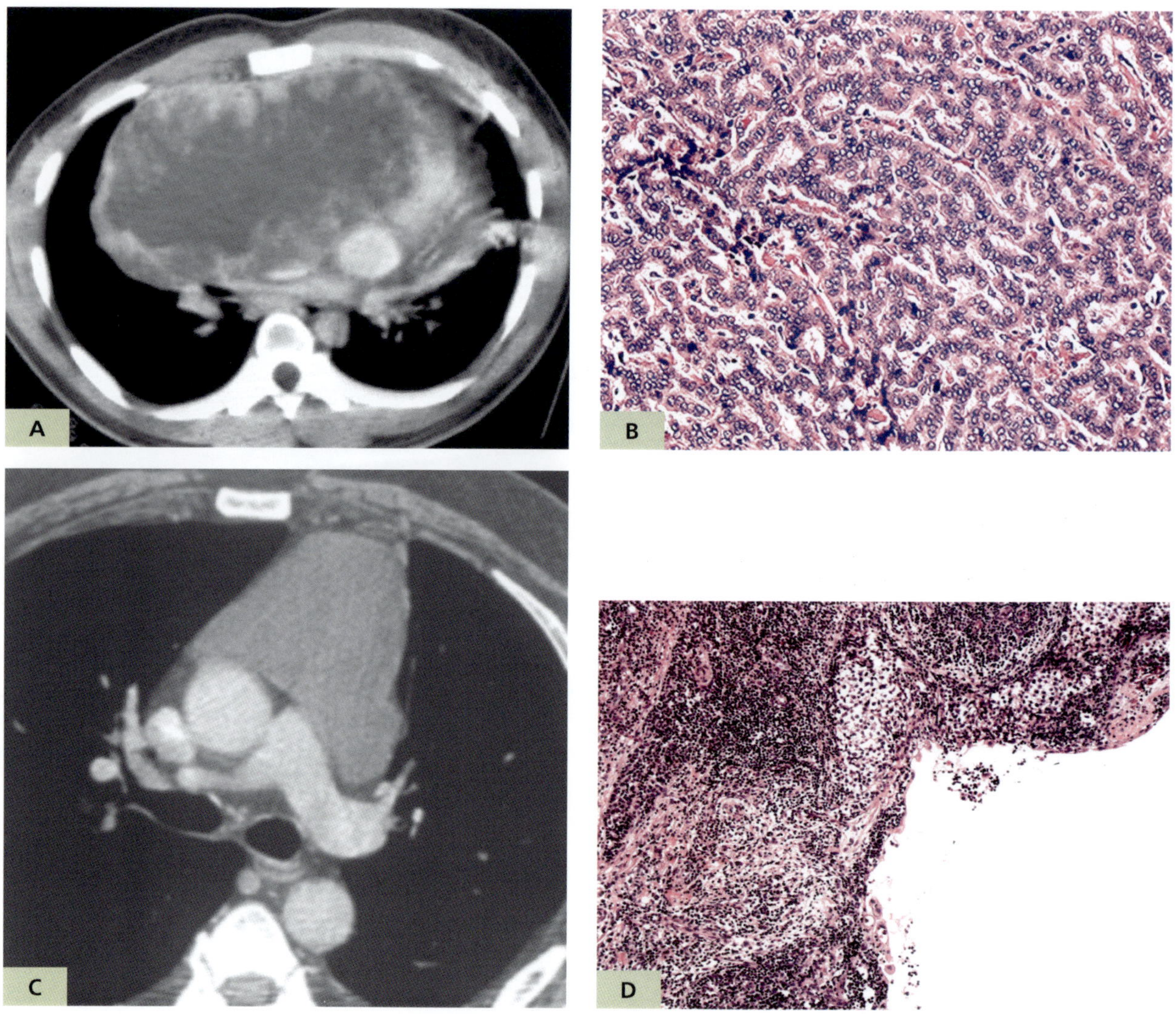

FIGURE 4.15 Several true neoplasms in the mediastinum may undergo cystification and be confused with thymic cysts. Examples include thymic neuroendocrine carcinoma ("carcinoid") (A & B); intrathymic seminoma (C & D); and thymoma (E & F). *(Continued)*

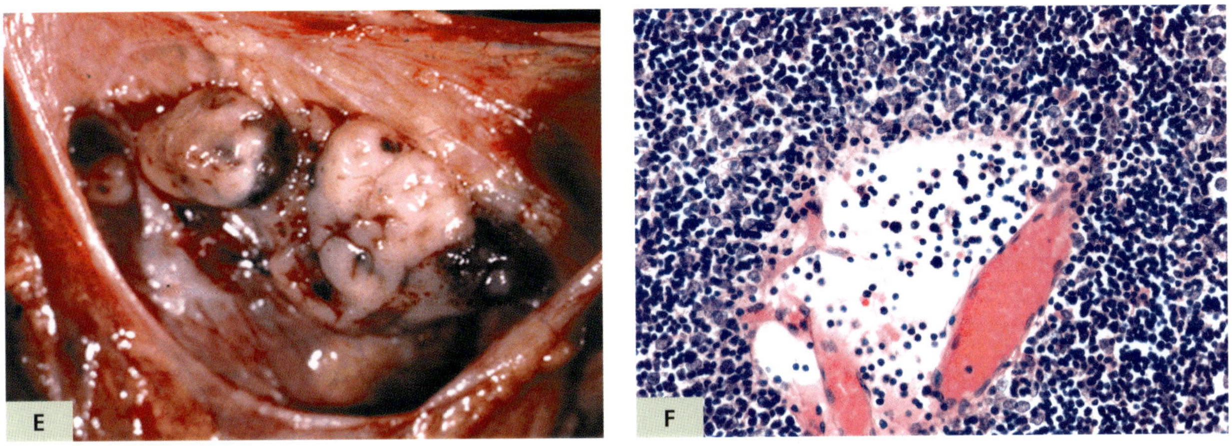

FIGURE 4.15 *(Continued)*

Moran et al. have described three examples of well-differentiated ovarian serous carcinoma that selectively metastasized to the anterior mediastinum (526). The microscopic images of the secondary lesions were remarkably similar to that of MTC, except for the focal presence of an atypical papillary epithelial component. The latter was immunoreactive for CA-125, in keeping with the Mullerian origin of the tumors.

TUMEFACTIVE SARCOIDOSIS AND SARCOIDAL REACTIONS

Sarcoidosis is a relatively common illness, and it principally manifests itself with thoracopulmonary lesions **(Figure 4.16)** (527,528). Occasionally, one may encounter examples of this disorder that produce large, localized masses—probably representing agglomerated lymph nodes **(Figure 4.17)**—in the mediastinum or other anatomic locations. The terms "tumefactive" or "tumoral" sarcoid have been used in reference to that scenario (529–531). As true of "ordinary" sarcoidosis, microscopic examination of affected tissue shows numerous non-caseating granulomas that efface the lymph node architecture **(Figure 4.18)**.

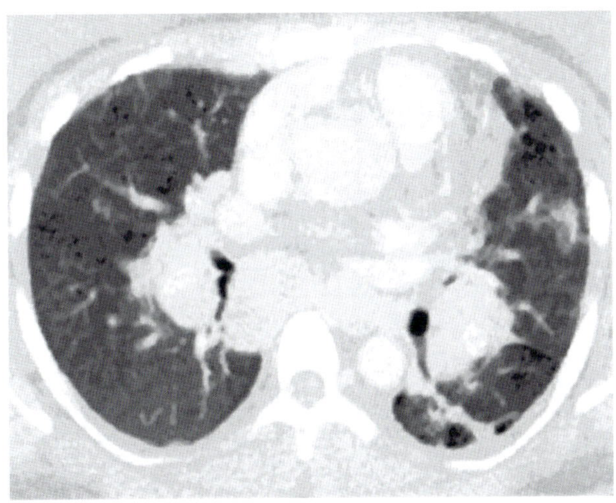

FIGURE 4.16 Several masses can be seen concurrently in the mediastinum and lung fields in florid sarcoidosis, imitating the image of a neoplastic process.

Neoplastic differential diagnostic alternatives must be considered in the specific context

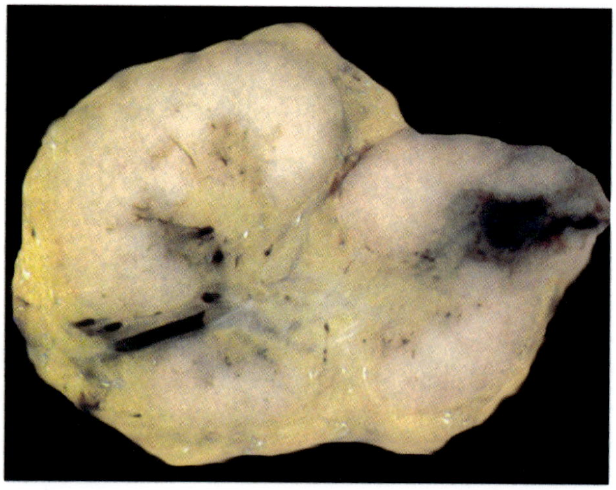

FIGURE 4.17 Sarcoidal masses in the thorax are typically based in lymph nodes.

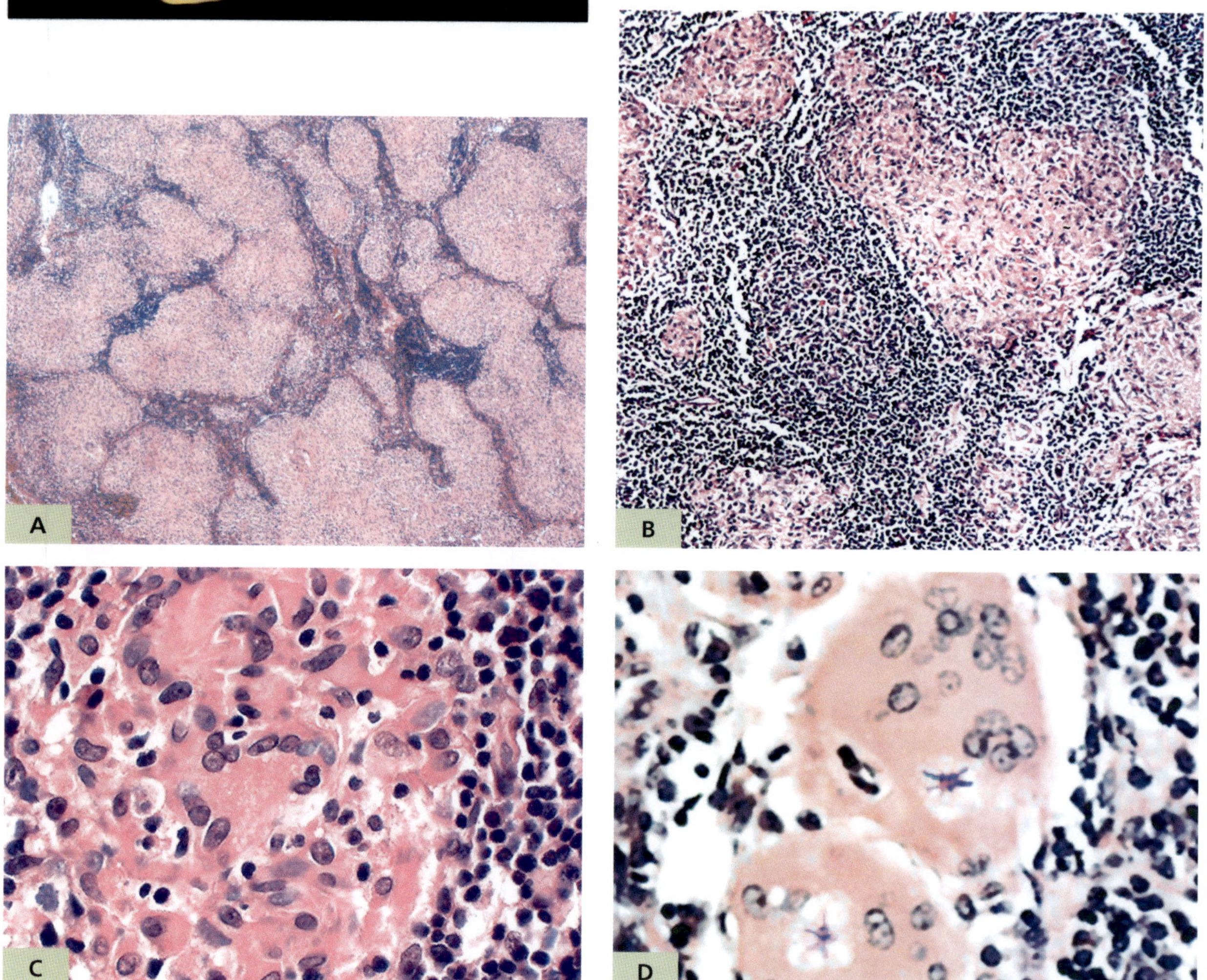

FIGURE 4.18 Sarcoid effaces lymph nodal architecture, replacing it with noncaseating epithelioid granulomas (A–C). These may contain "asteroid" bodies, as highlighted here with the phosphotungstic acid-hematoxylin stain (D).

of suspected mediastinal sarcoidosis. In particular, prominent granulomatous inflammation may be seen in connection with *Hodgkin's lymphoma*, not only in regional nonneoplastic lymph nodes but in the tumor tissue itself **(Figure 4.19)** (532–534). Merchant and coworkers have posited that the granulomatous lesions in some of these cases may represent a reaction to antineoplastic chemotherapy (534).

Thus, it would seem prudent to look carefully for Reed–Sternberg cells and their variants—perhaps with the aid of CD30 immunostains—in cases of "sarcoid" in elderly patients and in those with unusually large mediastinal

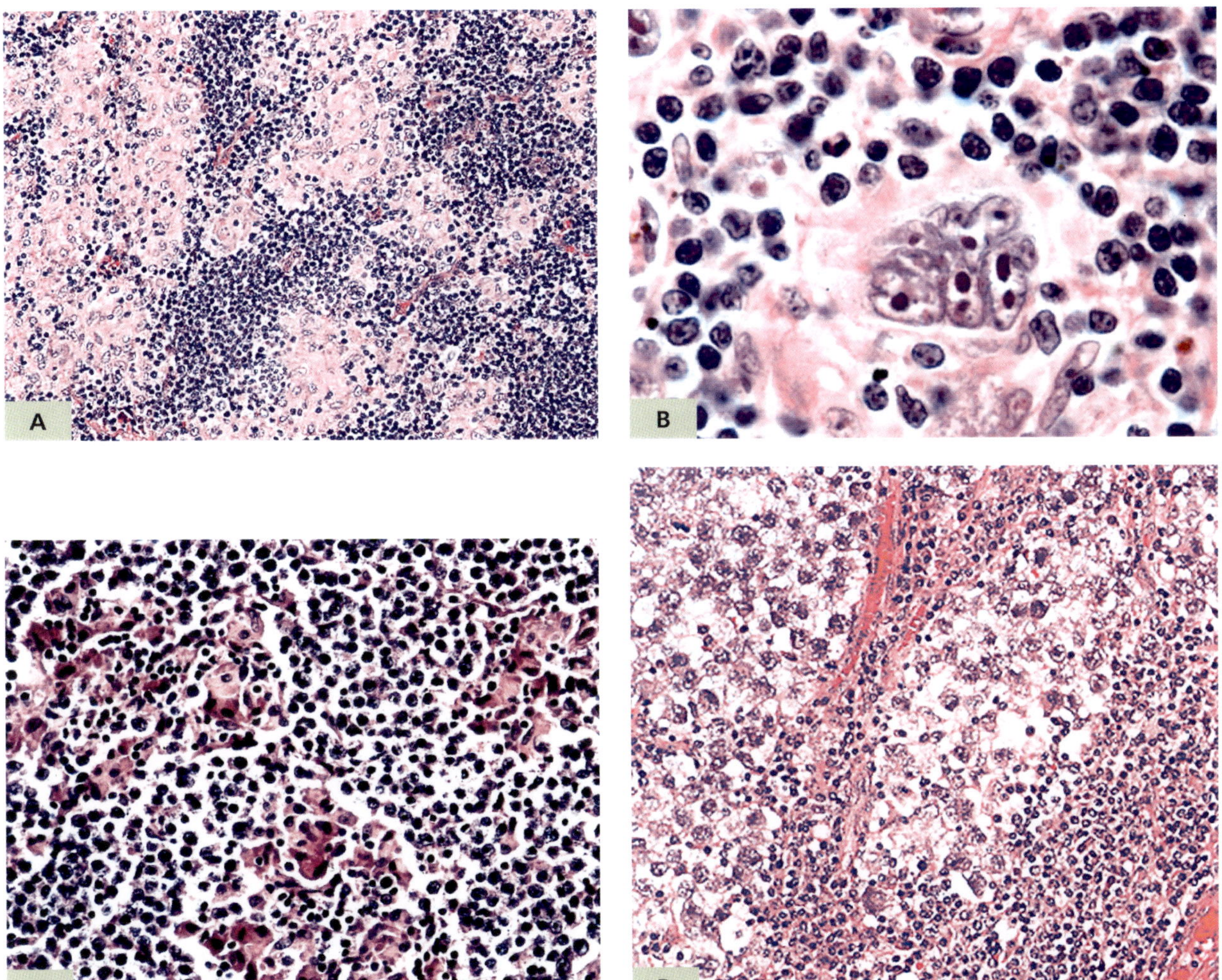

FIGURE 4.19 Epithelioid, sarcoid-like granulomas may be seen microscopically in association with true thoracic neoplasms as well, including, but not limited to, Hodgkin's lymphoma (A & B) and seminoma (C & D).

masses. That is particularly true if "B" symptoms (e.g., fever, night sweats) are present (533). Unfortunately, there are still no discriminatory and "proactive" serologic or immunohistochemical markers for sarcoidosis itself.

Primary *carcinomas of the lung* also may be accompanied by a prominent sarcoid-like reaction in the regional lymph nodes, even if the nodes are uninvolved by metastases (535,536). The mechanism for this association is unknown, but it argues strongly for direct tissue sampling of pulmonary masses for diagnostic purposes.

THYMIC HYPERPLASIA

Asymptomatic children and adults alike may be found to have large anterior mediastinal masses in chest radiographs that are obtained for unrelated reasons **(Figure 4.20)** (537–539). In a very small proportion of all such cases, resection of the lesion demonstrates only morphologically normal thymic tissue **(Figure 4.21)**, and the diagnostic designation of "true thymic hyperplasia" (TTH) is appropriate in these circumstances. It may represent an idiopathic sporadic disorder but has sometimes followed endocrine disorders such as hyperthyroidism, Addison's disease, and acromegaly; administration of antineoplastic chemotherapy; or severe burns (540,541). Only exceptionally does the glandular enlargement itself cause respiratory compromise (538).

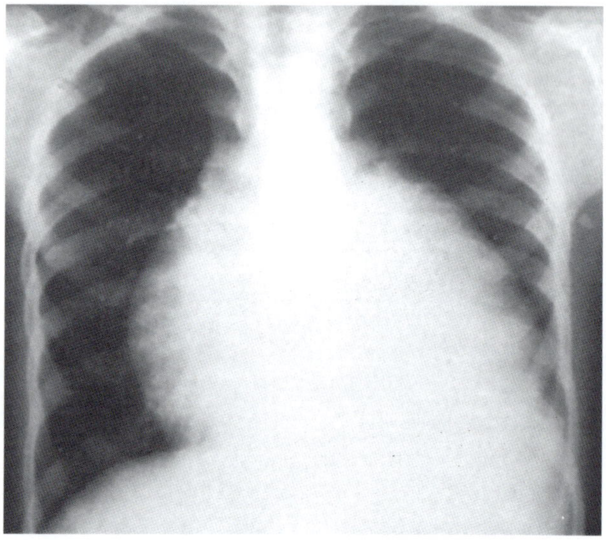

FIGURE 4.20 "True" thymic hyperplasia is represented by enlargement of a histologically unremarkable thymus gland, sometimes to a remarkable extent.

The clinical diagnosis of TTH is difficult, mainly because biopsies of the enlarged gland show no histologic abnormalities. In that context, one could not exclude the possibility that a truly pathological lesion had been missed through sampling bias. Therefore, formal excision of the thymus is ultimately felt to be the safest intervention. Alternatively, an old clinical test of the diagnosis rests on the administration of a brief course of high-dose corticosteroids. If the thymic mass shrinks markedly with that treatment, TTH is likely to be present (541).

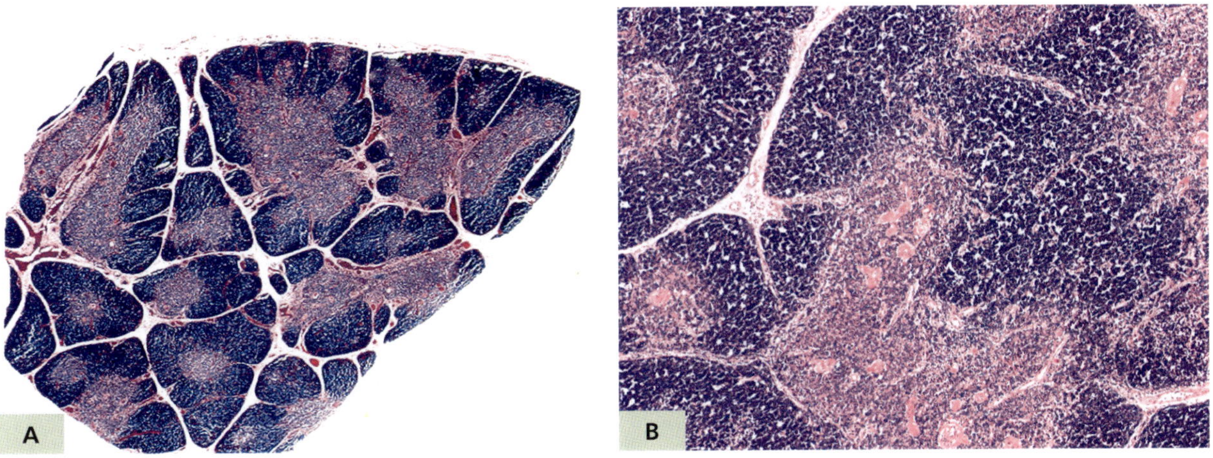

FIGURE 4.21 A & B: Histological examination of true thymic hyperplasia shows normal thymic architecture with no abnormalities in either the cortex or medulla.

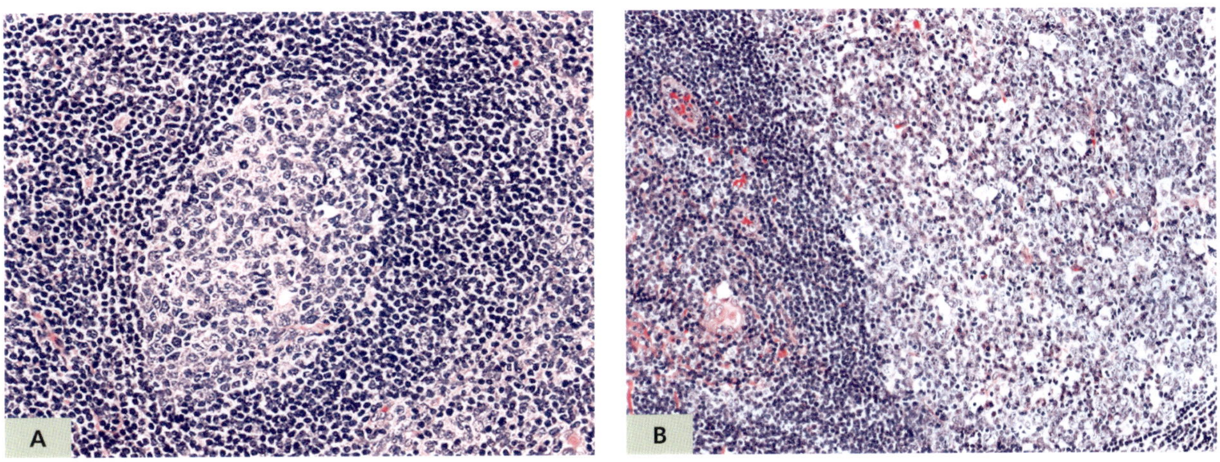

FIGURE 4.22 A & B: Intrathymic lymphoid hyperplasia (ILH) differs from "true" thymic hyperplasia by the presence in the former condition of lymphoid follicles and germinal centers. ILH is often associated with myasthenia gravis.

TTH differs from intrathymic lymphoid hyperplasia (ILH), in which germinal centers are present microscopically **(Figure 4.22)**. The latter condition is virtually always associated with myasthenia gravis (541,542), whereas TTH is not.

A particular danger that is associated with both TTH and ILH concerns their possible confusion with *lymphocyte-predominant thymoma* **(Figure 4.23)** or *lymphoblastic* lymphoma **(Figure 4.24)** if only fine-needle aspiration

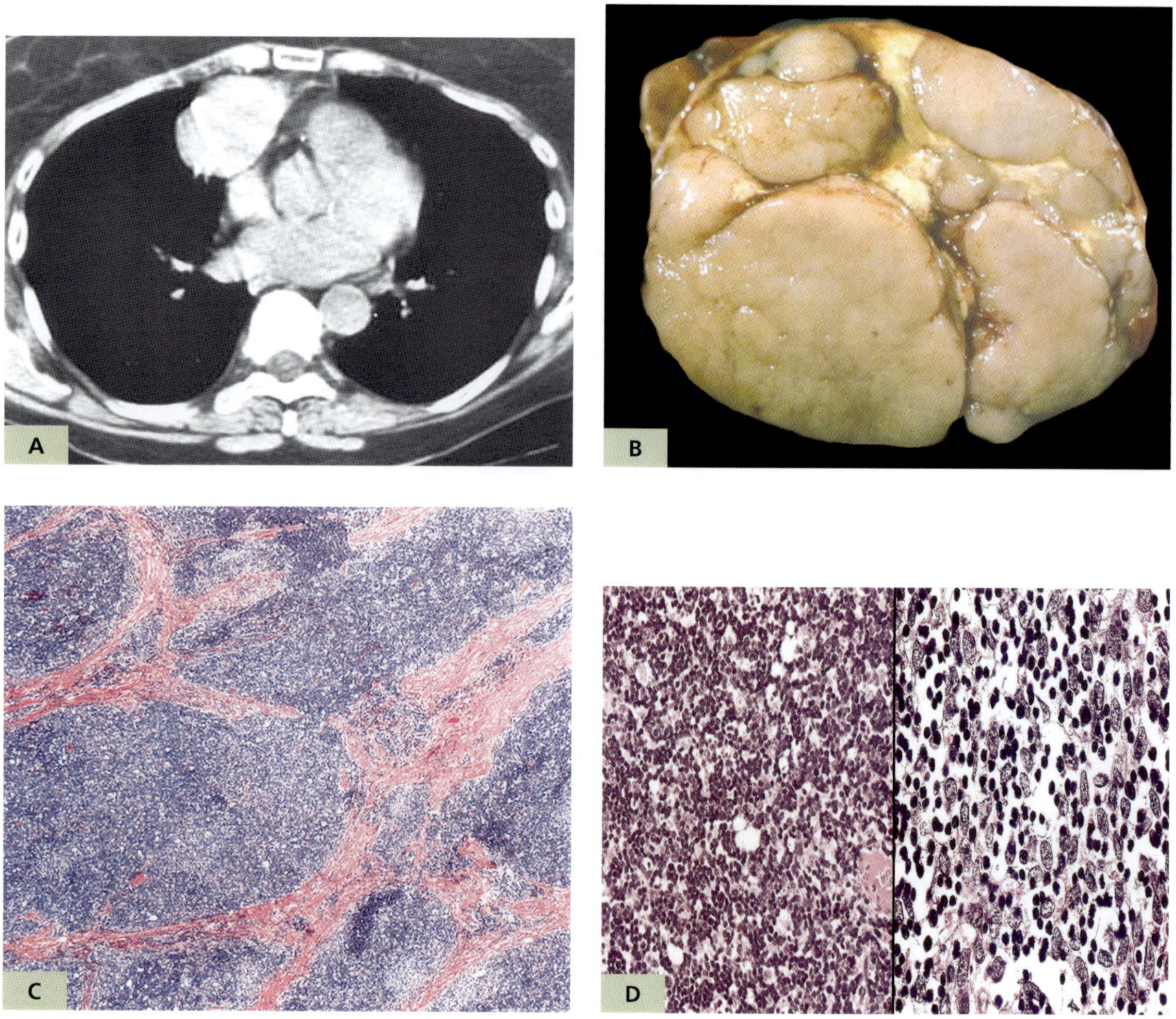

FIGURE 4.23 Lymphocyte-predominant thymoma (LPT) (A) differs from thymic hyperplasias because it shows abnormal thymic architecture. Fibrous bands transect this neoplasm at gross (B) and microscopic (C) levels, and LPT shows dispersed populations of both thymic epithelial cells and lymphocytes (D).

biopsies or small needle-core biopsies of the thymus have been obtained. That is so because the cytological, histological, immunohistochemical, and flow-cytometric profiles of thymic hyperplasias can overlap considerably with those of selected thymic epithelial neoplasms and lymphoblastic malignancies in evaluations of limited tissue samples (543).

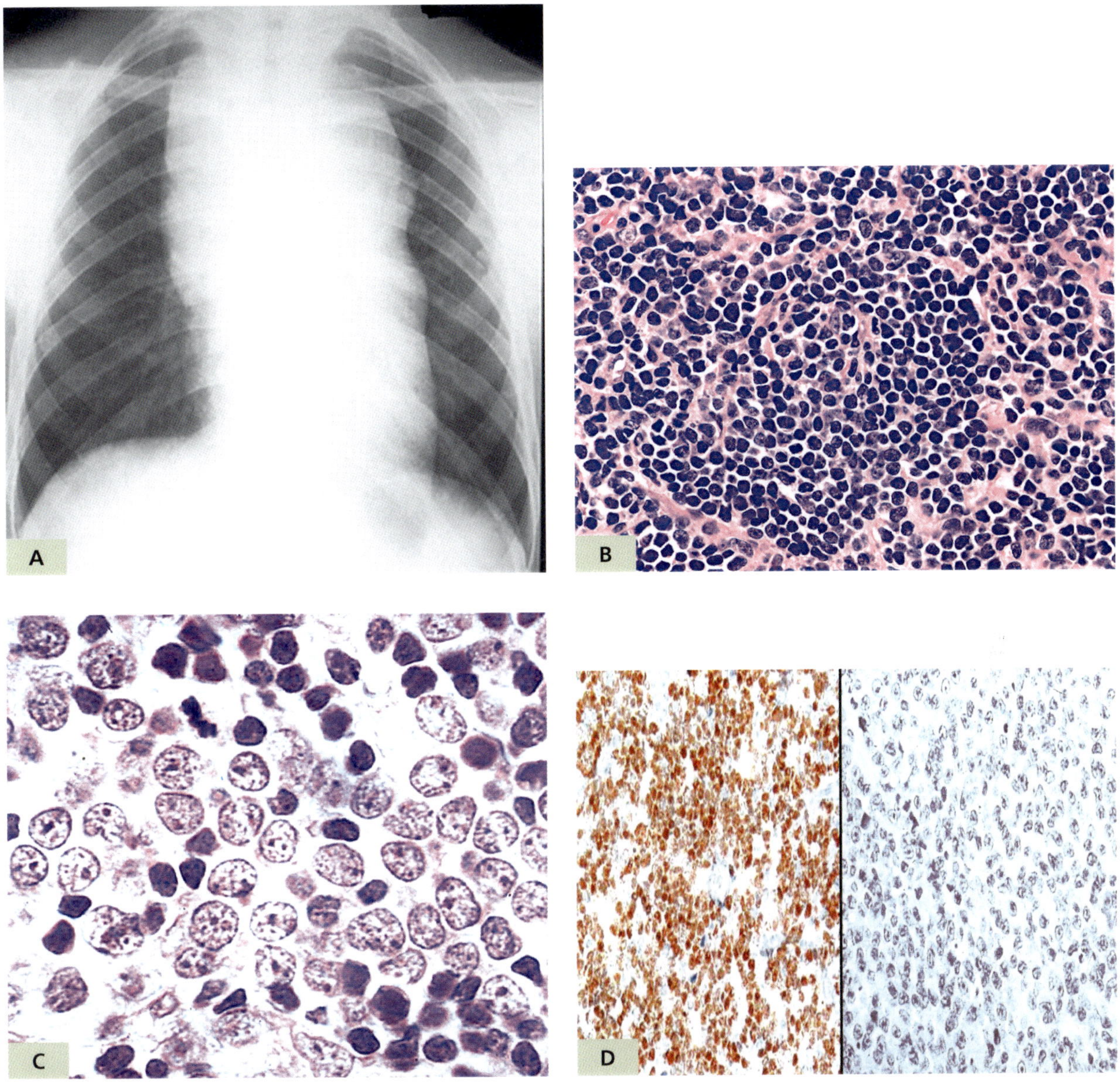

FIGURE 4.24 Lymphoblastic lymphoma (LBL) may be imitated microscopically by either intrathymic lymphoid hyperplasia (ILH) or lymphocyte-predominant thymoma (LPT). However, ILH would not be expected to produce a mass lesion that was comparable to that of LBL (A), and LBL is comprised of a more monomorphic population of atypical lymphoid cells with folded nuclear contours (B & C). LPT and LBL share a capacity to be immunoreactive for terminal deoxynucleotidyl transferase (D, left), but LBL lacks keratin-positive constituents (D, right), which are present in LPT.

OTHER PSEUDONEOPLASTIC MEDIASTINAL LESIONS

In similarity to their ability to affect either the lung or pleura, ***Rosai–Dorfman disease*** (544–546), ***extramedullary hematopoiesis*** (455,547–552), and ***Castleman's disease*** (321,322,324,325) may present themselves as masses in the mediastinum as well. Differential diagnosis in such cases is identical to that which has been outlined in other sections of the foregoing text.

Part II
Cardiovascular Pathology

5

Pseudoneoplastic Lesions of the Heart and Blood Vessels

- HAMARTOMAS AND CHORISTOMAS OF THE HEART
  - Rhabdomyomatous Hamartomas
  - Fibromatous Hamartoma ("Cardiac Fibroma")
  - Endodermal Choristoma (Formerly "Mesothelioma") of the Interatrial Septum
- LIPOMATOUS HYPERTROPHY OF THE HEART
- MESOTHELIAL-MONOCYTIC INTRACARDIAC EXCRESCENCES
- INTRACARDIAC INFLAMMATORY PSEUDOTUMORS
- INTRACARDIAC PAPILLARY ENDOTHELIAL HYPERPLASIA
- ATYPICAL LYMPHOID INFILTRATES OF THE MYOCARDIUM
  - Severe Viral Myocarditis and Cardiac Allograft Rejection
  - Florid "Quilty" Lesions in Cardiac Allografts
  - Rosai–Dorfman Disease (Sinus Histiocytosis With Massive Lymphadenopathy)
  - Intracardiac Castleman's Disease
  - Tumefactive Extramedullary Hematopoiesis in the Myocardium

Secondary tumors—usually representing metastatic melanomas, breast carcinomas, and lung cancers—are the most often-encountered neoplasms of the heart (553–556). Truly primary cardiac neoplastic proliferations are very uncommon. Most of them are benign, with the majority being atrial myxomas (557–561); those particular lesions are seen with sufficient frequency that surgical pathologists are familiar with their morphologic characteristics (562). Malignancies arising in the endocardium, myocardium, or pericardium are exceedingly rare; nevertheless, fibrosarcomas, myxofibrosarcomas (MFSs), rhabdomyosarcomas, angiosarcomas, neurogenic sarcomas, malignant fibrous histiocytomas (MFHs), liposarcomas, leiomyosarcomas, extraosseous osteosarcomas, synovial sarcomas, non-Hodgkin's lymphomas, and malignant mesotheliomas have indeed been observed in such sites (553,559–561).

There is a small number of tumefactive intracardiac disorders that are capable of simulating neoplasms at both clinical and pathologic levels. Hamartomas, other developmental anomalies, inflammatory conditions, and selected hyperplasias and hypertrophies of various tissue elements are included in this group. This chapter also considers pseudoneoplastic lesions of the large blood vessels. All of the processes discussed herein are listed in **Table 5.1**, along with their principal differential diagnoses.

TABLE 5.1 Neoplastic Mimics of the Heart and Blood Vessels, and the Lesions That They Simulate

HEART

- Rhabdomyomatous hamartoma (True rhabdomyoma & rhabdomyosarcoma)
- Fibromatous hamartoma (Fibrosarcoma & myxofibrosarcoma)
- Endodermal choristoma ("mesothelioma") (Metastatic carcinoma)
- Lipomatous cardiac hypertrophy (Lipoma & liposarcoma)
- Mesothelial-monocytic intracardiac excrescences (Metastatic adenocarcinoma)
- Inflammatory pseudotumor (Inflammatory myofibroblastic tumor; inflammatory malignant fibrous histiocytoma; calcifying fibrous tumor)
- Atypical lymphoid infiltrates of the myocardium
  - Severe viral myocarditis (Lymphoma)
  - Severe allograft rejection (Posttransplant lymphoproliferative disease (PTLD))
  - Florid "quilty" lesions in cardiac allografts (PTLD)
  - Rosai–Dorfman disease (Lymphoma)
  - Castleman's disease (Lymphoma)
- Extramedullary hematopoiesis (Granulocytic sarcoma)

PERICARDIUM

- Pericardial mesothelial hyperplasia (Mesothelioma)
- Viral pericarditis (Lymphoma)
- Organizing/vascularizing pericarditis (Angiosarcoma)
- Constrictive pericarditis (Desmoplastic mesothelioma)
- Pericardial fat pad (Lipoma & liposarcoma)
- Castleman's disease (Lymphoma)
- Extramedullary hematopoiesis (Granulocytic sarcoma)

BLOOD VESSELS

- Inflammatory aortic aneurysm (Desmoid; low-grade fibrosarcoma)
- Plasma cell granuloma of carotid artery (Inflammatory myofibroblastic tumor; inflammatory malignant fibrous histiocytoma)

1. Aneurysmal bone cyst-like lesion of carotid artery (Giant cell tumor of soft parts)

   Tumefactive Wegener's granulomatosis (Lymphoma)

HAMARTOMAS AND CHORISTOMAS OF THE HEART

At least three tumefactive lesions of the heart were originally described with the assumption that they represented truly neoplastic proliferations; however, with the passage of time and the accrual of clinicopathologic details on these disorders, it now appears that they are hamartomatous growths. The conditions in question include rhabdomyomatous hamartoma (RH, so-called cardiac "rhabdomyoma"), fibromatous hamartoma, and endodermal choristoma of the atrioventricular (AV) septum (formerly called "mesothelioma of the atrioventricular node").

RHABDOMYOMATOUS HAMARTOMAS

So-called rhabdomyomas of the heart are well known in the context of the tuberous sclerosis complex (TSC; Bourneville's disease), a multiorgan phakomatosis that also potentially affects the kidneys, lungs, central nervous system, and skin (556,563–565). Cardiac lesions occur in up to 50% of patients with TSC. They may be single or multiple and are characteristically nodular, measuring from 1 mm to several cm in maximal dimension. These masses may project into one of the four cardiac chambers or be entirely intramural (**Figure 5.1**). RHs are present from birth, and they have been seen in TSC patients who died soon after delivery (563–565).

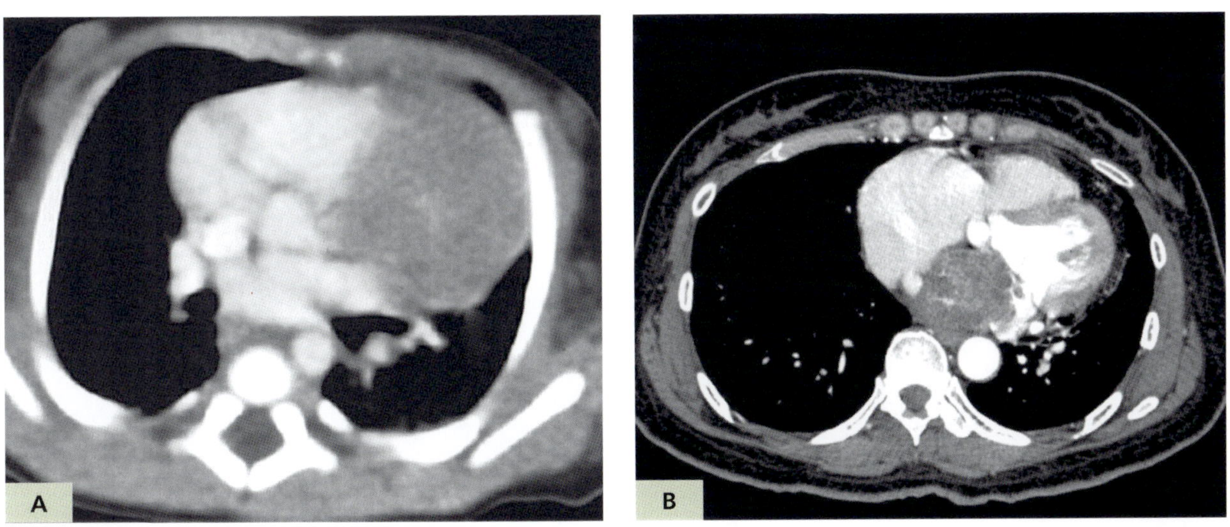

FIGURE 5.1 A & B: Computed tomography of the thorax shows masses of variable size that distort the myocardium in cases of rhabdomyomatous cardiac hamartoma.

As summarized by McAllister and Fenoglio (556), RHs may also develop sporadically, outside the context of TSC. Most patients with sporadic lesions are asymptomatic, and the masses are discovered incidentally during cardiac angiography or echocardiography done for other reasons. Nonetheless, a minority presents with symptoms and signs of congestive heart failure that are attributable to the effects of the hamartoma on myocardial contractility. Most non-TSC-related RHs affect individuals who are 25 years old or younger. Therapeutic intervention is necessary only if the lesions interfere with cardiac function, and there have been no documented reports of malignant transformation in RH.

Macroscopically, RHs are tan–pink, homogeneous, solid nodules that exhibit a vaguely fascicular substructure **(Figure 5.2)**. They have a variable interface with the surrounding myocardium and do not exhibit internal necrosis or hemorrhage.

Histologic examination shows broadly lobulated aggregates of large polygonal myogenic cells that focally show mature cardiac-type cytoplasmic cross-striations. Nuclei are generally centrally located, with evenly distributed chromatin and small chromocenters. Nuclear atypia and mitotic activity are not encountered in RHs **(Figure 5.3)**. A characteristic feature of "adult" rhabdomyomas in extracardiac locations, as well as RHs of the heart, is the presence of so-called spider cells (553,563–565) **(Figure 5.4)**. These are rhabdomyocytes in which artifactual retraction of the cytoplasm has occurred in a centripetal manner, leaving radially disposed strands that are attached to the plasmalemma and that resemble the legs of a spider.

The principal differential diagnostic considerations in cases of RH are represented by two other patterns of "rhabdomyoma" that are usually seen in other

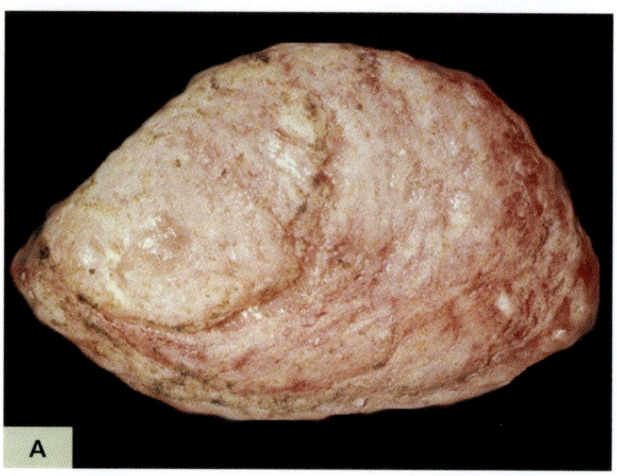

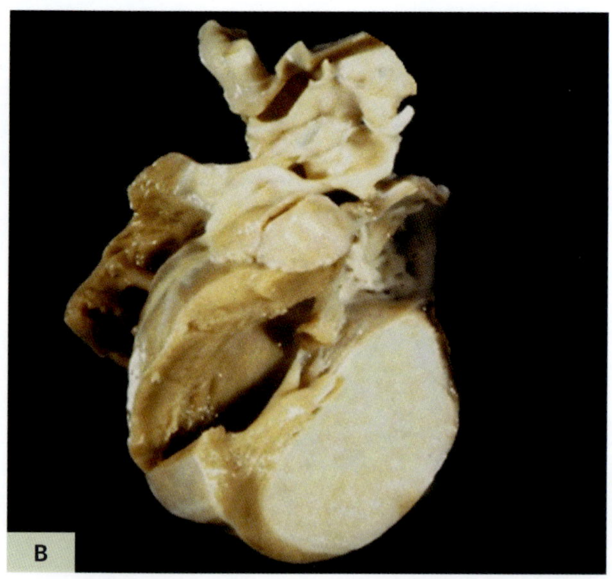

FIGURE 5.2 A & B: Rhabdomyomatous hamartomas of the heart are fleshy intramyocardial masses with indistinct borders.

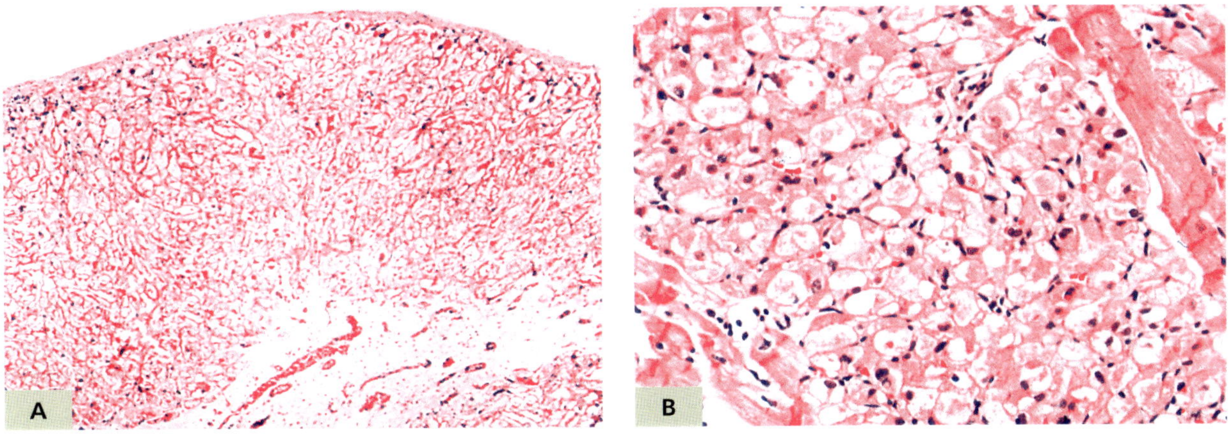

FIGURE 5.3 A & B: Large, cytologically bland epithelioid cells comprise intracardiac rhabdomyomatous hamartomas. They show variable cytoplasmic eosinophilia.

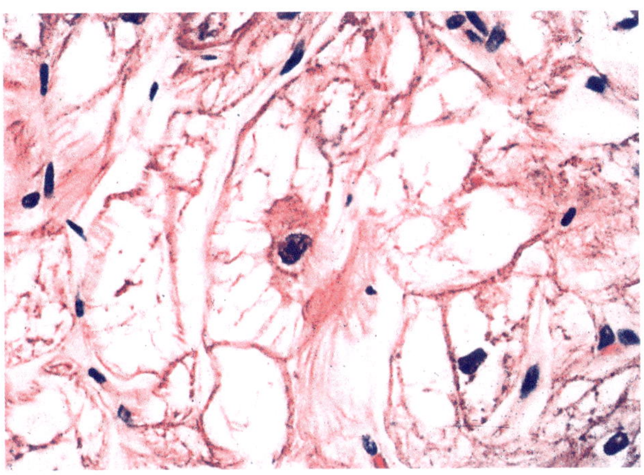

FIGURE 5.4 The most characteristic histological feature of rhabdomyomatous hamartoma is its content of "spider" cells. These are striated myocytes with a netlike cytoplasmic substructure against a lucent background, simulating the appearance of a spider. They are also present in "adult" type rhabdomyomas in extracardiac locations.

topographic locations—namely, the "fetal" and "juvenile" types (566–568) **(Figure 5.5)**. These lesions have also been reported rarely in the heart (569,570). They differ from RH in containing a predominance of more compact and fusiform rhabdomyocytes, which retain the cytoplasmic striations of normal striated muscle. RH, fetal rhabdomyoma, and juvenile rhabdomyoma all lack the degree of cellular anaplasia that is seen in cardiac rhabdomyosarcoma (571–580) **(Figure 5.6)**. In addition, the last of those lesions is immunoreactive for myogenin (572) **(Figure 5.7)**; that marker is typically lacking in rhabdomyomas, and especially in RH.

Selected examples of RHs might be confused with metastatic clear-cell carcinomas or melanomas (581,582) **(Figure 5.8)**. In comparison with the latter neoplasms, however, the immunophenotype of RHs is distinctive. It features reactivity for desmin, muscle-specific actin, and myoglobin **(Figure 5.9)** but

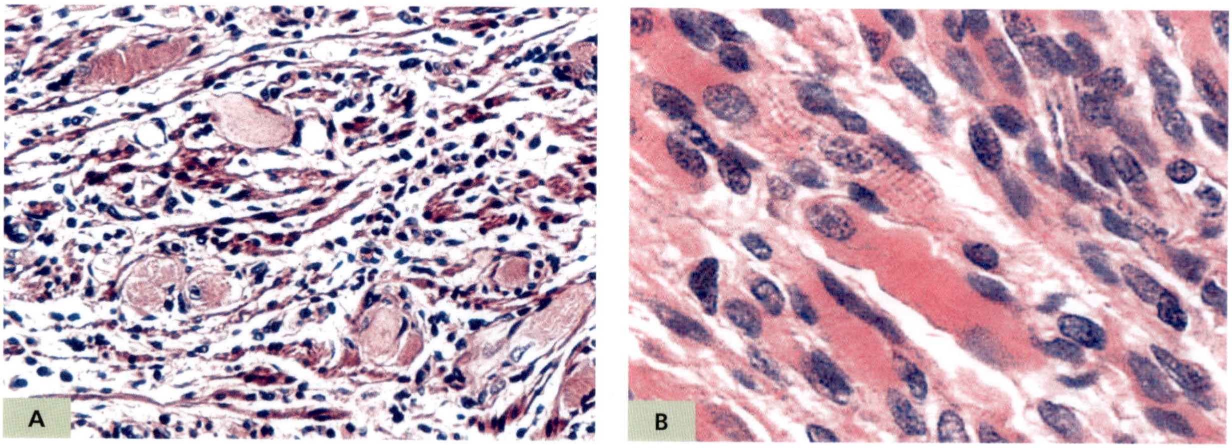

FIGURE 5.5 Fetal-type rhabdomyomas are also rarely found in the heart (A). These differ from rhabdomyomatous hamartomas by containing more elongated myocytes showing clear-cut cytoplasmic cross-striations (B). In addition, fetal rhabdomyomas are partially constituted by bland, nondescript, compact polygonal and fusiform cells.

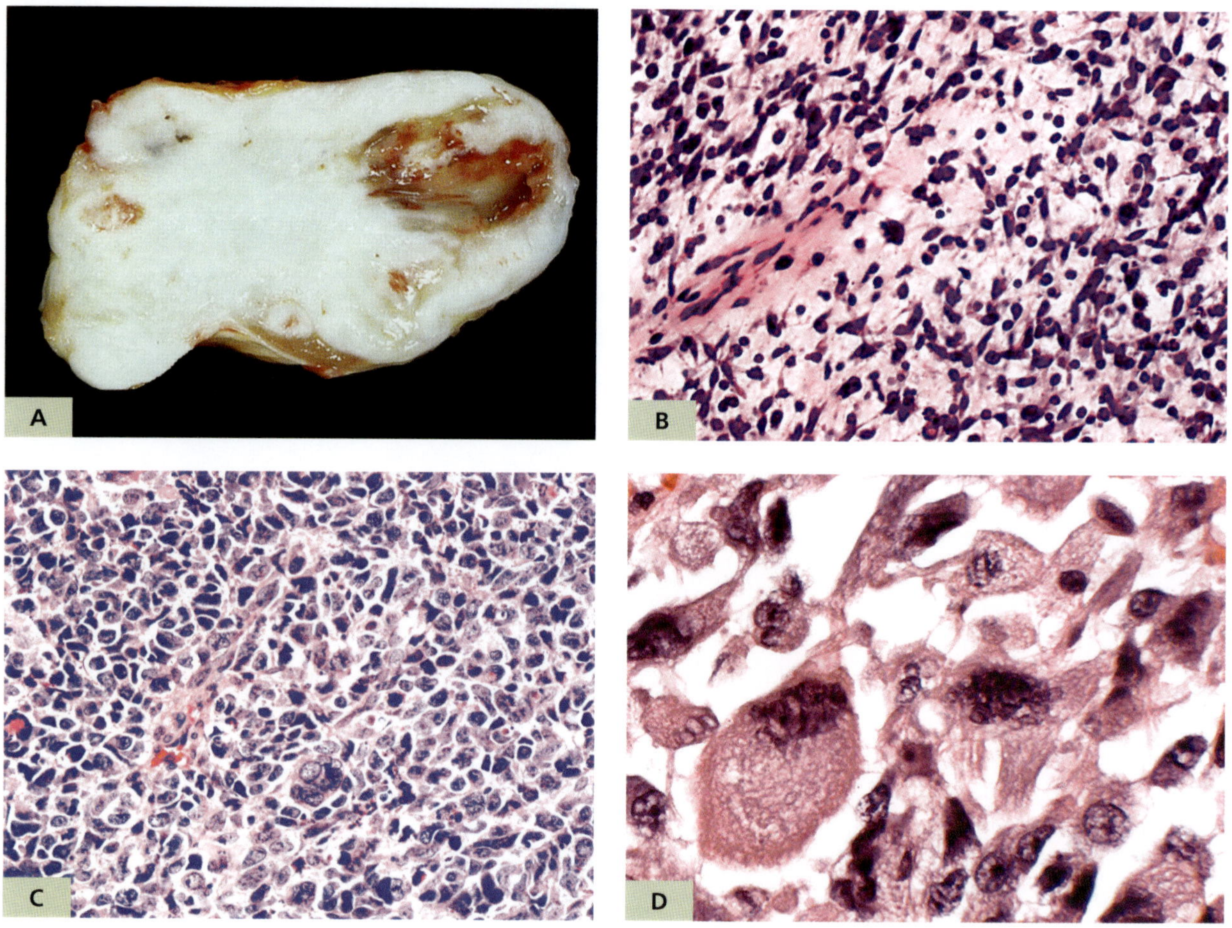

FIGURE 5.6 Intracardiac rhabdomyosarcomas (A and B) efface normal cardiac structure markedly (A) are comprised of a population of round or spindle cells with obvious nuclear pleomorphism and atypicality (B–D).

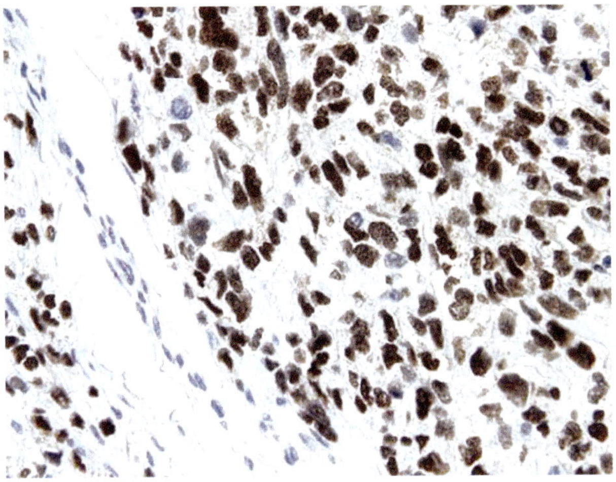

FIGURE 5.7 Myogenin is often present in rhabdomyosarcomas immunohistologically. That marker is not expected in rhabdomyomatous hamartomas or rhabdomyomas.

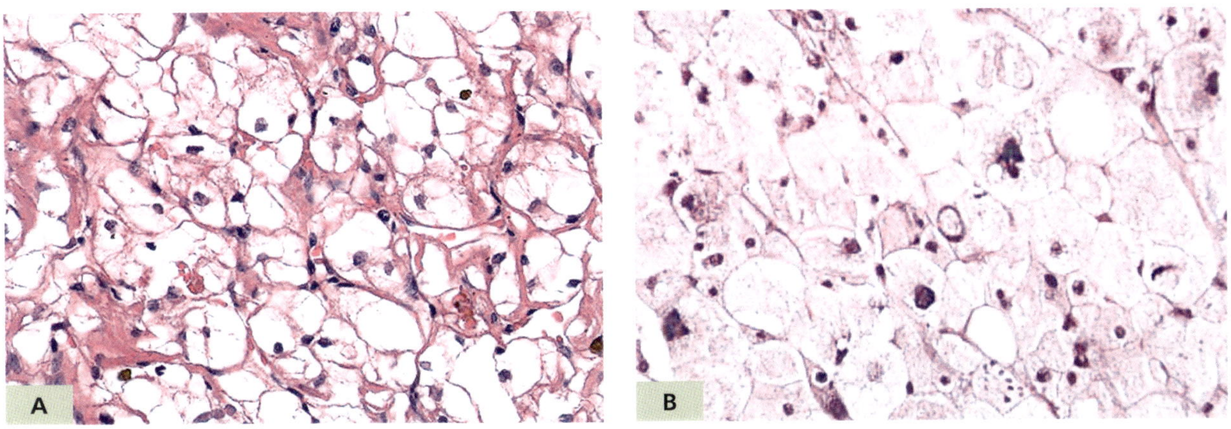

FIGURE 5.8 Metastatic clear-cell carcinomas (A, renal cell carcinoma) and "balloon" [clear]-cell melanomas (B) in the myocardium may partially simulate the clear "spider" cells of rhabdomyomatous hamartoma.

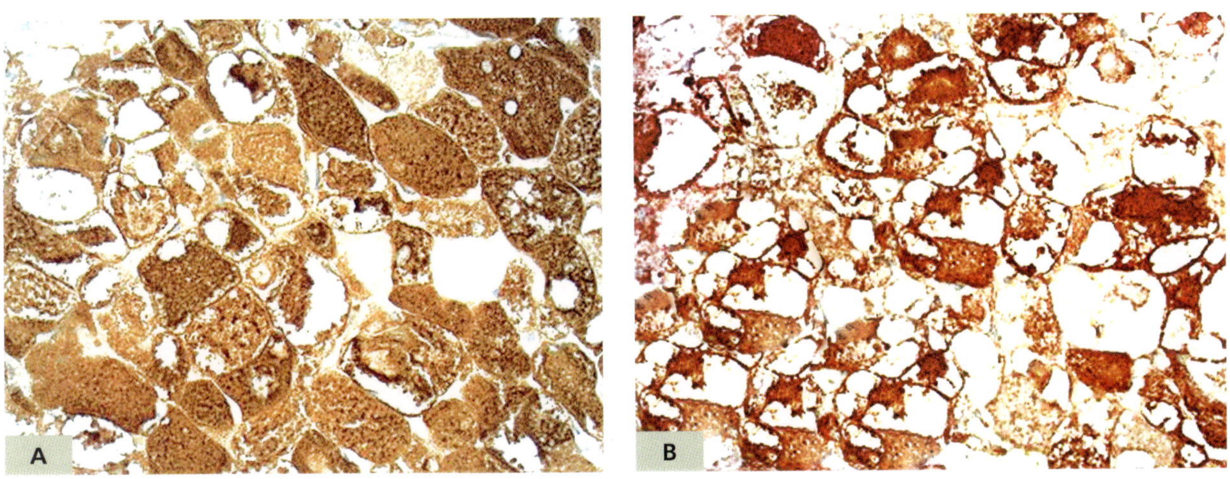

FIGURE 5.9 Immunoreactivity is present for myoglobin (A) and desmin (B) in rhabdomyomatous hamartoma. Those determinants are not seen in metastatic carcinomas or melanomas.

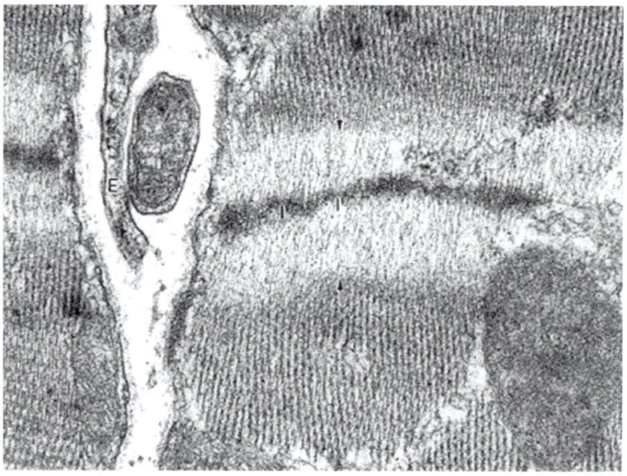

FIGURE 5.10 Well-represented sarcomeric substructure is apparent ultrastucturally in rhabdomyomatous hamartoma.

does not include labeling for keratin or S100 protein (567,569). Similarly, well-developed sarcomeric development is seen in RHs ultrastructurally (563) (**Figure 5.10**), distinguishing them from the other cited diagnostic possibilities. Lastly, RH usually becomes manifest in children, who would not be expected to have metastatic carcinomas or melanomas.

FIBROMATOUS HAMARTOMA ("CARDIAC FIBROMA")

In contrast to papillary fibroelastomas of the cardiac valves (**Figure 5.11**), which represent malformations that are essentially never confused with true

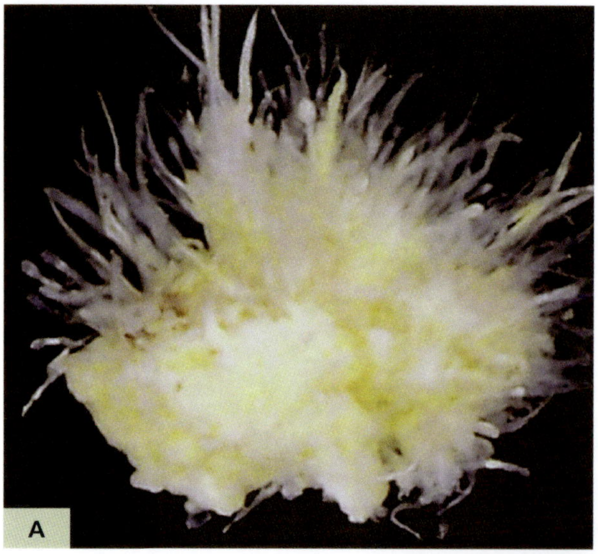

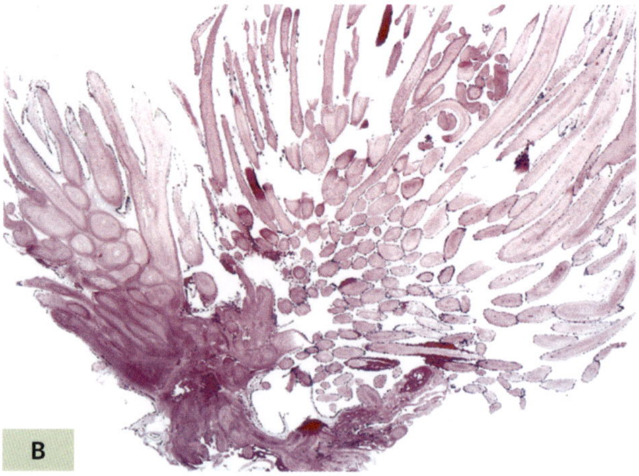

FIGURE 5.11 Despite its name, papillary fibroelastoma is likely hamartomatous in nature. It is typically based on a cardiac valve (A), comprising a filiform proliferation of fibroelastic tissue (B–D). (*Continued*)

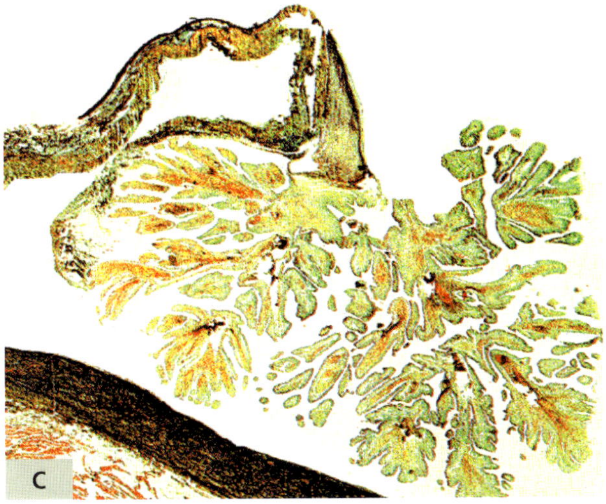

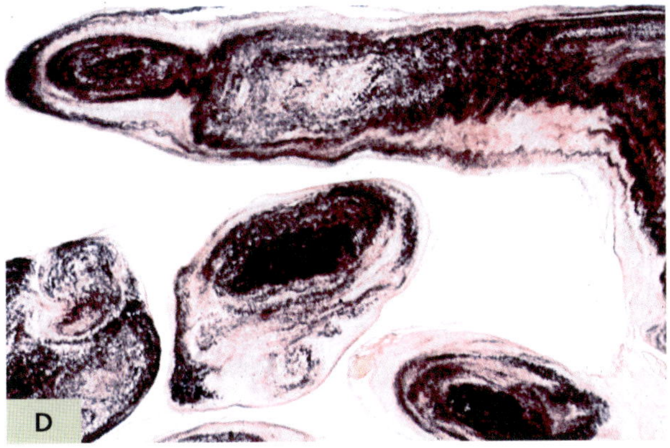

FIGURE 5.11 (*Continued*) The elastic tissue in fibroelastoma can be highlighted with the Verhoeff–van Gieson stain (C & D).

neoplasms by pathologists (583–585), intramyocardial fibromas (IMFs) do have an ability to imitate neoplastic lesions. IMFs are usually detected in young children who present with congestive heart failure or arrhythmias, but some of them are asymptomatic until well into adulthood (556,559,586–590). They may be seen in any of the four cardiac chambers, varying in size from <1 to several centimeters in maximal dimension **(Figure 5.12)**. When it is necessary, surgical resection is curative.

Microscopically, IMF is constituted by a population of variably dense and bland fusiform fibrocytes, embedded in a densely collagenized stroma. Some lesions show a fascicular arrangement of the spindle-cells, whereas others manifest a "patternless pattern" of growth **(Figure 5.13)**. An interdigitating interface with the surrounding myocardium is usually present, and there is no nuclear atypia, mitotic activity, or necrosis in IMF. Foci of calcification are common and helpful in differential diagnosis. Immunostains show reactivity for vimentin and, sometimes, for alpha-isoform actin in the lesional spindle-cells, with no labeling for myoglobin, desmin, myogenin, or Myo-D1 (589).

Differential diagnoses for IMF are limited. One is the ***cardiac mesenchymal hamartoma***, another recently described malformative cardiac lesion that contains not only fibrous tissue but cardiac muscle, smooth muscle, fat, and nerve fibers (591). As such, that lesion itself may be confused with a *monodermal teratoma* **(Figure 5.14)**. Other diagnostic alternatives are intracardiac *fibrosarcoma* (FS) and *MFS* (592–595). Those malignant neoplasms have most often been encountered in the atria, where they cause symptoms because of interference

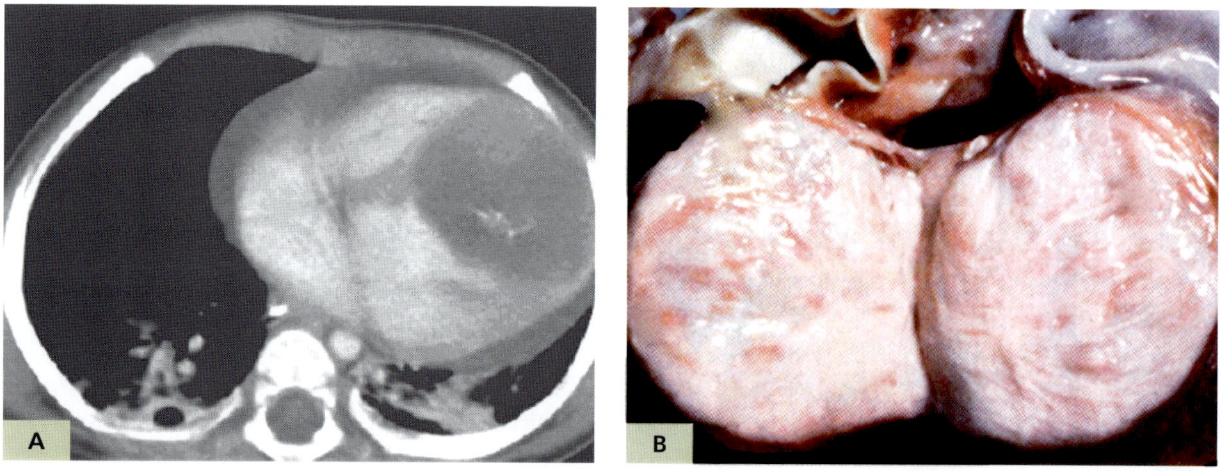

FIGURE 5.12 A & B: Intracardiac fibroma produces a mass composed of confluent, variably-mature collagenized tissue.

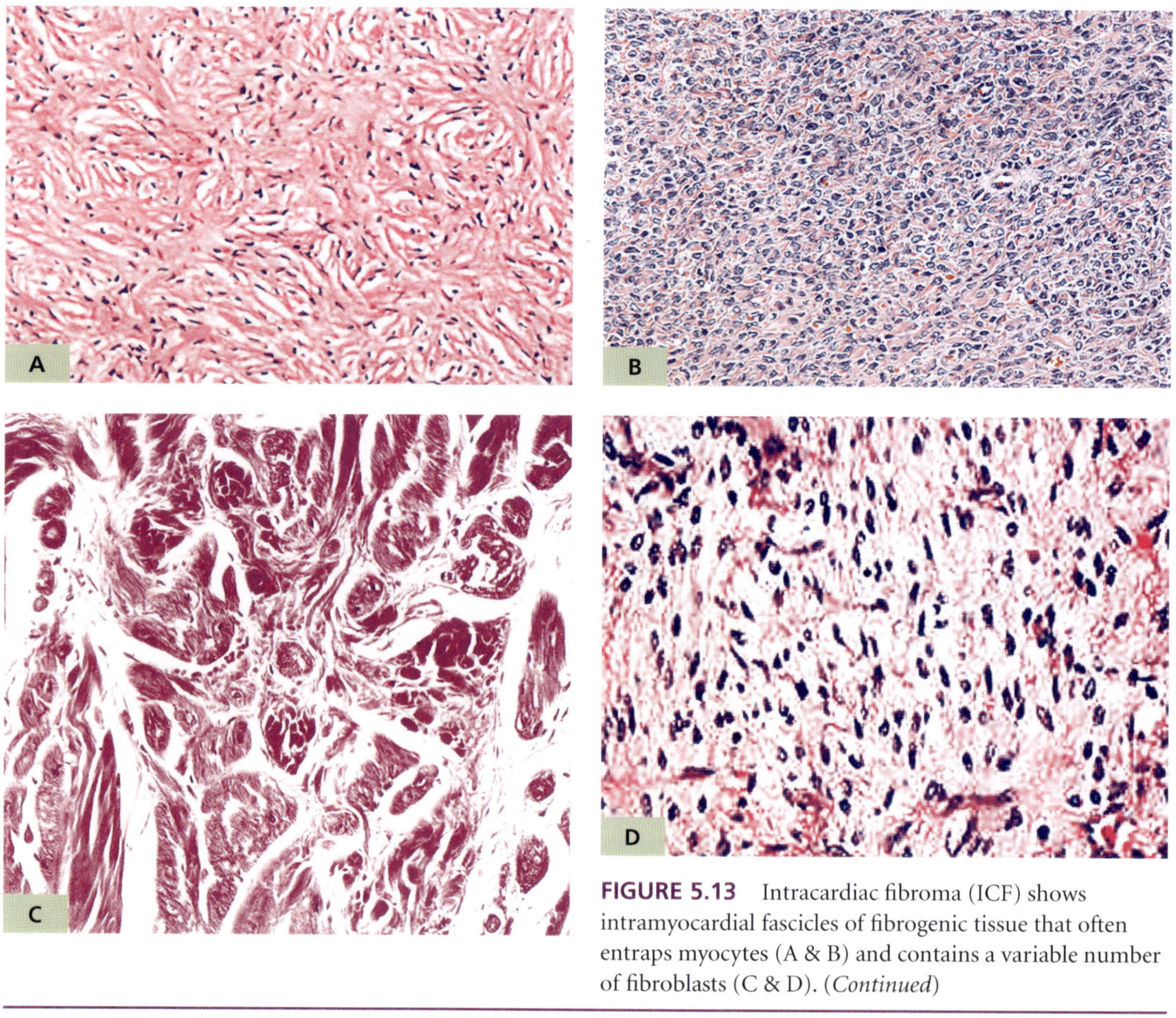

FIGURE 5.13 Intracardiac fibroma (ICF) shows intramyocardial fascicles of fibrogenic tissue that often entraps myocytes (A & B) and contains a variable number of fibroblasts (C & D). (*Continued*)

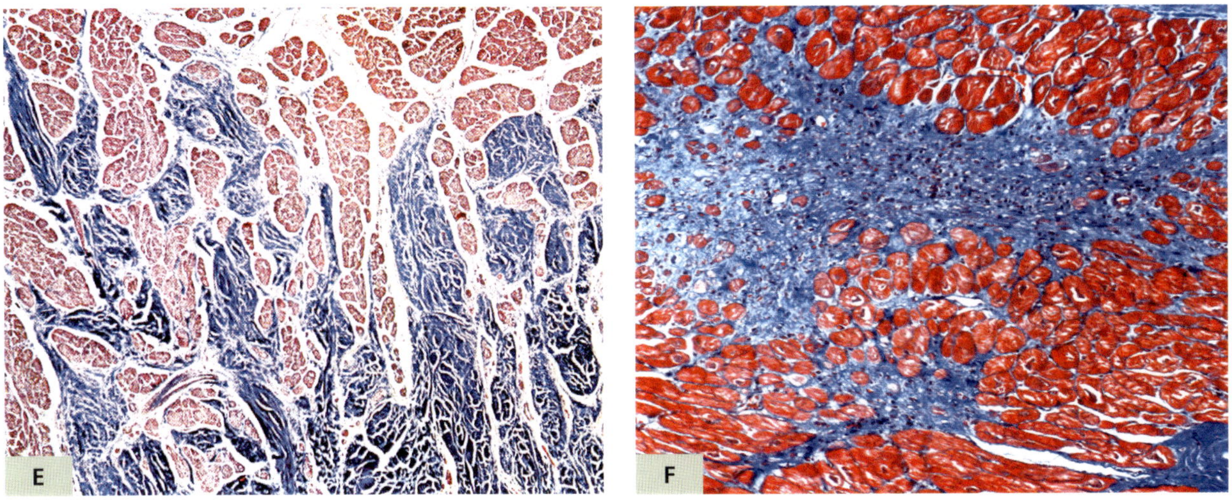

FIGURE 5.13 (*Continued*) The collagenous matrix in ICF can be stained blue with the Masson trichrome method (E & F).

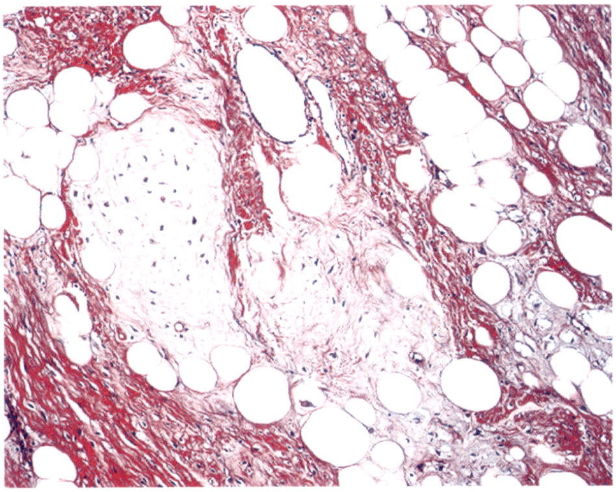

FIGURE 5.14 Mesodermal mesenchymal hamartoma is probably related nosologically to intracardiac fibroma. The former of those lesions is constituted by a mixture of banal fibroblasts, adipocytes, and collagenous matrix.

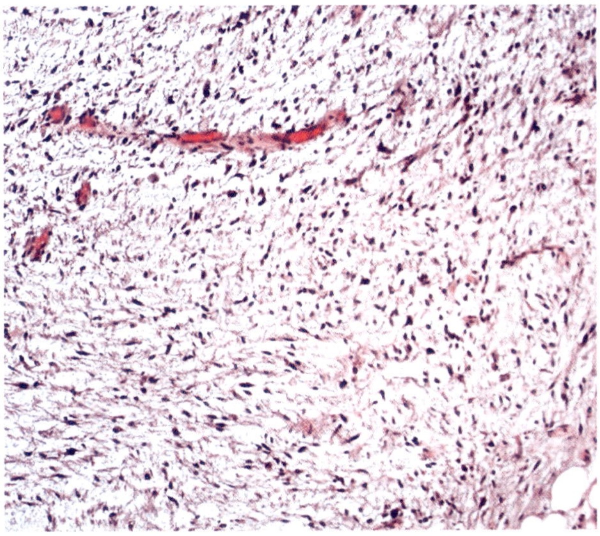

FIGURE 5.15 Low-grade myxofibrosarcoma (LGMF), shown here, may rarely affect the myocardium and might be confused with intracardiac fibroma (ICF). Nonetheless, LGMF effaces the myocardium rather than entrapping it as ICF does. Moreover, LGMF shows a higher level of cellularity and nuclear atypia.

with AV valvular function (593–595). Both FS and MFS show a higher degree of cellularity than that of IMF; the former two lesions also manifest at least some nuclear atypia and mitotic activity, and MFS has a uniformly myxoid stroma that is not seen in IMF **(Figure 5.15)**.

ENDODERMAL CHORISTOMA (FORMERLY "MESOTHELIOMA") OF THE INTERATRIAL SEPTUM

Several reports have been made of a fascinating lesion of the interatrial septum in the region of the AV node. It was initially felt to be a form of benign "mesothelioma" and, if it was identified at all macroscopically, it was usually composed of an agglomeration of minuscule cysts (596–601). Patients with this abnormality have spanned all age groups, and there is no predilection for either gender.

It is notable that several cases of AV "mesothelioma" have involved infants who had concomitant developmental anomalies in other organs. These have included isolated cardiac valvular atresia, coarctation of the aorta, patent ductus arteriosus, ventricular septal defects, Meckel's diverticulum of the terminal ileum, patent omphalovitelline duct, pulmonary hypoplasia, and diaphragmatic agenesis (599). We also have seen an association with congenital dyshormogenetic goiter in one case.

Symptoms from "mesothelioma of the AV node" (MAV) are typically related to abnormalities in cardiac conduction, manifested by syncope, bradycardia, or sudden death, and these problems usually become evident early in life (598,599). Thus, this lesion is a rare but potential cause of heart block in children. Obviously, it needs treatment if the affected patients are symptomatic, but pacemakers are usually implanted in *all* cases of known MAV because of the risk of a sudden tachyarrhythmia or asystole. Nevertheless, the reality of the situation is that MAV is only exceptionally identified during life (600).

Histologically, MAV is composed of variably sized nests of bland polygonal cells in the interatrial myocardium. Many of these cellular aggregates contain central lumina, whereas others may exhibit a squamoid appearance or take on a solid configuration. The cell nests are usually grouped in a locally organoid fashion, but occasionally they may demonstrate a more randomly disposed architecture (599,601) **(Figure 5.16)**. Nuclei are compact with evenly dispersed chromatin, and cytoplasm is amphophilic or eosinophilic and relatively abundant. There is no nuclear atypia or mitotic activity.

Immunohistochemical studies have shown that "mesothelioma" of the AV node does not, in fact, have the phenotype of mesothelial cells. Instead, it commonly exhibits reactivity for carcinoembryonic antigen (CEA) and tumor-associated glycoprotein-72 (TAG-72 [also known as CA72.4]; recognized by the monoclonal antibody B72.3), as seen in activated or neoplastic glandular epithelial cells (599,601). Electron microscopy has confirmed the epithelial

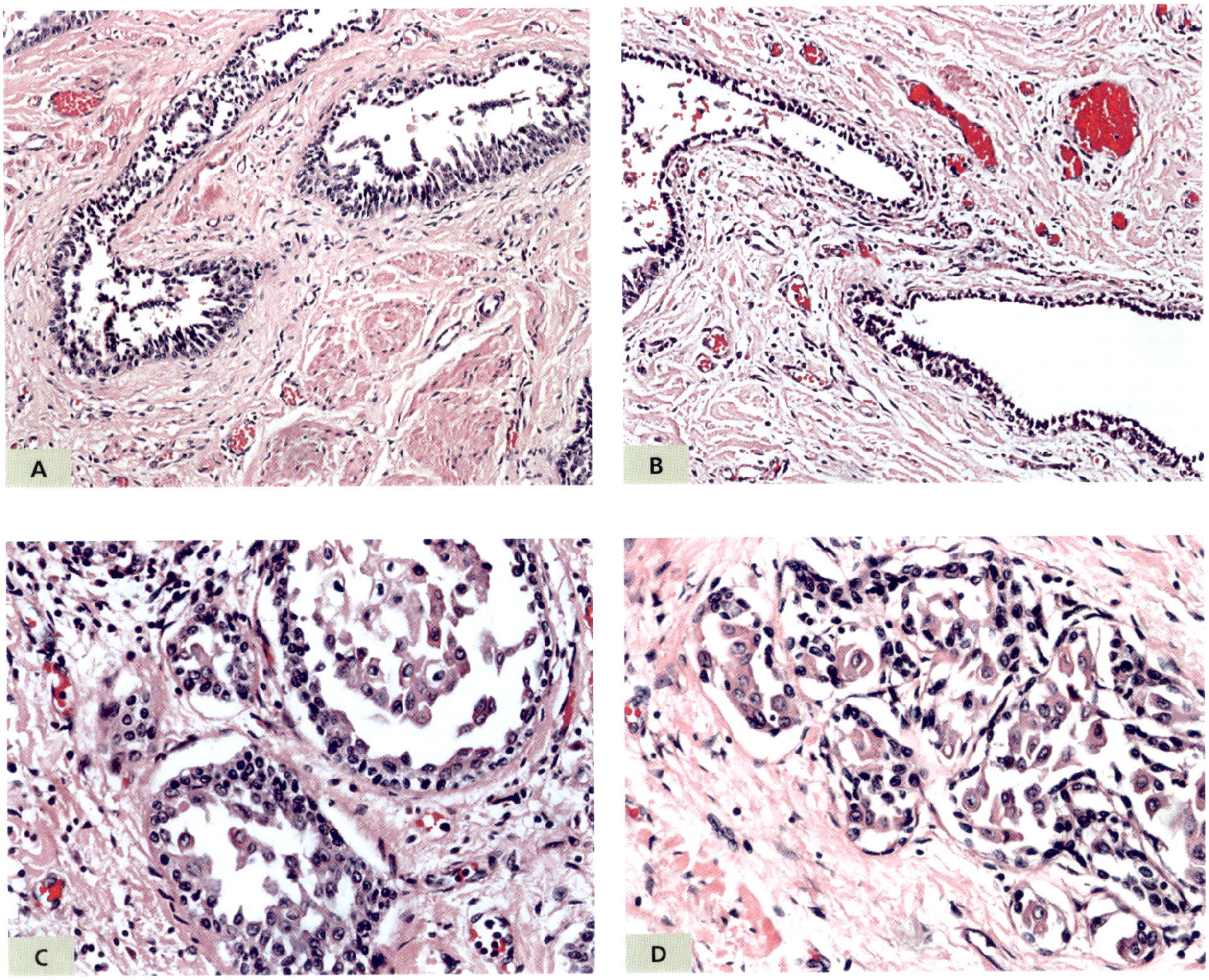

FIGURE 5.16 A–D: Endodermal choristoma of the myocardium comprises multiple microcysts in which micropapillary arrays are present. The latter structures may show modest cellular atypicality.

nature of the lesion and shown that it manifests attenuated surface microvilli resembling those of endodermal tissues (597) **(Figure 5.17)**. Thus, on the whole, it would appear best to relabel MAV as an ***intracardiac endodermal choristoma*** (IEC).

Differential diagnosis concerns the exclusion of *metastatic adenocarcinoma* (602). This is facilitated by attention to the bland cytologic attributes of IEC, as well as to the fact that most affected individuals are very young and therefore unlikely to have an epithelial malignancy. Furthermore, metastatic carcinoma in the myocardium and epicardium manifests grossly visible nodules **(Figure 5.18)**, in contrast to the macroscopically-unobtrusive nature of IEC. Carcinomas also exhibit a greater degree of nuclear atypicality.

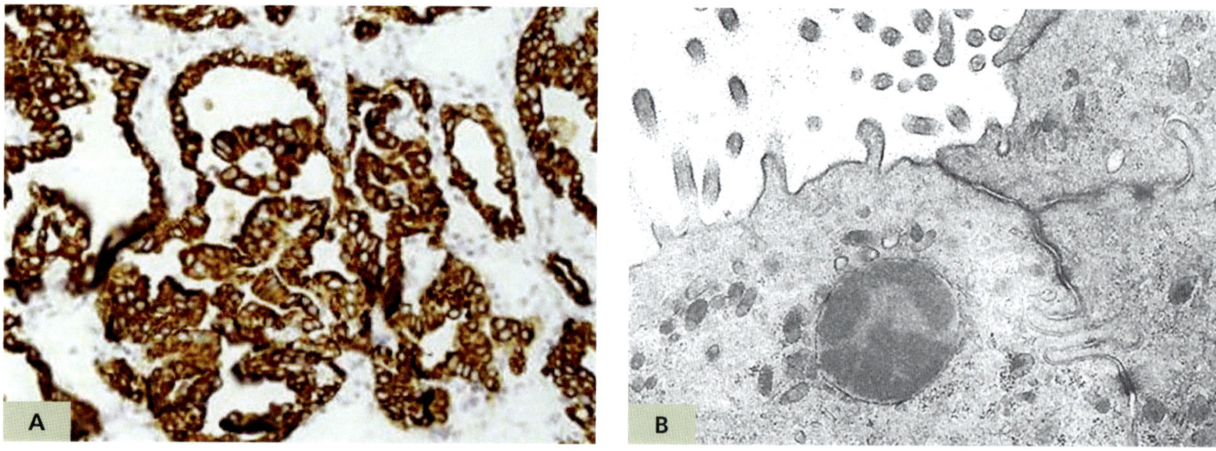

FIGURE 5.17 Endodermal choristomas of the heart (ECH) can be labeled immunohistochemically with MOC-31, a generic marker for glandular epithelial differentiation (A). By electron microscopy, the cells of ECH demonstrate short, blunt, plasmalemmal microvilli, indicating the presence of glandular rather than mesothelial features (B).

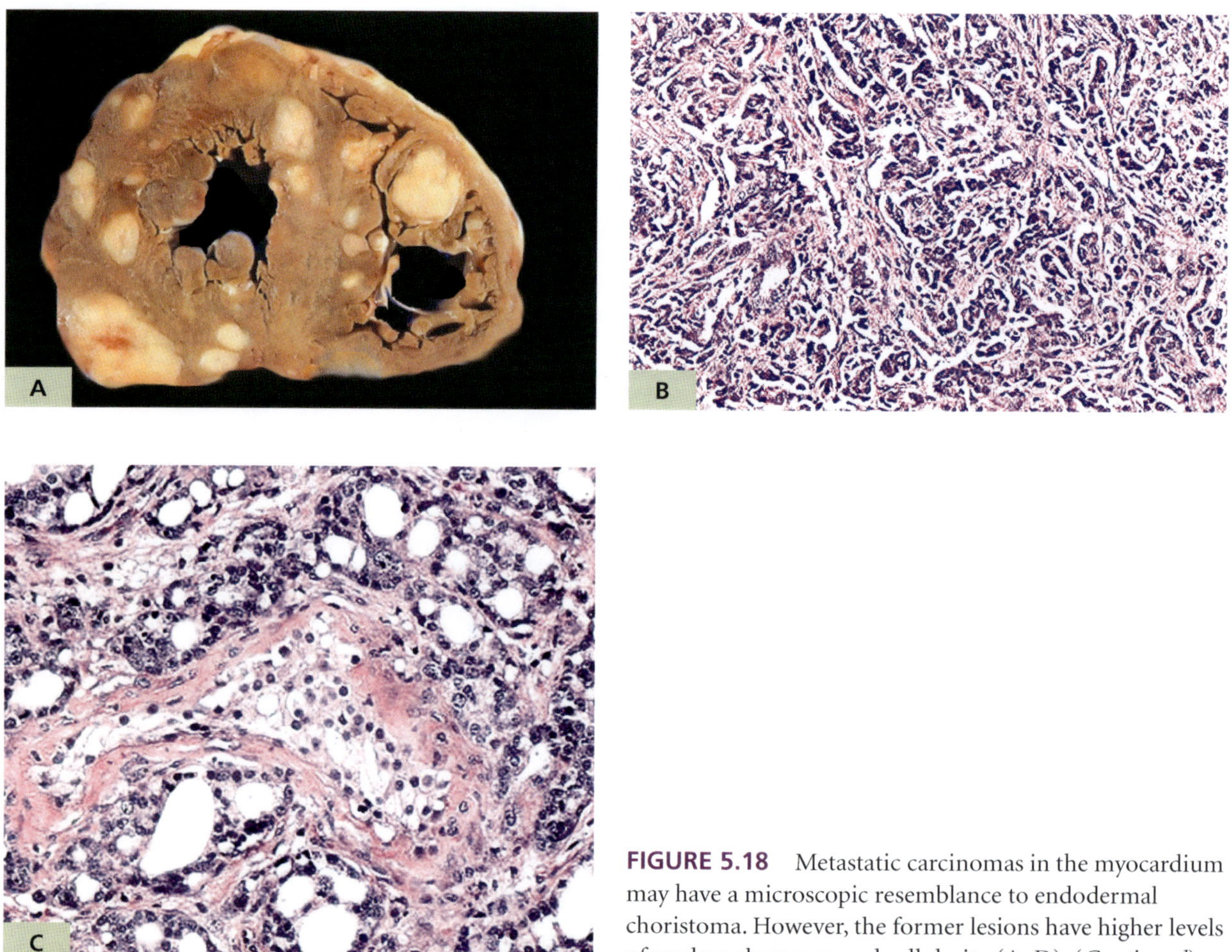

FIGURE 5.18 Metastatic carcinomas in the myocardium may have a microscopic resemblance to endodermal choristoma. However, the former lesions have higher levels of nuclear aberrancy and cellularity (A–D). (*Continued*)

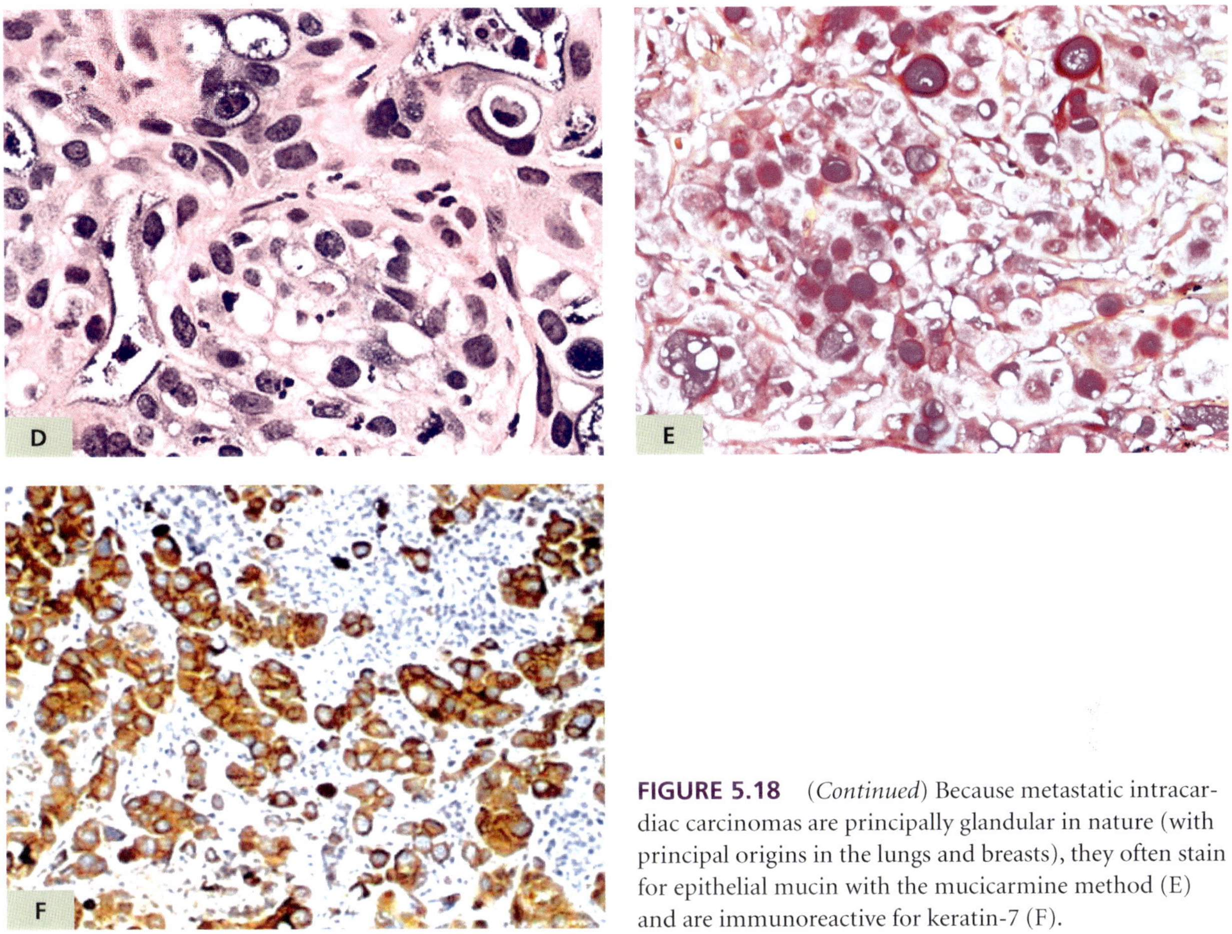

FIGURE 5.18 (*Continued*) Because metastatic intracardiac carcinomas are principally glandular in nature (with principal origins in the lungs and breasts), they often stain for epithelial mucin with the mucicarmine method (E) and are immunoreactive for keratin-7 (F).

LIPOMATOUS HYPERTROPHY OF THE HEART

True *lipomas* and *liposarcomas* of the myocardium—which assume the form of well-demarcated accumulations of adipose tissue (577,603–605)—may be confused with a condition known as "lipomatous hypertrophy" (LH) of the heart. The latter disorder is seen increasingly with advancing age in obese adults and probably represents participation by intracardiac lipocytes in the systemic storage of excess fat (606–614).

LH most commonly manifests itself as a fusiform tumefactive mass in the interatrial septum, usually measuring >2 cm (**Figure 5.19**). Multiple lesions may be present in the muscular walls of other chambers as well, potentially overlapping macroscopically with the condition known as "arrhythmogenic fatty metamorphosis/dysplasia" of the myocardium (612). LH may likewise produce a variety of complex supraventricular arrhythmias, as well as AV block and sudden death (608,609). Although it was known principally to autopsy pathologists in the

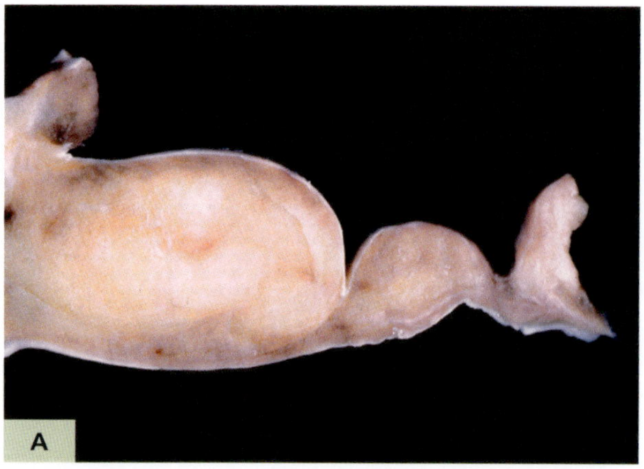

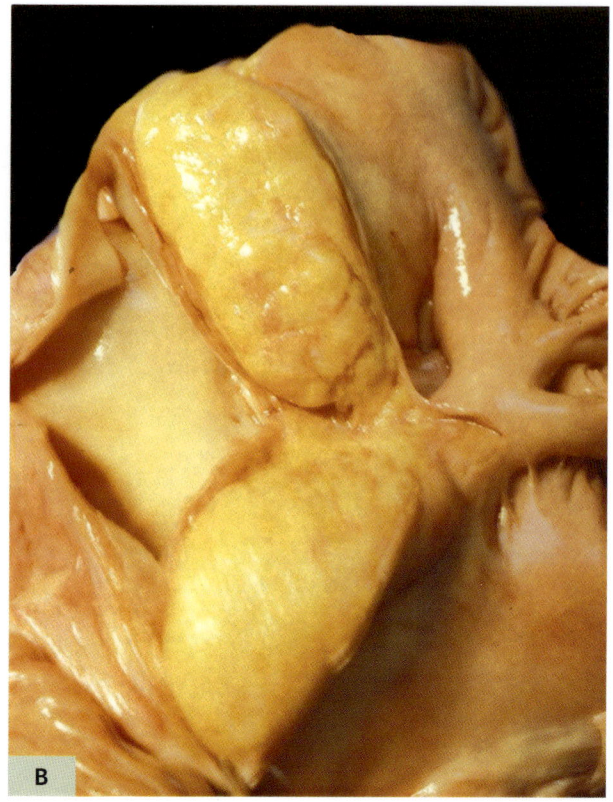

FIGURE 5.19 A & B: Lipomatous hypertrophy of the heart typically affects the interatrial septum, which is expanded and distorted by the deposition of adipose tissue.

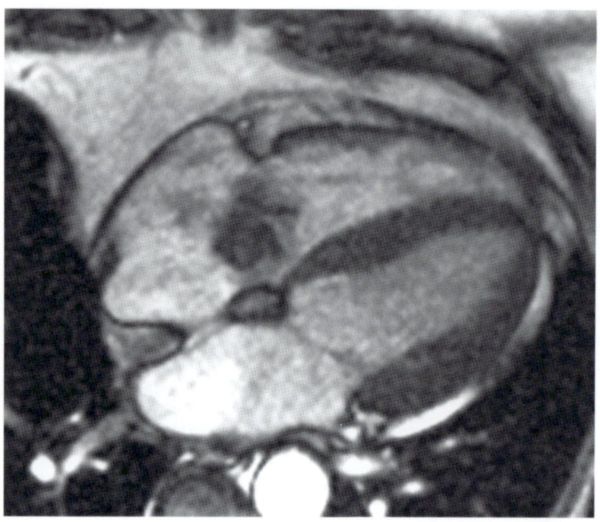

FIGURE 5.20 The difference in attenuation between lipomatous hypertrophy of the heart and the myocardium is apparent in this magnetic resonance image.

past, modern cardiovascular imaging techniques have allowed for the diagnostic recognition of LH during life (**Figure 5.20**). In the event that they are symptomatic, the lipoma-like deposits may now be electively removed surgically (607).

LH is typically poorly circumscribed and it lacks fibrous encapsulation. Histologically, it is composed of an admixture of mature fat, fetal fat, and hypertrophied cardiac myocytes (**Figure 5.21**). The presence of fetal fat (**Figure 5.22**) is a hallmark of LH, and its recognition is helpful in distinguishing LH from true cardiac *lipomas* and *liposarcomas* (**Figure 5.23**). The latter lesions are usually located in the wall of the left or right atrium but not within the interatrial septum. Furthermore, by definition, liposarcoma should contain lipoblasts that are cytologically atypical (604,605) (**Figure 5.24**), and which contain multiple

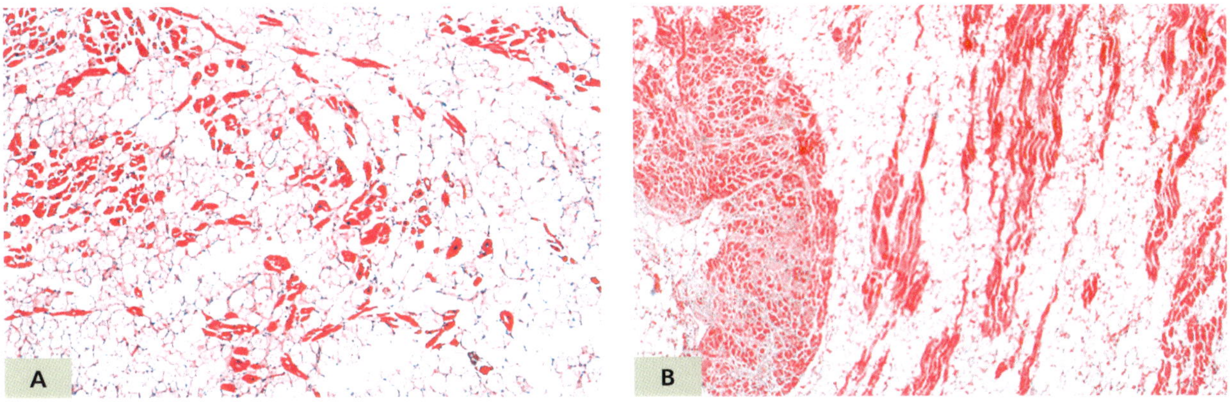

FIGURE 5.21 A & B: Myocytes are entrapped by adipose tissue in lipomatous hypertrophy of the heart. These images overlap with those seen in "arrhythmogenic right ventricular dysplasia."

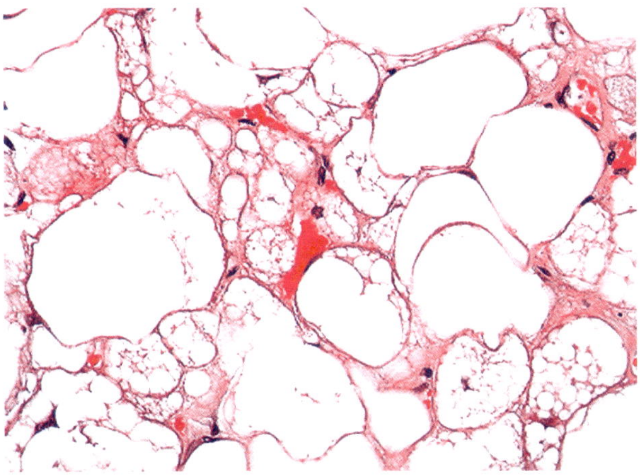

FIGURE 5.22 Fetal fat is present in lipomatous hypertrophy of the heart, in contrast to other fat-containing intracardiac lesions.

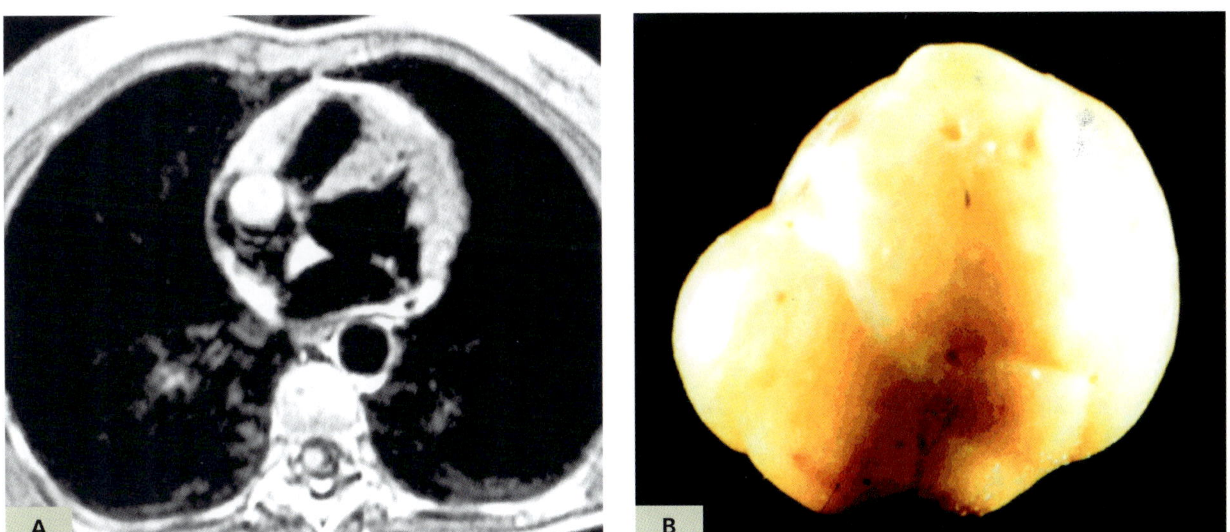

FIGURE 5.23 A & B: Intracardiac lipoma may occur in any of the four chambers of the heart and has a more globose gross appearance than does lipomatous hypertrophy.

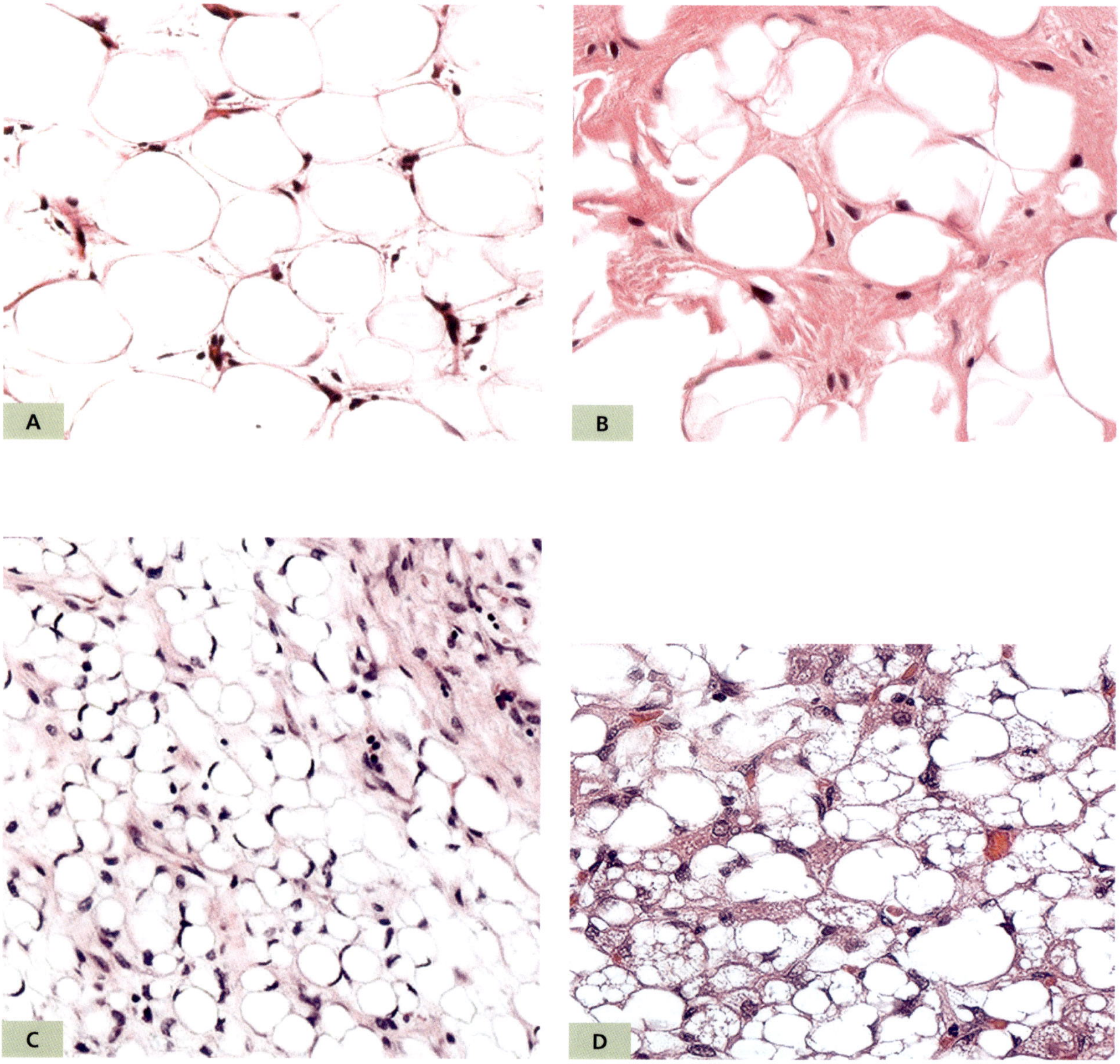

FIGURE 5.24 Cardiac lipomas comprise mature fat cells (A & B), unlike liposarcomas in which variable numbers of signet ring cell and "mulberry" lipoblasts are present (C & D).

vacuoles that indent the nucleus. This profile differs from that of fetal fat cells, which tend to be univacuolar with round or oval nuclei. True cardiac lipomas are well-circumscribed fatty neoplasms composed of mature fat cells without interspersed fetal fat or admixed myocytes (614). They are usually located on the epicardial surface but have been seen in the atrial and ventricular myocardium as well.

MESOTHELIAL-MONOCYTIC INTRACARDIAC EXCRESCENCES

Veinot et al. (615) initially described several examples of a lesion that was previously reported to resemble histiocytoid (epithelioid) hemangiomas in the cardiovascular system (616,617). Aggregated evidence has since suggested that such lesions are best regarded as a type of artifactually produced pseudotumor. Additional examples of cardiac ***mesothelial-monocytic intracardiac excrescences*** (MICE) have been reported in patients from 5 to 76 years of age (618–621). All have been incidental findings; some have been found to be free-floating in the cardiac chambers, attached to cardiac valves or found with right ventricular endomyocardial biopsy specimens. Other locations for MICE have included the pericardial sac and the ascending aorta (621).

The lesions range in size from <1 mm up to 3 cm in diameter. All have been solitary. Grossly, they are dark red or brown and are frequently associated with an obvious thrombus.

Histologically, the excrescences are composed of two cell types, set in a background of fibrin (**Figure 5.25**). The first type comprises cytologically bland histiocytes, often present in sheets, in which representatives of the second cell type—which is more cuboidal in shape—are enmeshed. The latter elements form cords and pseudoglandular spaces, and they show central oval nuclei, dispersed or slightly vesicular chromatin, small nucleoli, and a moderate amount of amphophilic cytoplasm (615,618).

Immunohistochemical analysis of MICE shows that one population of the constituent cells is keratin-negative but expresses CD68—supporting a histiocytic/monocytic nature—whereas the more cuboidal and pseudoglandular component demonstrates the converse of that immunophenotype (615,619) (**Figure 5.26**). Ultrastructural studies (**Figure 5.27**) and additional immunohistologic assessments for such markers as calretinin, WT-1 protein, and podoplanin indicate that the keratin positive cells show mesothelial differentiation.

An initial hypothesis regarding the origin of MICE held that they might represent a form of mesothelial hyperplasia (615). This reaction was thought to possibly relate to previous cardiac catheterization, because 75% of the patients in one series had such a history.

An additional premise was put forward by Courtice and coworkers (618), as a result of the examination of material found in extracorporeal bypass pumps and adherent to pericardial drains. Based on their study, in which cardiac MICE were observed in the filters of 82% of bypass pumps and 13% of drains, those authors suggested that the lesions were produced during cardiac surgery.

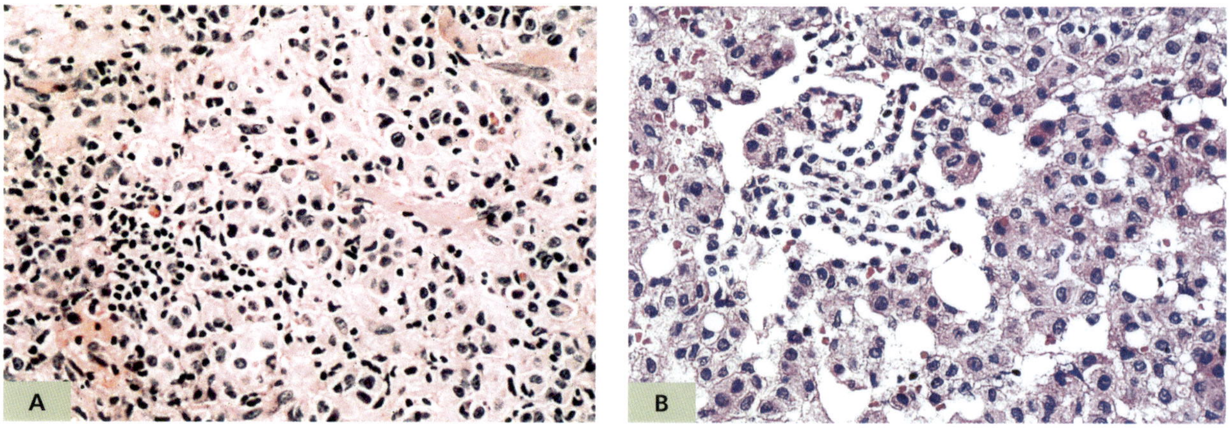

FIGURE 5.25 A & B: Mesothelial-monocytic intracardiac excrescences (MICE) are mixed aggregates of mesothelial and histiocytic cells enmeshed in fibrin, with a variable number of inflammatory cells.

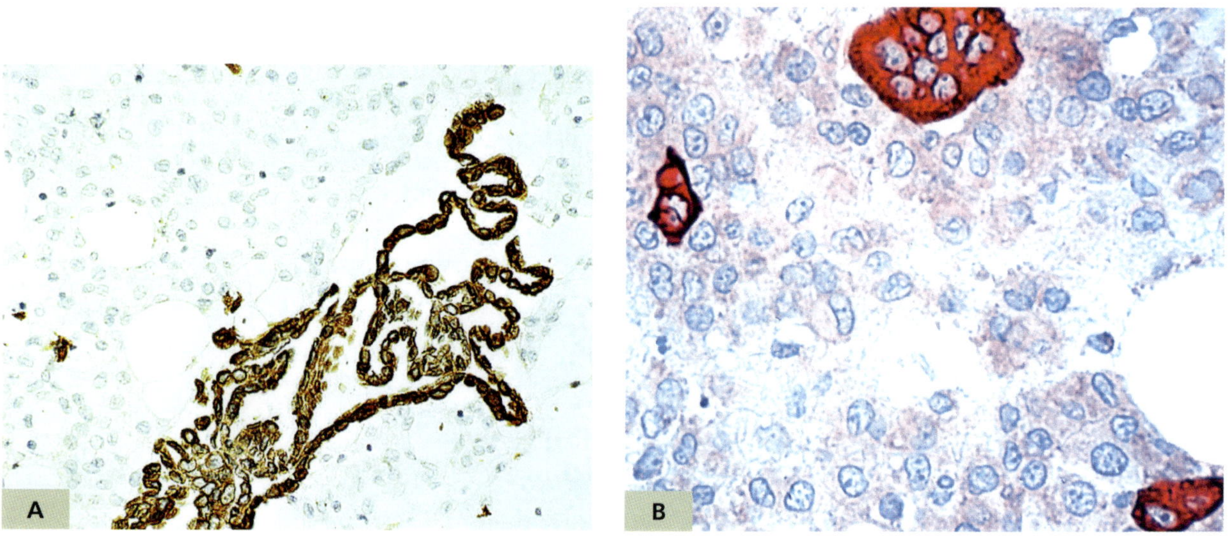

FIGURE 5.26 The histiocytes in mesothelial-monocytic intracardiac excrescences can be labeled for CD68 (A) or CD163 immunohistologically. In contrast, mesothelial components are reactive for keratin (B), WT1, podoplanin, mesothelin, and calretinin.

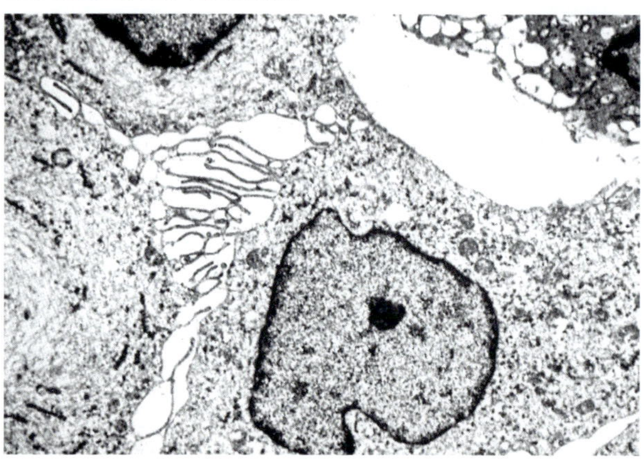

FIGURE 5.27 Electron microscopy of mesothelial-monocytic intracardiac excrescences demonstrates elongated plasmalemmal microvilli in their mesothelial elements.

The formation of MICE was attributed to compaction of friable mesothelial strips, other tissue, cellular debris, and fibers on cardiotomy suction tips. The agglomerated masses could then be transported around and from the operative site, and thus be found by either the surgeon or the pathologist. This hypothesis is attractive, but it does not account for MICE found in right ventricular endomyocardial biopsy specimens. Thus, rare examples of this lesion may instead result from perforation of the right ventricle and subsequent displacement of mesothelial cells into the cardiac chambers. Along with fibrin, previously circulating macrophages, and rare inflammatory cells, MICE probably again form in the latter scenario by cellular coalescence to yield a pseudoneoplasm (618,619).

The lack of histologic attachment to underlying tissues and the absence of supporting stroma highlight the fact that the fibrin meshwork of MICE is not only a prominent feature of these lesions but is also probably an essential element in their formation and adherence to other tissues. The absence of stroma also argues against a capacity for MICE to enlarge themselves, other than by increased adherence of cells to the fibrinous matrix.

The importance of MICE lies in the potential for their misdiagnosis as *metastatic adenocarcinoma* (614), particularly in those examples that exhibit a prominent pseudoglandular component comprising cuboidal mesothelial cells. This mistake can be avoided by an awareness of their clinical presentation, in which MICE are incidental and unexpected, as well as by their biphasic cytologic features and characteristic immunophenotype. All of those points represent consistent differences from the typical features of metastatic carcinomas (622).

INTRACARDIAC INFLAMMATORY PSEUDOTUMORS

Rare reports of polyclonal intracardiac inflammatory pseudotumor (IIPT)—as distinct from "inflammatory myofibroblastic tumor" (IMT)—have been made. Children, adolescents, and young adults have typically been affected by this lesion (619,623–625). In one remarkable case, a 17-year-old boy with IIPT also had leukocytoclastic vasculitis, polyarteritis, and inferior vena caval thrombosis (626).

Grossly, these lesions measure up to 3 cm in greatest dimension, and are typically smooth-surfaced and sessile. They are attached to the atrial or ventricular walls by a broad base, with projection into the lumina of the cardiac chambers (**Figure 5.28**). The interface between an IIPT and the surrounding myocardium is usually indistinct.

The histologic profile of cardiac inflammatory pseudotumor (**Figure 5.29**) is no different than that of the same lesion in other topographic sites, as described in several foregoing chapters of this book. Therefore, its details will not be recounted at this point. The differential diagnosis of IIPT focuses not only on IMT, which is a clonal lesion with potential immunoreactivity for the *ALK*-1 gene product (627,628), but also on *true sarcomas* of the heart such as inflammatory *MFH* (629–632) (**Figure 5.30**). The obvious nuclear atypia that is seen in sarcomas is sufficient unto itself to exclude the possibility of inflammatory pseudotumor.

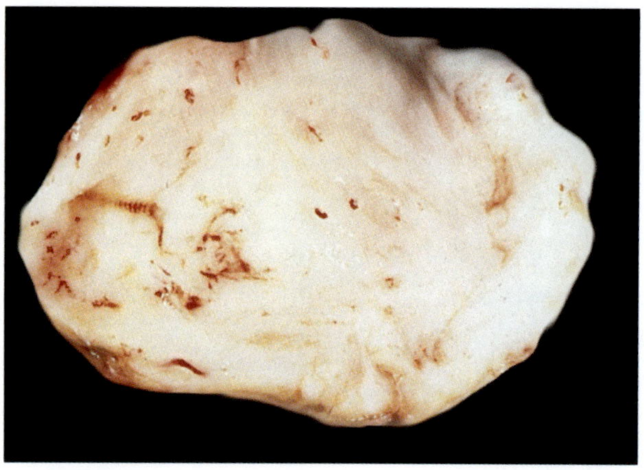

FIGURE 5.28 "True" inflammatory pseudotumors of the heart are fleshy, sessile masses that can be seen in any cardiac chamber.

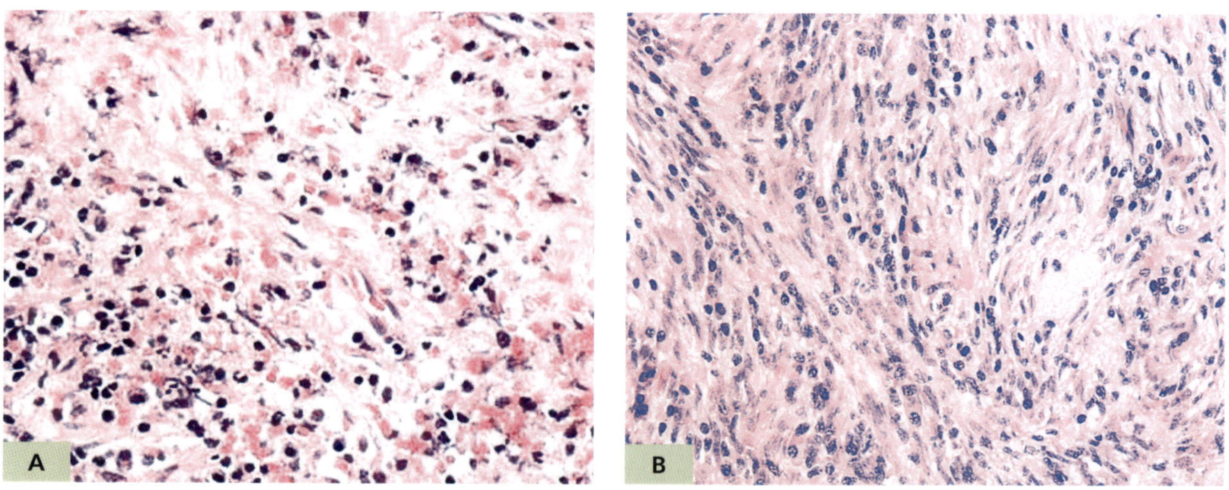

FIGURE 5.29 "True" inflammatory cardiac pseudotumors comprise a mixture of lymphocytes, plasma cells, fibroblasts, and stromal collagen (A & B).

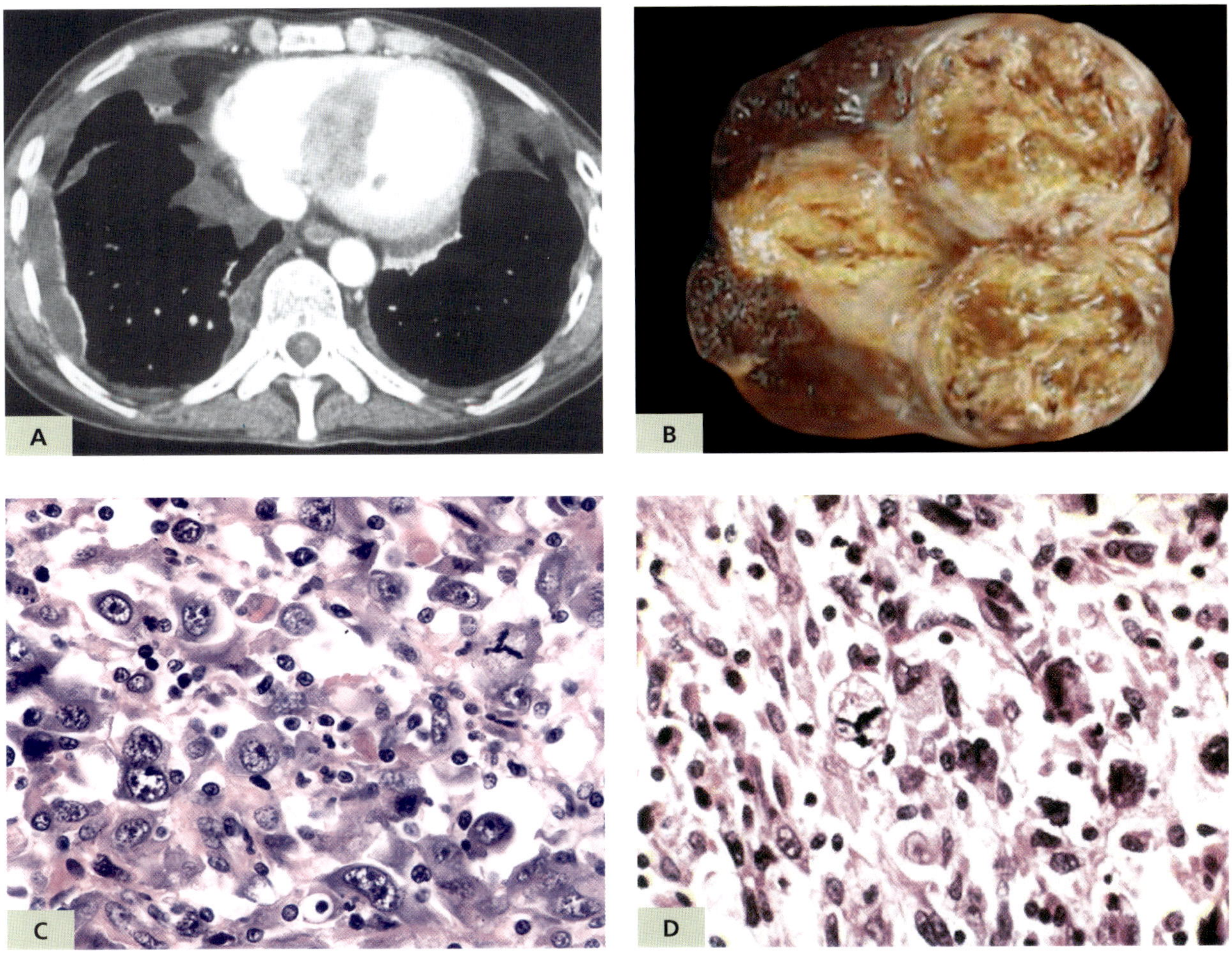

FIGURE 5.30 Inflammatory malignant fibrous histiocytoma. Sarcomas of the heart may demonstrate similarities to inflammatory pseudotumors (IPTs) radiologically (A), but they are more infiltrative than IPTs (B) and show higher levels of cellular pleomorphism and nuclear atypia (C & D).

Examples of IIPT in which an abundance of lymphocytes and plasma cells is seen can be mistaken for lymphoreticular neoplasms such as *dendritic-cell tumors*, *malignant lymphomas*, and *plasmacytoma* (630–633) **(Figure 5.31)**. The attributes of lymphoid lesions will be discussed in the next section of this chapter. With respect to dendritic cell tumors (DCTs)—of which we have seen only one intracardiac case—they have distinctive immunophenotypes that are not shared by IIPTs. Follicular DCT is reactive for CD21 and CD35 **(Figure 5.32)**, whereas interdigitating DCT expresses S100 protein and fascin (630). None of those markers are seen in IIPT.

Another subcategory of IIPT is that which shows marked sclerosis of the stroma and paucicellularity. That image may be confused with either of two true cardiac neoplasms; namely, *sclerotic solitary fibrous tumor* (634) and *calcifying fibrous tumor* (CFT) (635,636) **(Figure 5.33)**. Both of the latter two entities are immunoreactive for CD34, unlike IIPT. In addition, CFT contains psammomatoid microcalcifications (636), which are lacking in inflammatory pseudotumors.

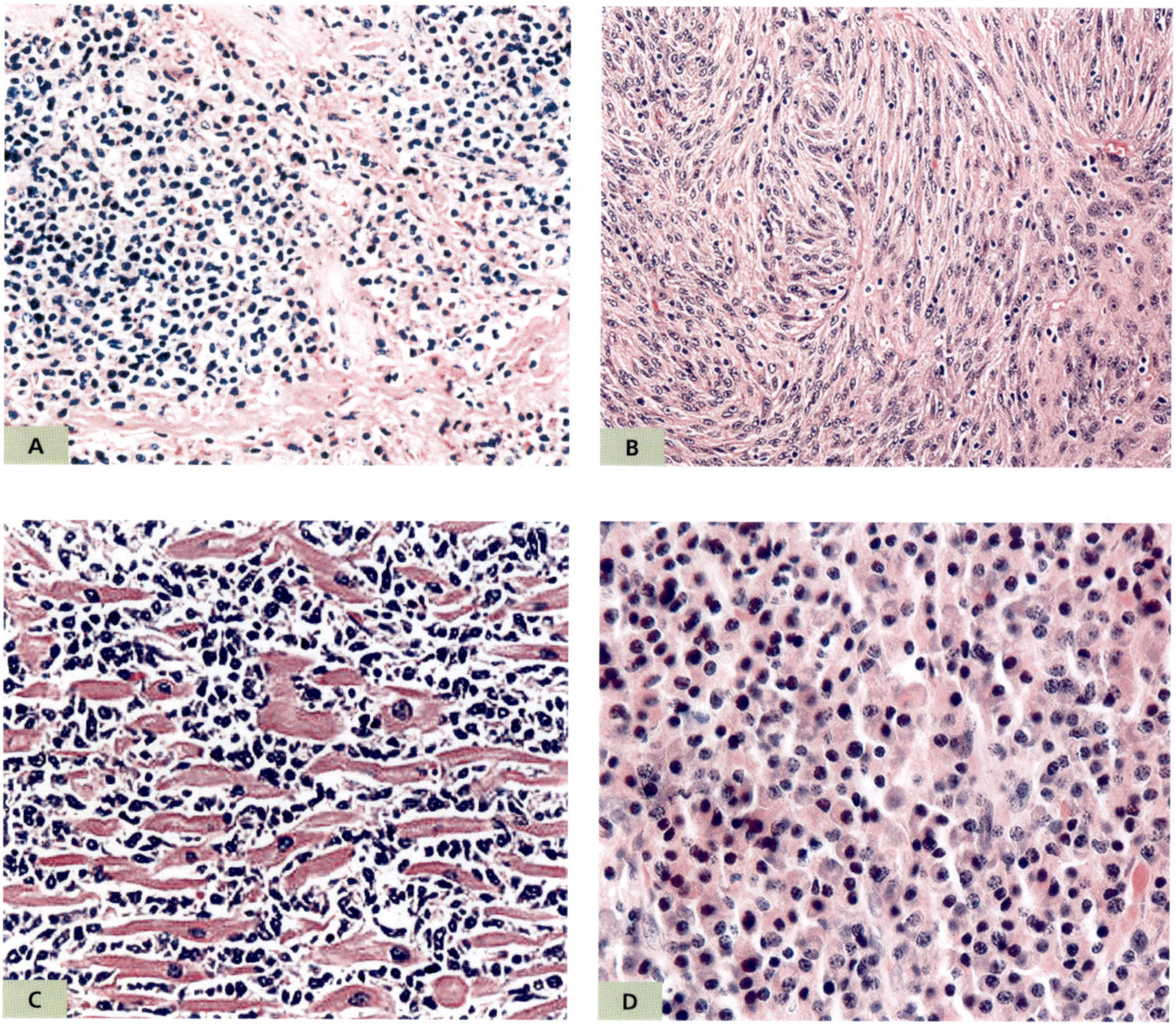

FIGURE 5.31 "True" inflammatory pseudotumors containing abundant inflammatory cells (A) can be confused histologically with dendritic-cell neoplasms (B), non-Hodgkin's lymphomas (C), and plasmacytomas (D) in the heart.

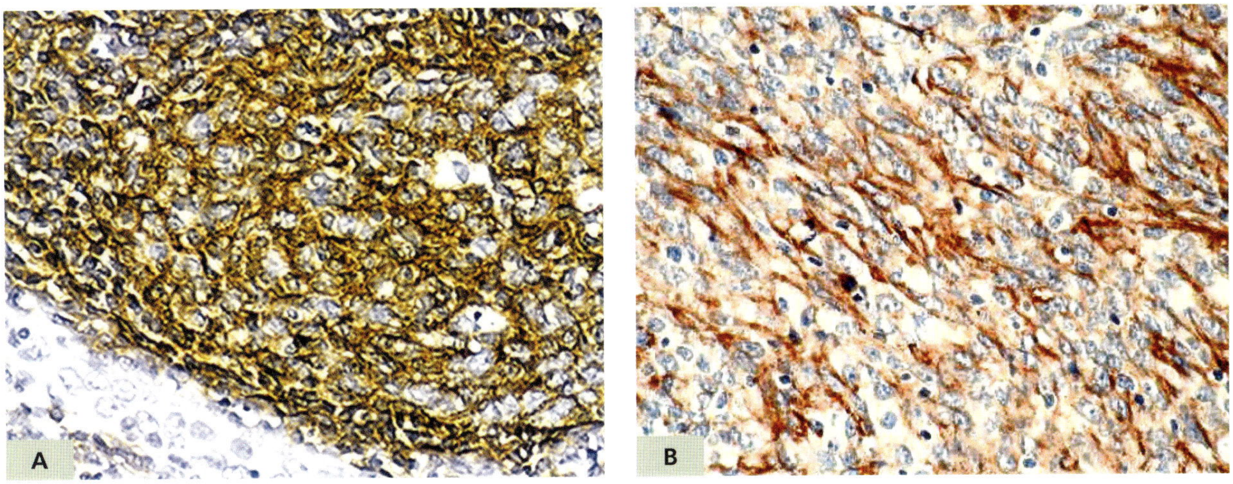

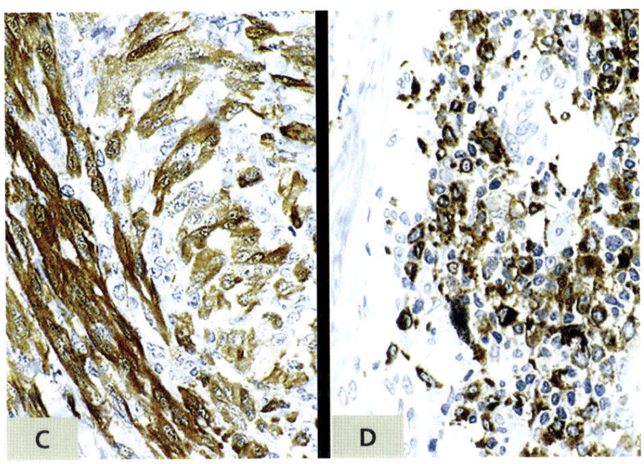

FIGURE 5.32 Follicular dendritic-cell sarcomas of the heart are immunoreactive for CD21 (A), CD35 (B), or both. Interdigitating dendritic-cell sarcomas are labeled for S100 protein (C, left) and fascin (D, right).

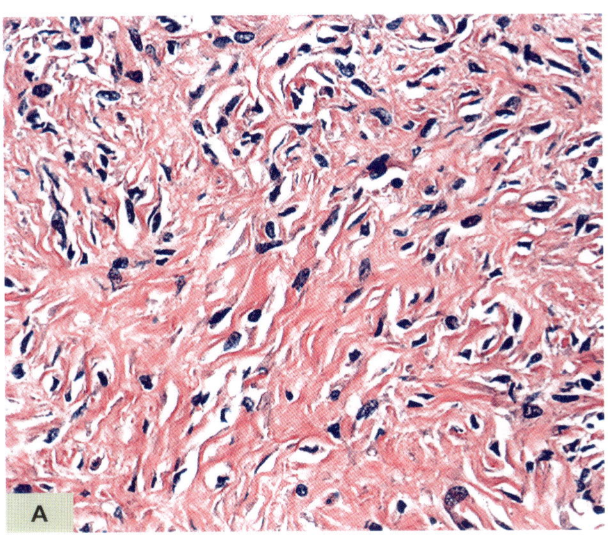

FIGURE 5.33 Sclerotic solitary fibrous tumor (SSFT) (A) may resemble sclerotic inflammatory pseudotumors. *(Continued)*

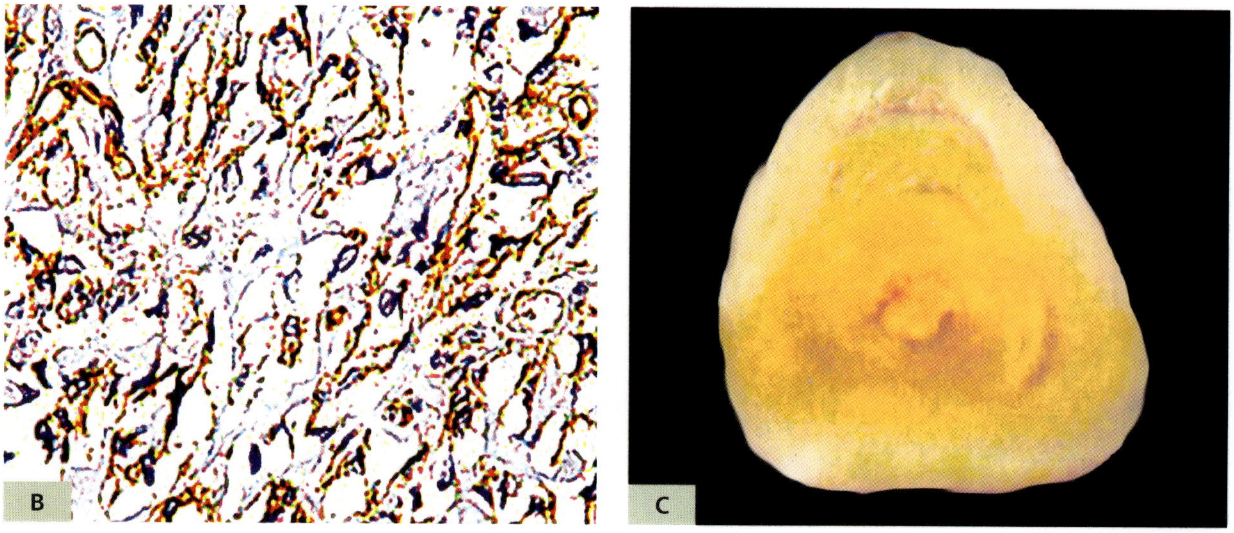

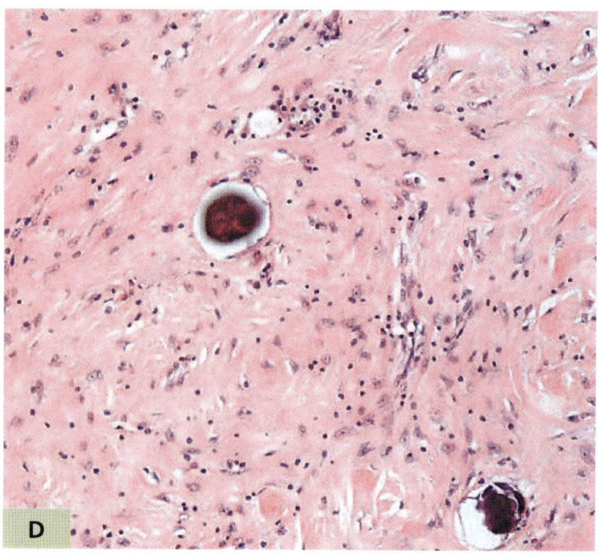

FIGURE 5.33 *(Continued)* However, SSFT is immunoreactive for CD34 (B) and CD99, but pseudotumors are not. Another possibility in differential diagnosis of cardiac pseudotumors is the calcifying fibrous tumor. It is relatively nondescript grossly (C), but microscopically shows the presence of psammomatoid calcifications in a densely fibrous background (D). All of these lesions can be seen in the epicardium.

INTRACARDIAC PAPILLARY ENDOTHELIAL HYPERPLASIA

Masson originally described a peculiar proliferative change in the lumina of hemorrhoids (637), which mimicked the histologic appearance of angiosarcoma. That phenomenon has also been reported in the chambers of the heart (especially the atria), in relation to preexisting mural thrombi (638,639). It is felt to be a consequence of endoluminal reendothelialization and recanalization. The currently preferred designation for this change is that of "papillary endothelial hyperplasia" (PEH) or, more simply, "Masson's lesion" (640,641).

Microscopically, this condition is typified by the formation of racemose channels inside a preformed vascular space, reflecting the recanalization of a fibrinocellular thrombus. The new endoluminal spaces are lined with cytologically bland endothelial cells that often form small papillary structures (641) (**Figure 5.34**). Physiological mitotic figures may be observed. However, there is never any extension of the cellular proliferation into adjacent parenchyma, nor is nuclear atypia present, as expected in true *angiosarcoma* (642) (**Figure 5.35**). The fibrinous nature of the intravascular "struts" in intracardiac PEH can be demonstrated with a Masson trichrome stain or the Mallory–Heidenhain method, both of which label them bright red. In contrast, vascular neoplasms have a variably fibrous stroma that stains blue.

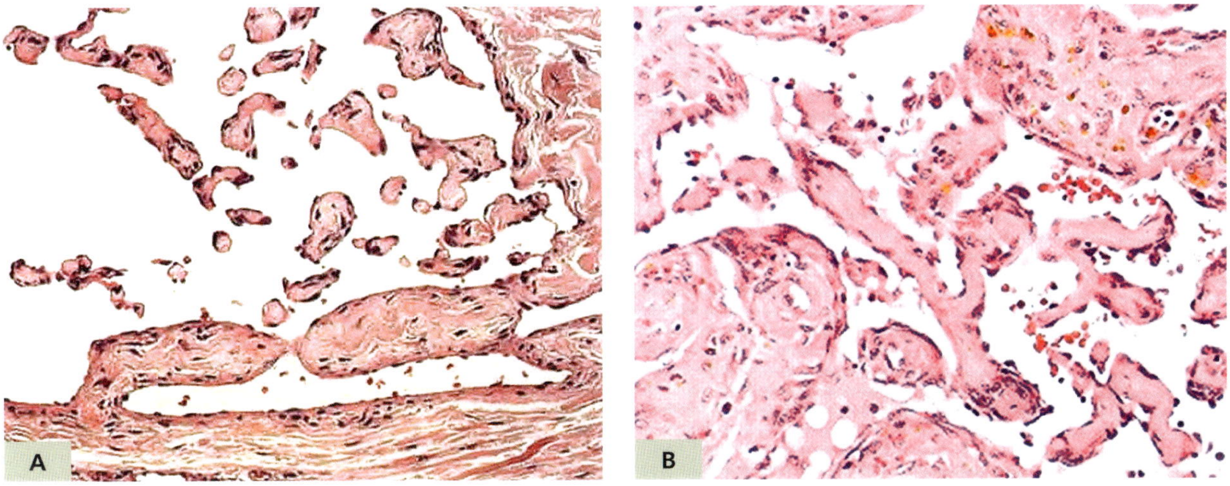

FIGURE 5.34 A & B: Papillary endothelial hyperplasia (PEH) is the result of recanalization of thrombi in the cardiac chambers. Its racemose architecture can imitate the general pattern of angiosarcomas.

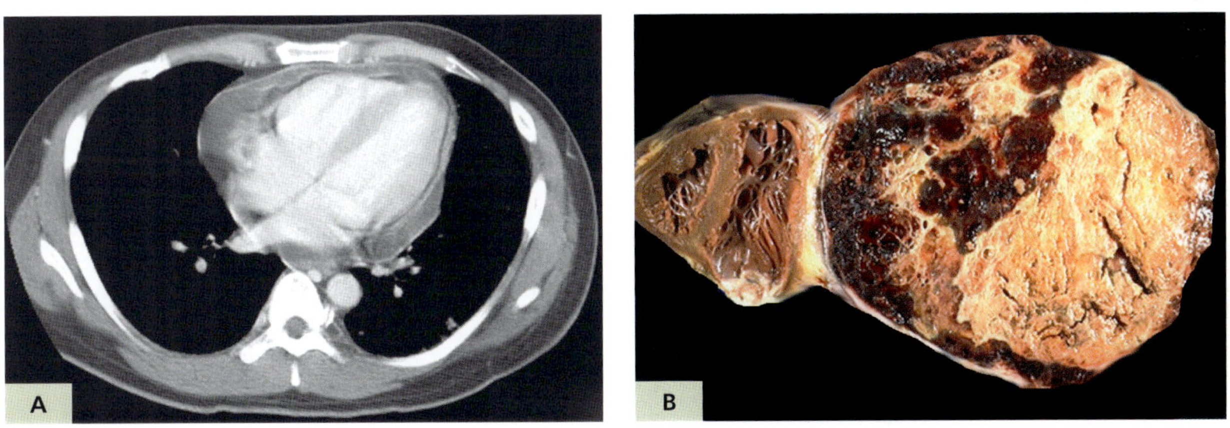

FIGURE 5.35 In contrast to papillary endothelial hyperplasia, true intracardiac angiosarcoma is a destructive mass-forming neoplasm (A & B) *(Continued)*

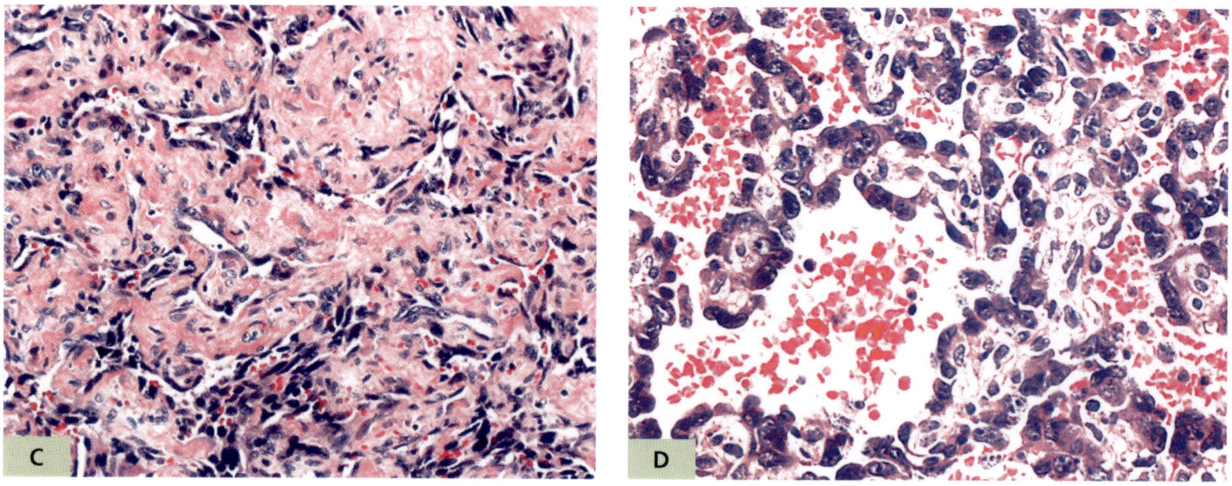

FIGURE 5.35 *(Continued)* with obvious cellular pleomorphism and nuclear atypicality (C & D).

ATYPICAL LYMPHOID INFILTRATES OF THE MYOCARDIUM

There are several conditions wherein lymphoid infiltrates may be seen in the myocardium that simulate the histologic appearance of cardiac lymphoma. In endomyocardial biopsies, these often present diagnostic problems.

SEVERE VIRAL MYOCARDITIS AND CARDIAC ALLOGRAFT REJECTION

Viral myocarditis (principally due to *Coxsackie* viruses, HIV, or Epstein–Barr virus [EBV]) often becomes manifest with rapidly declining cardiac output and cardiomegaly **(Figure 5.36)**, as well as symptoms and signs of congestive heart failure (643–645). Fever and other constitutional symptoms may be evident, and patients of all ages are potentially affected.

Endomyocardial biopsy is often undertaken in such cases to establish a histologic diagnosis, and sometimes to justify immunosuppressive therapy (643–646). Although most problems regarding the histologic diagnosis of myocarditis revolve around its distinction from variants of normal cardiac microstructure (647), some examples of diffuse and severe myocarditis may resemble the image of cardiac involvement by a lymphoproliferative process (648) **(Figure 5.37)**. This is particularly true when the lymphoid cells form partially confluent infiltrates of cytologically atypical, mitotically active, "activated" lymphocytes. By definition, light microscopic muscle-cell damage and necrosis are present in myocarditis, but similar patterns of such myocyte injury can also be associated with hematopoietic malignancies (649–651).

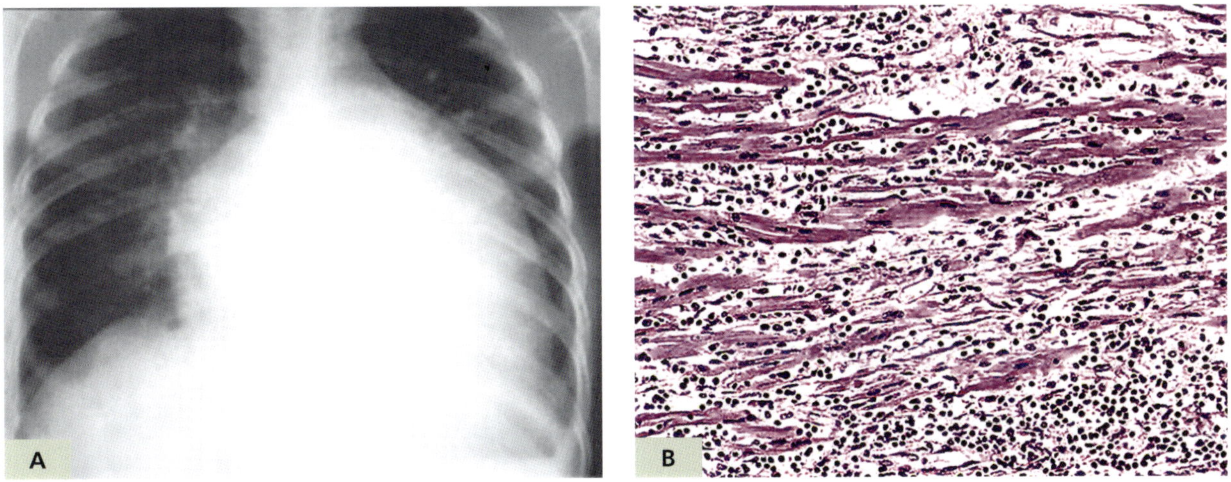

FIGURE 5.36 Severe viral myocarditis commonly causes marked cardiomegaly (A). Myocardial biopsies show a dense infiltrate of lymphocytes that may imitate the histological appearance of a lymphoma or leukemia (B).

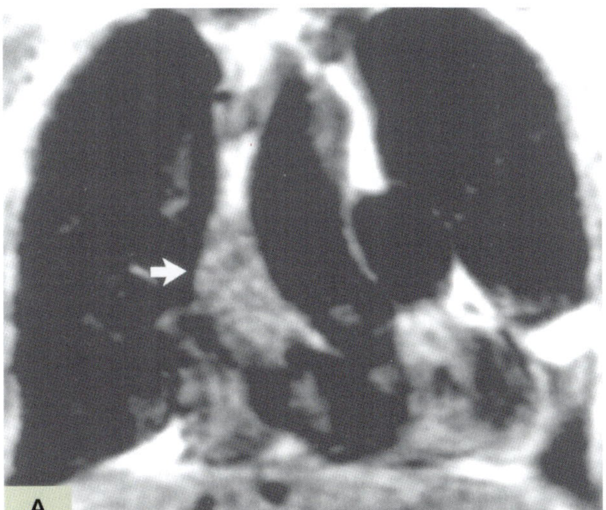

FIGURE 5.37 Intracardiac lymphoma may or may not produce enlargement of the heart (A). It is manifest by multifocal mass-forming infiltrates that may affect any chamber of the heart as well as the epicardium (B–D). *(Continued)*

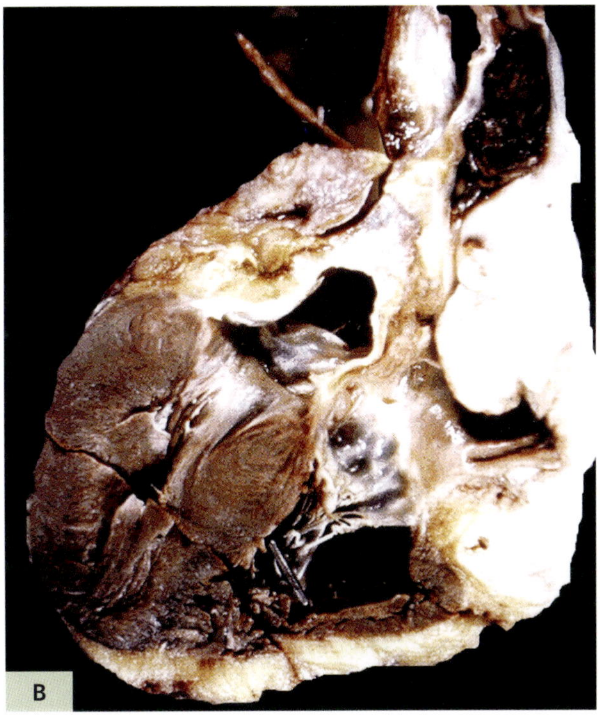

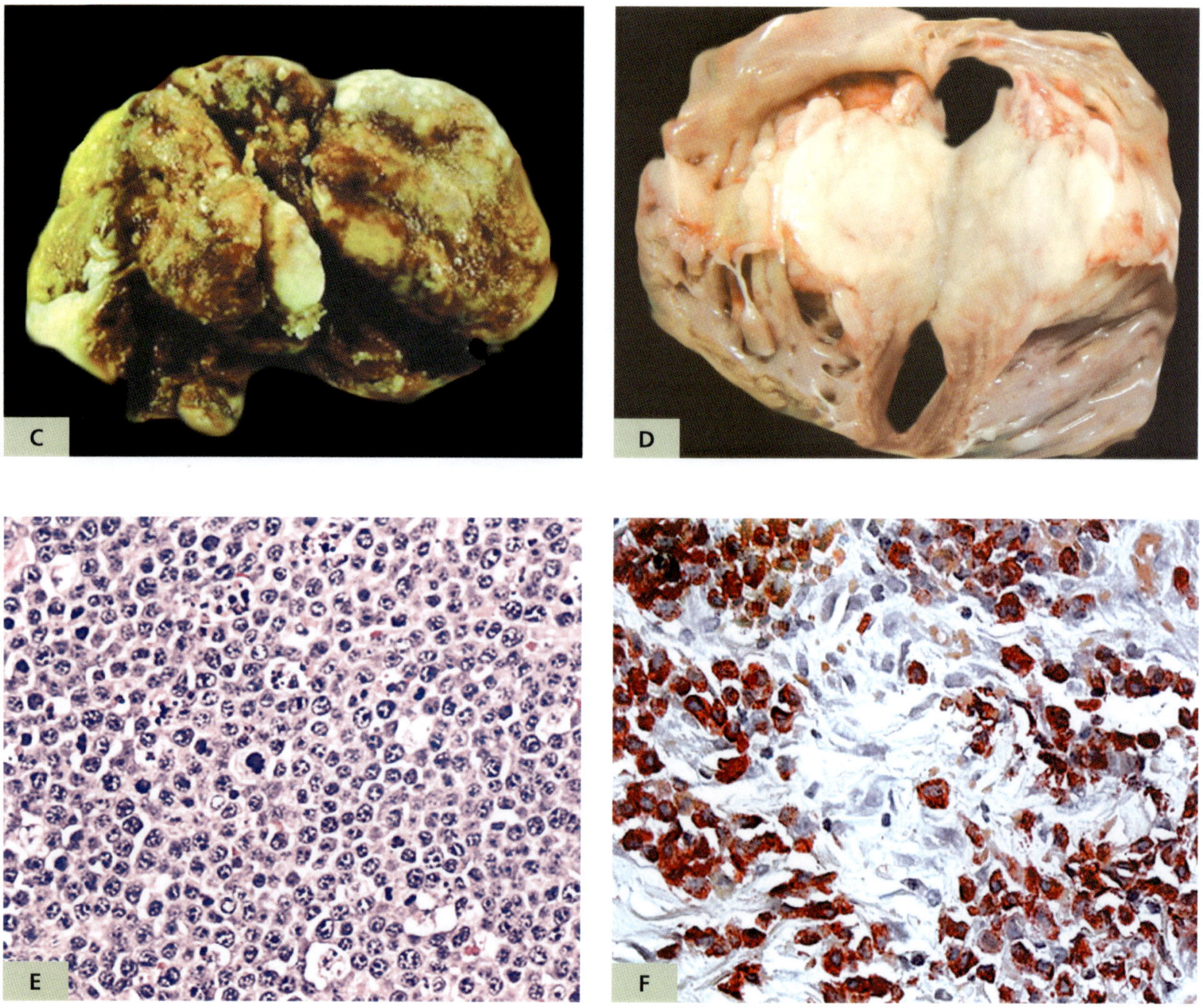

FIGURE 5.37 *(Continued)* The neoplastic cells are usually larger than mature lymphocytes (E), and are immunoreactive for CD45 (F).

A history of previous lymphoma is certainly helpful in suggesting the correct diagnosis, but adjuvant studies may be necessary for definitive pathologic interpretation when the heart is the primary and presenting site of involvement by lymphoid malignancies. The atypical but benign lymphoid infiltrates of "usual" viral myocarditis are composed of T-cells (649), whereas the majority of cardiac lymphomas are B-cell tumors. Those B-lymphocytes that may be apparent in cases of myocarditis are polytypic for light-chain and heavy-chain immunoglobulins by immunohistology or molecular pathologic evaluation (e.g., using the polymerase chain reaction). In cases of suspected leukemic involvement of the myocardium, immunostains for myeloid determinants (e.g., myeloperoxidase, CD34, or CD68) and the chloroacetate esterase (Leder) stain **(Figure 5.38)** may also be helpful diagnostically (648,652). Cardiac involvement by acute lymphoblastic leukemia-lymphoblastic lymphoma is supported by immunoreactivity for CD10, CD99, or terminal deoxynucleotidyl-transferase (TdT) (653), all of which are lacking in the lymphocytes in myocarditides.

Recipients of heterotopic cardiac allografts and patients with the AIDS also can develop B-cell lymphoproliferative lesions of the myocardium that are "driven" by EBV (e.g., posttransplant lymphoproliferative disease—PTLD) (651,654). It can be particularly troublesome to separate histologically dense but polyclonal examples of such disorders from monoclonal neoplastic proliferations; molecular studies designed to assess the presence of episomal viral DNA can be valuable in such instances (654).

In severe allograft rejection, which may feature striking infiltrates of atypical lymphocytes **(Figure 5.39)**, a conjoint lack of immunoreactivity for CD20, CD43, and EBV latent membrane protein has been observed (616). In contrast, histologically similar PTLDs do express those markers reproducibly (655)

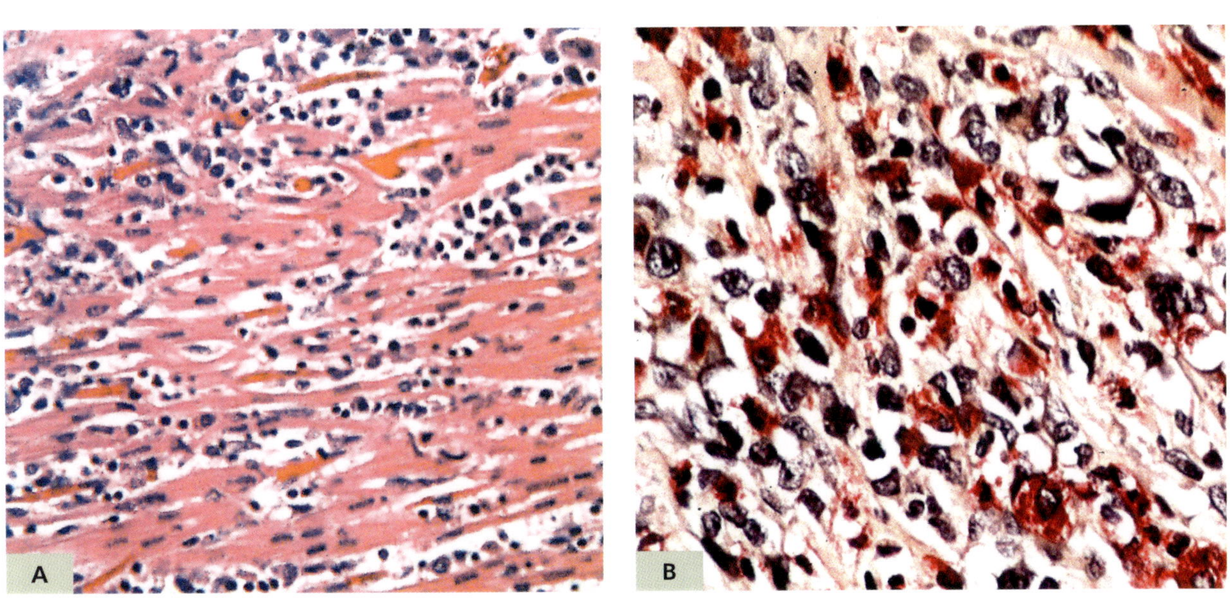

FIGURE 5.38 Another neoplasm that may be simulated by myocarditis is acute myelogenous leukemia (A). The lesional cells can be labeled histochemically for chloroacetate esterase (B) and immunohistologically for other myeloid markers.

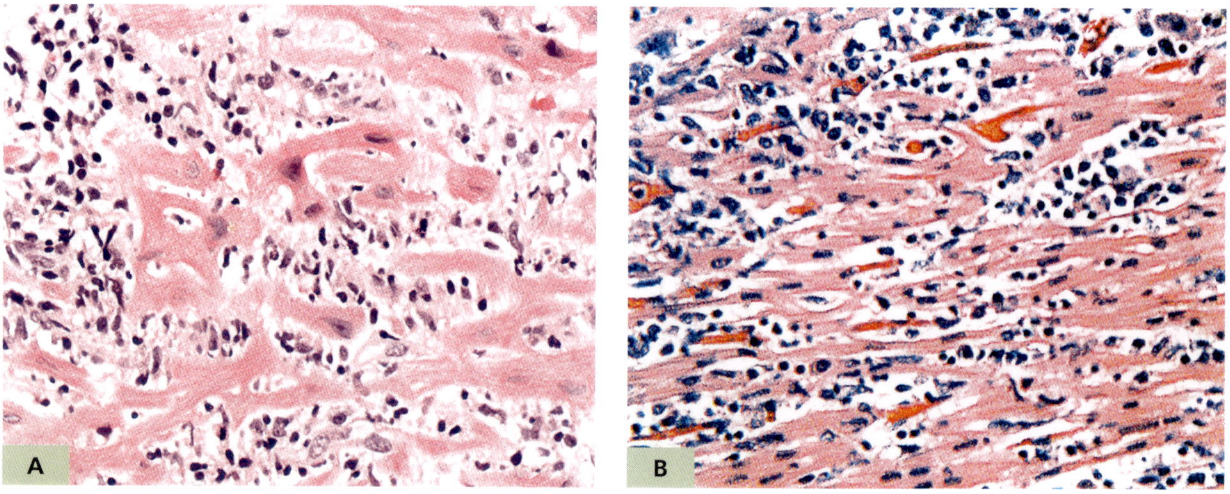

FIGURE 5.39 A & B: In transplanted hearts, severe rejection also has the potential to imitate a hematopoietic neoplasm histologically.

(Figure 5.40). T-cell-predominant and AIDS-related myocarditis can be identified with positive immunostains for CD3, CD5, CD7, CD43, and CD54RO in the lesional lymphocytes, or with HIV-p24 protein in the infiltrating lymphocytes and cardiac interstitial cells (656).

FLORID "QUILTY" LESIONS IN CARDIAC ALLOGRAFTS

Approximately 10% of patients who have undergone cardiac transplantation develop a peculiar and brisk lymphocytic infiltrate in the endocardial surface of the allograft. This phenomenon has been named endocardial lymphocytic infiltrate (ELI) or the "Quilty" lesion, after the first patient who exhibited such a tissue response. It may be so florid that the possibility of PTLD again may enter into differential diagnosis (646,649,657–659) **(Figure 5.41)**. This may be particularly problematic in regard to those Quilty lesions in which significant involvement of the underlying myocardium occurs. ELIs are typically small (1–2 mm) nodular aggregates of lymphocytes (occasionally with small numbers of plasma cells), punctuated by thin-walled dilated blood vessels. However, as just mentioned myocardial extension of the lymphoid cells may be seen in selected instances, and it may be associated with myocyte damage. There is little mitotic activity or apoptosis in the cells of ELIs, and immunoblasts are uncommon in them (649,657). These attributes differ from those of most cases of PTLD, as well as overt cardiac lymphomas.

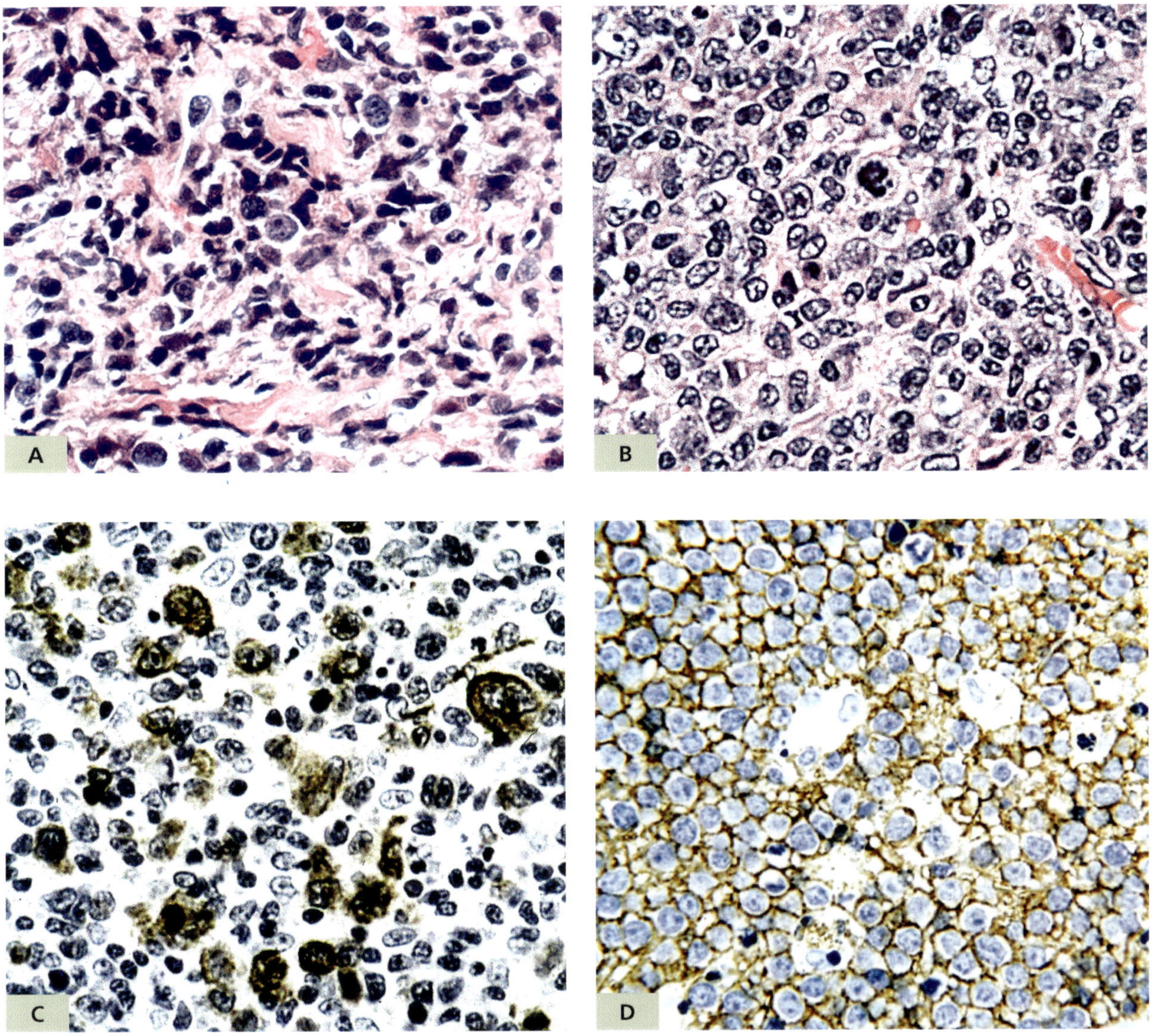

FIGURE 5.40 The principal diagnostic alternative to severe rejection is posttransplant lymphoproliferative disease (PTLD). It comprises variably atypical lymphoid cells that permeate and may efface the myocardium (A & B). Immunostains in PTLD are reactive for CD20 (C) and Epstein–Barr virus-latent membrane protein (D), whereas one sees positivity for CD3 and no viral proteins in the infiltrates of allograft rejection.

Immunohistology may prove useful in differential diagnosis in that it shows a preponderance of T-lymphocytes with only small numbers of B-cells in Quilty lesions (659) **(Figure 5.42)**. As stated above, such observations generally militate strongly against a diagnosis of neoplastic lymphoproliferations in the posttransplant setting. CD21 has also been shown to be expressed in the infiltrates of Quilty lesions and not in foci of cardiac rejection, so this may be another useful marker in some circumstances.

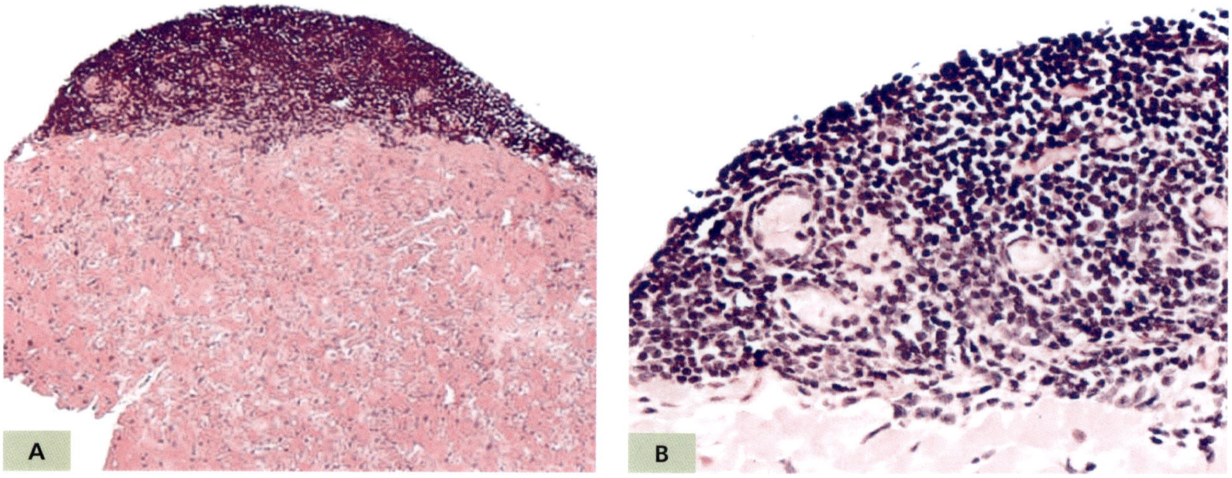

FIGURE 5.41 The Quilty effect is an idiosyncratic accrual of lymphocytes in the endomyocardium in allografted hearts. It may be sufficiently dense to raise the diagnostic possibility of a hematopoietic neoplasm (A & B).

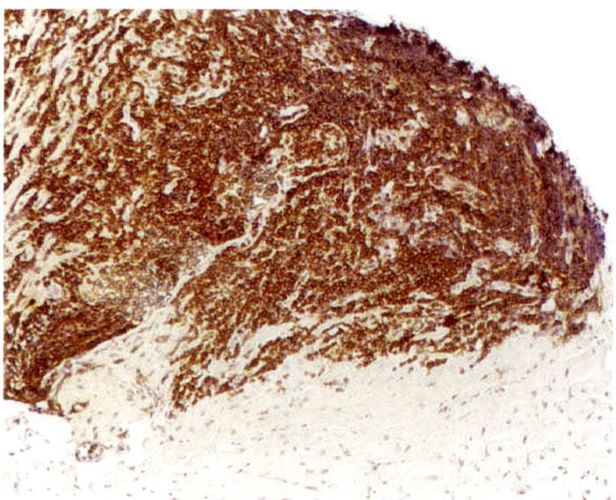

FIGURE 5.42 Whereas lymphomas of the heart are usually B-cell tumors, the Quilty lesion comprises lymphocytes that can be labeled for CD3—shown here—and other pan-T-cell determinants.

ROSAI–DORFMAN DISEASE (SINUS HISTIOCYTOSIS WITH MASSIVE LYMPHADENOPATHY)

A peculiar hematopoietic proliferation that principally affects lymph nodes—namely, sinus histiocytosis with massive lymphadenopathy (SHML; Rosai–Dorfman disease [RDD])—may also rarely involve the heart as a primary lesion (660–662). Despite the name of this condition, lymphadenopathy does not always coexist with extranodal disease. When it affects the myocardium, RDD appears to favor the atrial or ventricular muscle, involving it in a permeative as well as tumefactive fashion (662) (**Figure 5.43**). Complete surgical excision of the lesion is indicated, and cardiac transplantation may be necessary to adequately treat the condition.

Clinical evidence of associated immune dysfunction is often evident in SHML, including autoantibody formation, polyarthritis, immune-complex glomerulonephritis, asthma, and juvenile diabetes mellitus. Fever, night sweats, and weight loss can be present (663). RDD is nonneoplastic in nature, based on molecular data that indicate a polyclonal lymphoreticular composition. A familial form of the disorder has been linked to mutations in the SLC29A3 gene on the long arm of chromosome 10 (664).

Pathologic specimens of intracardiac RDD demonstrate dilated lymphatic spaces in which large pale histiocytes are situated, surrounded by lymphoid infiltrates that are punctuated by germinal centers and fibrous septa. The histiocytes demonstrate a peculiar tendency to engulf mature lymphocytes, a phenomenon known as "lymphemperipolesis" (663) **(Figure 5.44)**. The immunophenotype of the histiocytic elements in RDD is distinctive. It features prominent reactivity for S100 protein **(Figure 5.45)** and CD45 in the absence of CD1a. Labeling for CD68, lysozyme, MAC387, and alpha-1-antichymotrypsin may also be observed (665).

Differential diagnoses in cases of SHML potentially include *metastatic carcinoma*, *metastatic melanoma*, *Erdheim–Chester disease*, *large cell lymphoma*, and *Hodgkin disease* (663,665). The large tumor cells in the non-histiocytic conditions in that list differ from those in RDD immunohistologically, by their reactivity for keratin (in carcinoma); MART-1, PNL2, or tyrosinase (in melanoma) **(Figure 5.46)**; CD3 or CD20 (in non-Hodgkin's lymphomas); and

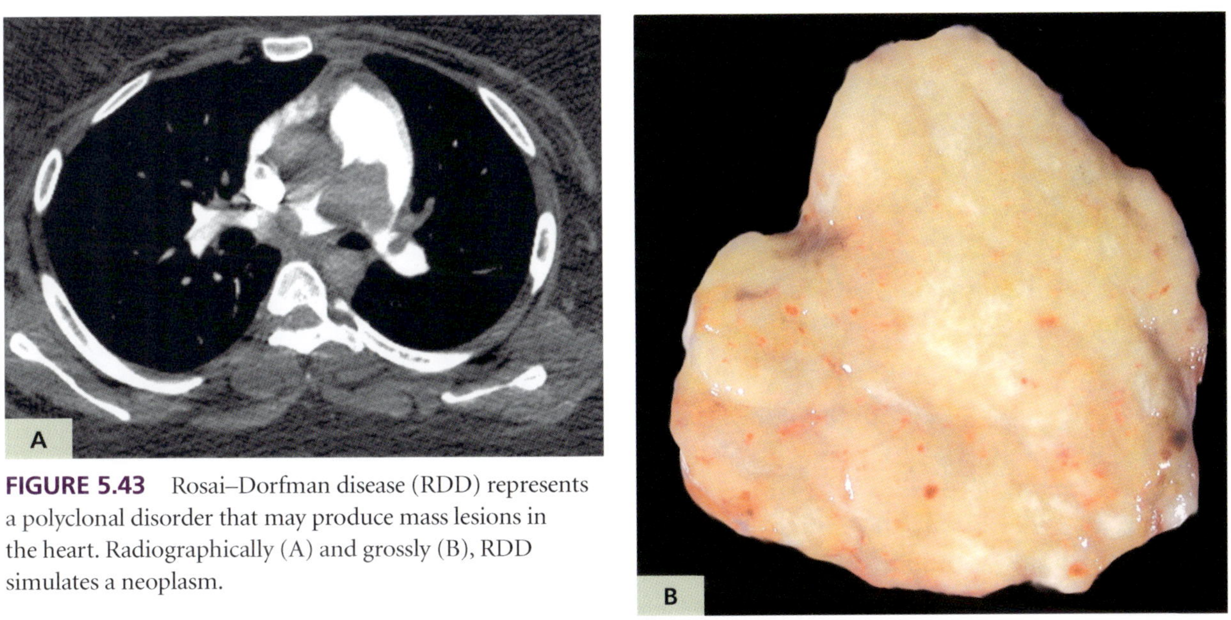

FIGURE 5.43 Rosai–Dorfman disease (RDD) represents a polyclonal disorder that may produce mass lesions in the heart. Radiographically (A) and grossly (B), RDD simulates a neoplasm.

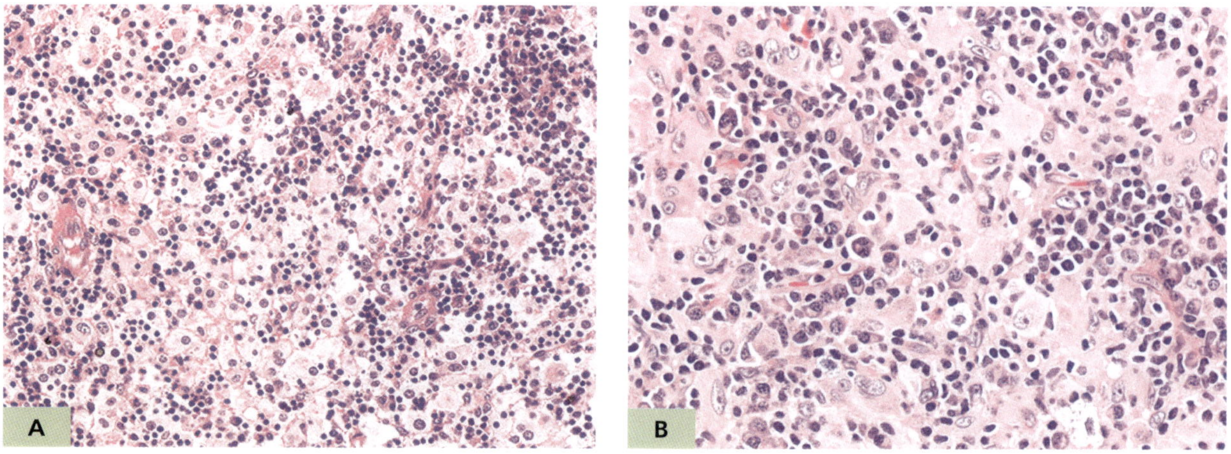

FIGURE 5.44 Cardiac Rosai–Dorfman disease (RDD) is constituted by a dense admixture of large histiocytes and lymphocytes (A). Intact intrahistiocytic lymphoid cells are commonly present (B), reflecting a phenomenon known as lymphemperipolesis.

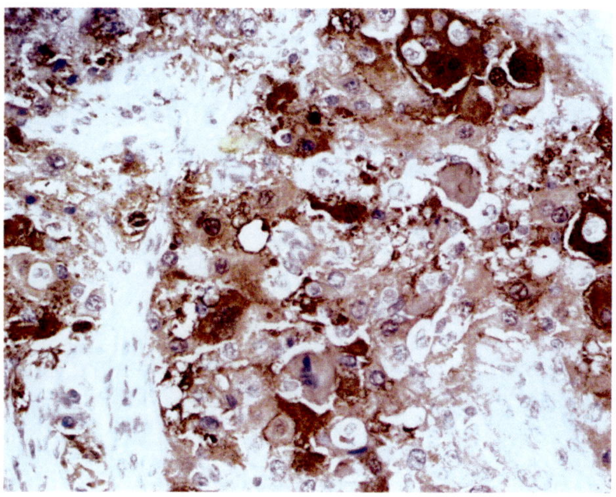

FIGURE 5.45 Rosai–Dorfman disease demonstrates consistent immunoreactivity for S100 protein in the lesional histiocytes. They are also positive for CD68 and CD163, but nonreactive for epithelial, melanocytic, and lymphocytic markers.

CD30 (in Hodgkin's lymphomas). Practically speaking, with the exception of Erdheim–Chester disease (666)—which is another nonneoplastic disorder comprising bland histiocytes—all of the other conditions also show much more cytologic atypicality than that seen in SHML. The histiocytes of Erdheim–Chester disease may also express s-100 protein, but in addition may express Factor XIIIa, generally not expressed on the histiocytes of SHML.

The clinical course of RDD is unpredictable. It has been noted that patients with more than one site of extranodal disease and obvious immune dysfunction often have significant morbidity and possible mortality from this condition (663). Treatment is individualized, with antineoplastic chemotherapy being used for those patients with serious organ dysfunction and unresectable masses.

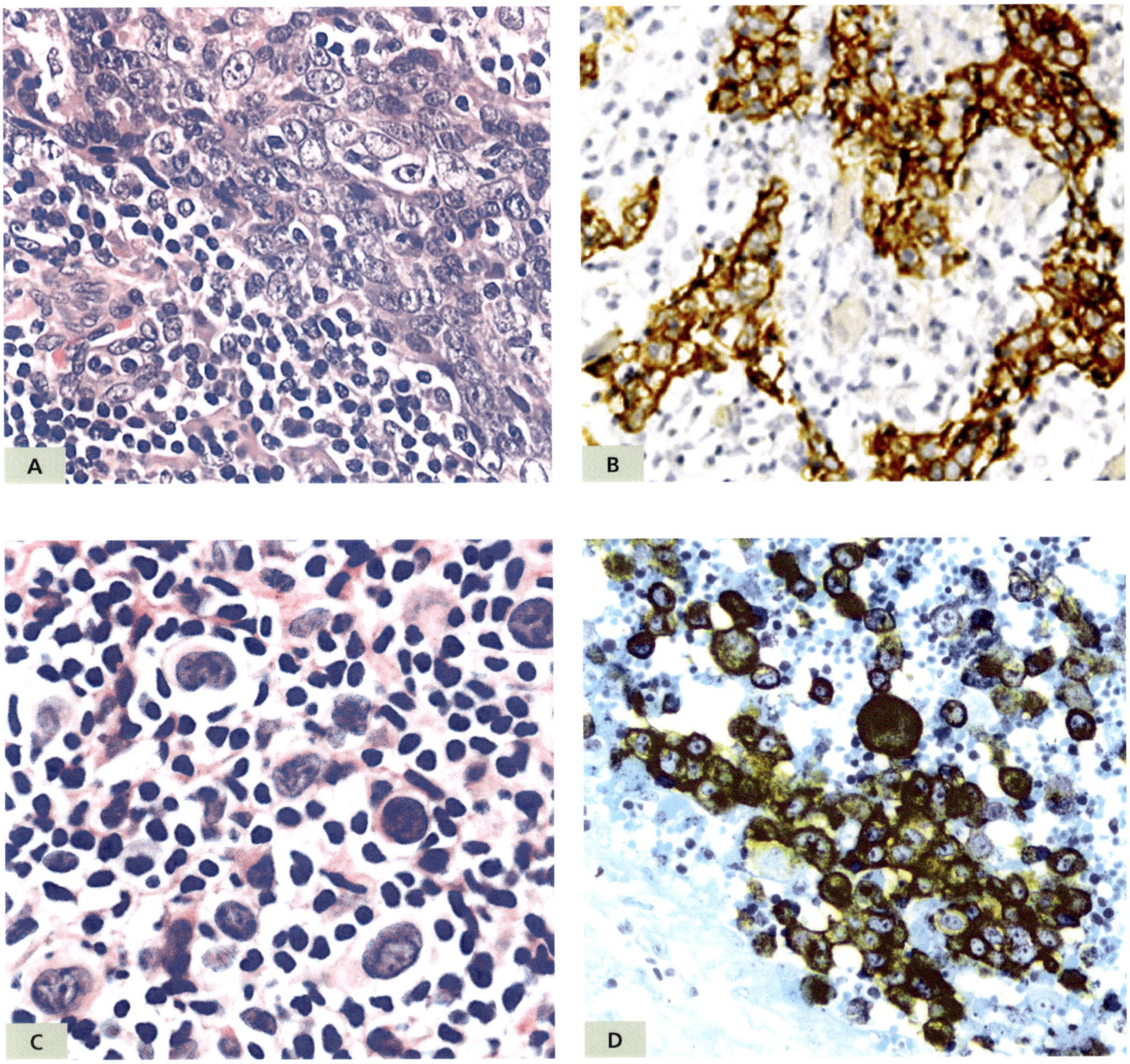

FIGURE 5.46 Differential diagnostic considerations in cases of cardiac Rosai–Dorfman disease include metastatic lymphoepithelioma-like carcinomas (A; stained for pankeratin, B); metastatic lymphocyte-rich melanoma (C; stained for tyrosinase, D); *(Continued)*

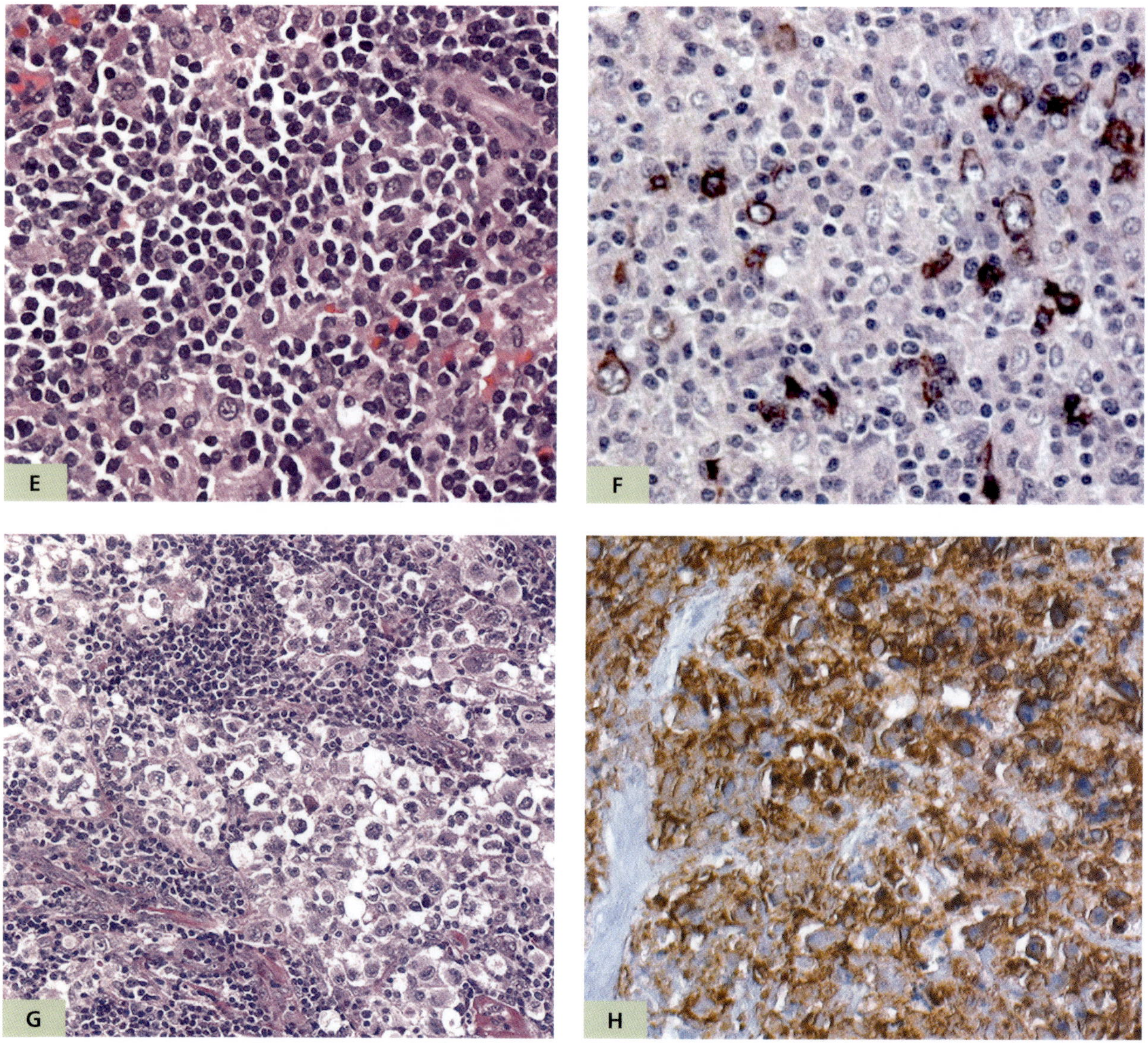

FIGURE 5.46 *(Continued)* T-cell-rich B-cell lymphoma (E; stained for CD20, F); and syncytial Hodgkin's lymphoma (G; stained for CD30, H).

INTRACARDIAC CASTLEMAN'S DISEASE

Castleman's disease (CaD) has only exceptionally been reported as an intracardiac lesion, where it favors the myocardium adjacent to the large coronary arteries (667,668). Two clinical forms of CaD are recognized—solitary and multicentric (669). The first variant is represented by a single mass that is typically asymptomatic. However, secondary symptoms and signs of coronary ischemia may be seen in reference to its presence in the heart. Multicentric CaD manifests itself with widespread lymphadenopathy, and hepatosplenomegaly can also be present. "B" symptoms such as fatigue, night sweats, fever, and anorexia are common in multicentric CaD (670). Despite these clinicopathologic similarities to malignant lymphomas, both types of CaD are constitutively polyclonal (671).

The histopathologic image of solitary CaD features the presence of germinal center-like structures with hyalinized vascular cores; these follicular units are surrounded by concentric arrays of lymphocytes, and plasma cells are relatively inapparent **(Figure 5.47)**. Capillary proliferation is evident in the tissue between the germinal centers, yielding the designation of "hyaline-vascular" CaD (669). Multicentric CaD shows more numerous hyperplastic lymphoid follicles with larger mantle zones, as compared with the hyaline vascular form. Confluent plasma cell infiltrates also are present in interfollicular areas of the lesion **(Figure 5.48)**, accounting for the term "plasmacellular CaD." Solitary CaD is causally idiopathic, but multicentric CaD is often associated with infection by human herpesviruses 6 and 8, with or without coinfection by HIV (672).

Localized-solitary CaD is cured by surgical excision in most anatomic sites. Nevertheless, in the heart it may occupy such a large volume of myocardium that complete resection is impossible (668). Cardiac transplantation may be needed in that circumstance.

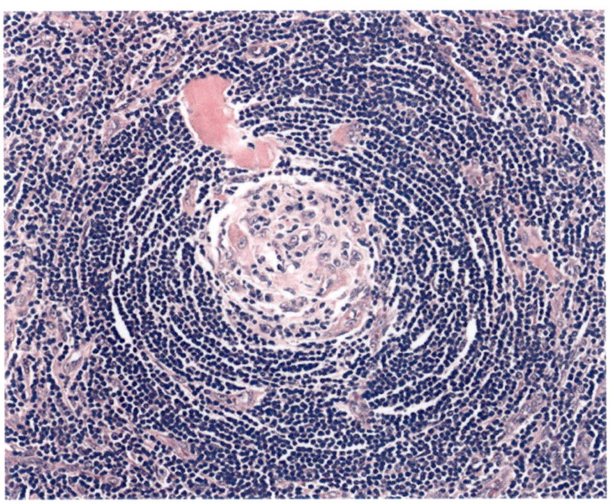

FIGURE 5.47 Angiofollicular lymphoid hyperplasia—also known as hyaline-vascular-type Castleman's disease—manifests caricatures of lymphoid germinal centers. These contain a hyalinized eosinophilic vascular core, and a concentrically arranged mantle of mature lymphocytes.

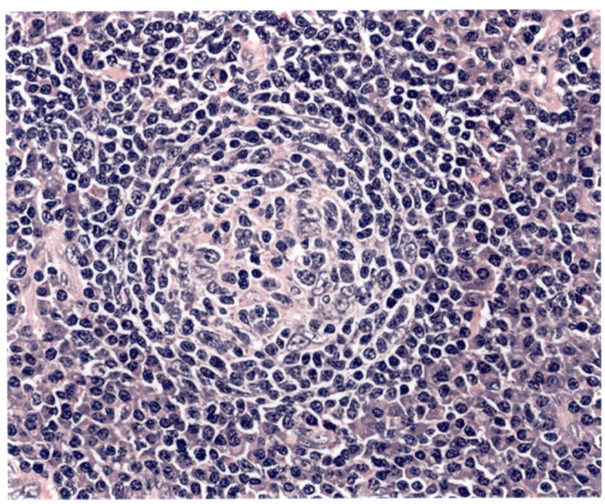

FIGURE 5.48 Another form of Castleman's disease (CaD) is the plasma-cell variant. It lacks the hyalinized vessels and stroma of hyaline-vascular CaD, is dominated by interfollicular plasma cell infiltrates, and has a tendency to be multifocal. Hence, it may in part simulate the appearance of marginal zone lymphoma or plasmacytoma.

Multicentric CaD can persist in several organ sites for a prolonged period of time and ultimately require antineoplastic treatment for adequate control. It also can be associated with Kaposi's sarcoma and the "POEMS" syndrome (polyneuropathy; organomegaly; endocrine dysfunction; monoclonal protein in serum or urine; and skin lesions [glomeruloid hemangiomas]) (670).

The differential diagnosis of cardiac CaD centers on exclusion of *follicular non-Hodgkin's lymphoma*. The latter possibility lacks the hyaline-vascular cores and plasma-cell infiltrates of CaD; it also shows diffuse immunoreactivity for bcl-6 protein **(Figure 5.49)** and CD10 in constituent lymphocytes, unlike the cell population of CaD (673).

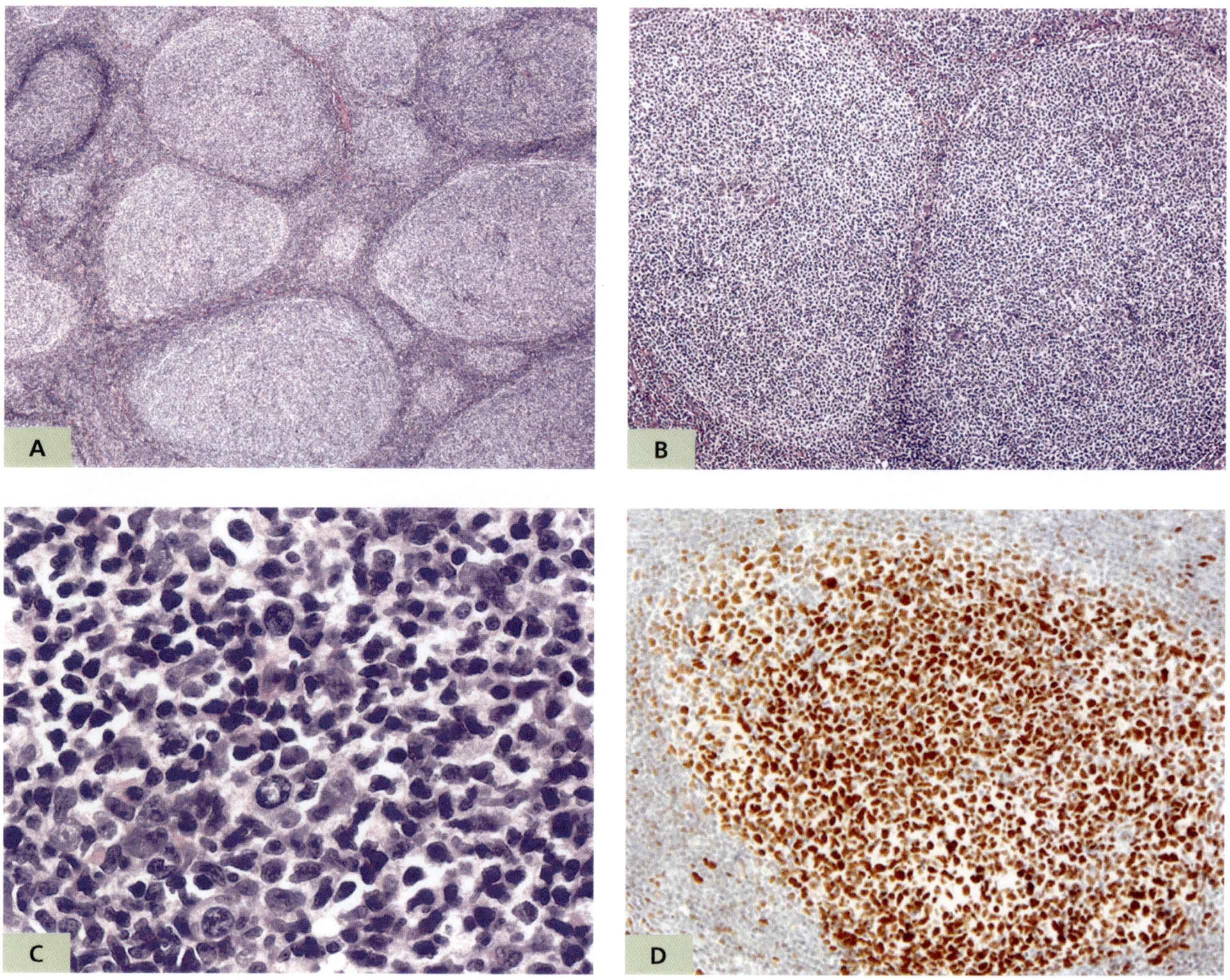

FIGURE 5.49 Follicular lymphoma (FL), with which Castleman's disease (CaD) can be confused, comprises congeries of abnormal lymphoid follicles without vascular cores (A & B), and has a constituent population of atypical lymphocytes with cleaved nuclear membranes (C). FL is immunoreactive for bcl-6 (D), as well as CD10 and bcl-2. Those features are not shared by CaD.

TUMEFACTIVE EXTRAMEDULLARY HEMATOPOIESIS IN THE MYOCARDIUM

In patients who have preexisting disorders of myelopoiesis—such as idiopathic myelofibrosis, chronic leukemias, constitutive hemoglobinopathies, severe hemolytic anemias, or Gaucher's disease—myeloid tissue that has been nascent since infancy can potentially reappear in extramedullary sites, including the heart (674). If the proliferation of such elements is sufficiently robust, it may produce discrete masses that imitate neoplasms macroscopically.

Fine-needle aspiration or needle biopsies of extramedullary hematopoiesis (EMH) demonstrate a variable mixture of erythroblasts, myeloid precursors, and megakaryocytes. These cell lines are usually recognizable as such by conventional morphological study (**Figure 5.50**); however, should confirmation of their identity be desired, the Leder (chloroacetate esterase) stain and immunostains for glycophorin-A, neutrophil elastase, myeloperoxidase, factor VIII-related antigen, and CD61 can be used (675).

In the myocardium, EMH has usually been observed as an incidental finding in or around healed myocardial infarcts (676,677). Goldman and Wurzel postulated that this may be true because of altered and prohematopoietic intramyocardial cytokine synthesis in dysfunctional cardiac tissue (676). Mass lesions represented by EMH have only been reported in the context of chronic myeloid leukemia (674).

Occasionally, infiltrates of EMH may be dominated by one of the three hematopoietic cell lines. In that eventuality, a resemblance to *granulocytic sarcoma* (tumefactive acute myelogenous leukemia) (675) (**Figure 5.51**) or *non-Hodgkin's lymphoma* (678–684) may be encountered. The latter condition is rather easily eliminated from consideration by immunostains for B- and T-cell markers as well as CD30 (675), all of which are absent in EMH. On the other hand, studies for cellular clonality may be necessary to separate granulocytic sarcoma from "lineage-imbalanced" EMH (**Figure 5.52**).

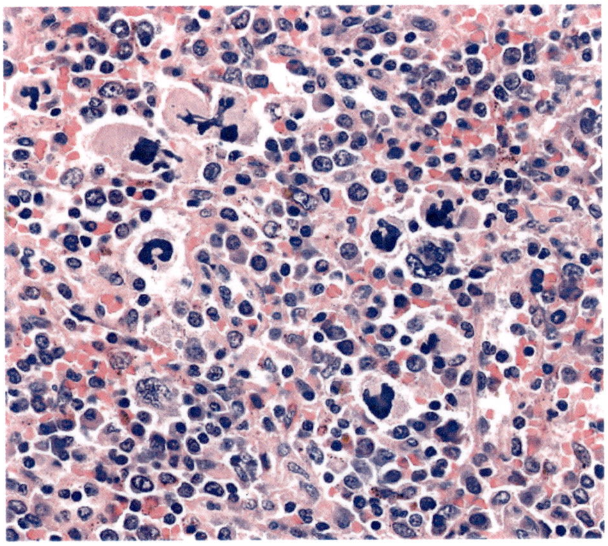

FIGURE 5.50 Extramedullary hematopoiesis can be observed as a diffuse infiltrate in the myocardium or as a tumefactive mass therein. It comprises cells with erythroid, myeloid, and megakaryocytic lineages, and typically develops in patients with disordered and insufficient hematopoiesis in the bone marrow.

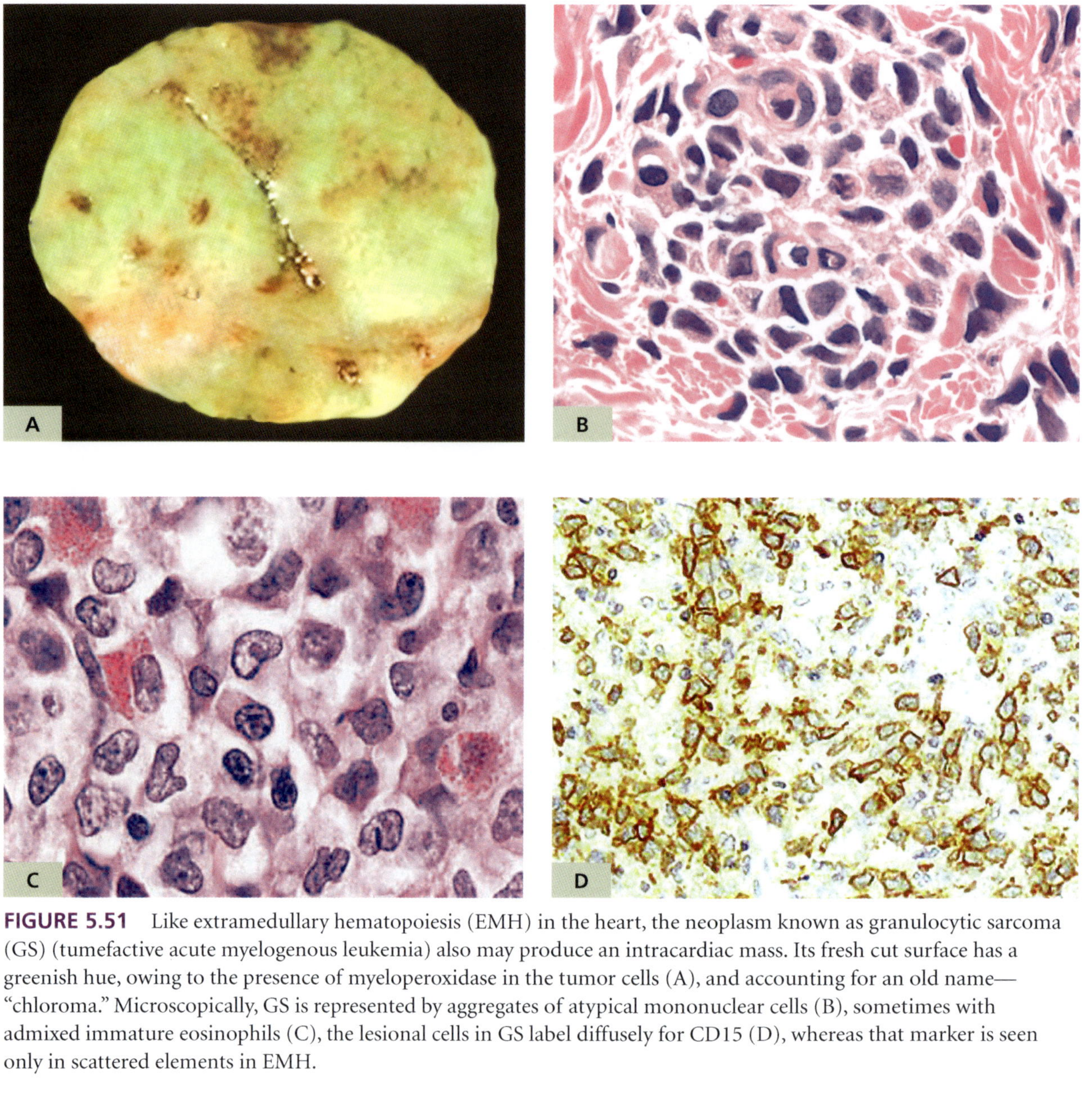

FIGURE 5.51 Like extramedullary hematopoiesis (EMH) in the heart, the neoplasm known as granulocytic sarcoma (GS) (tumefactive acute myelogenous leukemia) also may produce an intracardiac mass. Its fresh cut surface has a greenish hue, owing to the presence of myeloperoxidase in the tumor cells (A), and accounting for an old name—"chloroma." Microscopically, GS is represented by aggregates of atypical mononuclear cells (B), sometimes with admixed immature eosinophils (C), the lesional cells in GS label diffusely for CD15 (D), whereas that marker is seen only in scattered elements in EMH.

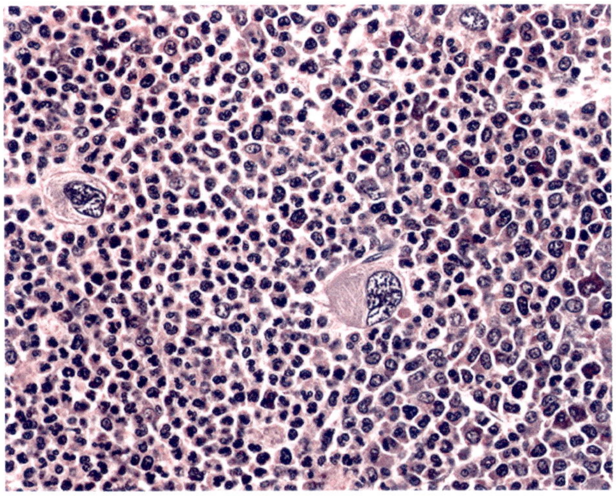

FIGURE 5.52 "Lineage-imbalanced" extramedullary hematopoiesis, which is dominated by one bone marrow lineage, as shown here, is particularly likely to be mistaken for granulocytic sarcoma.

6 Pseudoneoplastic Pericardial Lesions

- PERICARDIAL MESOTHELIAL HYPERPLASIA
- ATYPICAL VIRAL PERICARDITIS
- ORGANIZING AND VASCULARIZING SUBACUTE PERICARDITIS
- CONSTRICTIVE (FIBROSING) PERICARDITIS
- PSEUDOTUMORAL PERICARDIAL FAT PADS
- OTHER NEOPLASTIC MIMICS IN THE PERICARDIUM

PERICARDIAL MESOTHELIAL HYPERPLASIA

In likeness to reactions in other serosal surfaces, nonspecific or infectious pericarditis may incite florid mesothelial hyperplasia in association with a pericardial effusion (685). Focal lesions are typically inapparent on gross inspection of the external cardiac surface, but occasional examples of visible nodular hyperplasia have indeed been documented (686–688). In fact, rare examples may simulate the macroscopic appearance of *malignant mesothelioma* (689–694) because the inflammatory response in the pericardium creates a dense fibrofibrinous rind that involves both the visceral and parietal layers.

At a microscopic level, the distinction between reactive pericardial mesothelial hyperplasia and mesothelioma can also be challenging. Reactive benign mesothelial cells may acquire a striking degree of nuclear atypia **(Figure 6.1)**, with prominent nucleoli and nuclear pleomorphism. Moreover, the presence of nested entrapped mesothelial cells within a thickened pericardium may also simulate invasion (688).

In cytologic preparations, where one does not have the benefit of architectural landmarks, interpretation must rely on strict cytologic criteria for the separation of benign and malignant mesothelial proliferations (689,695,696). Numerous mitotic figures—especially if some are atypical—and any appreciable spindle cell growth favor the diagnosis of mesothelioma. Because one is dealing with mesothelial cells in each of the pathologic processes being considered, histochemical and immunohistochemical stains have little differential diagnostic

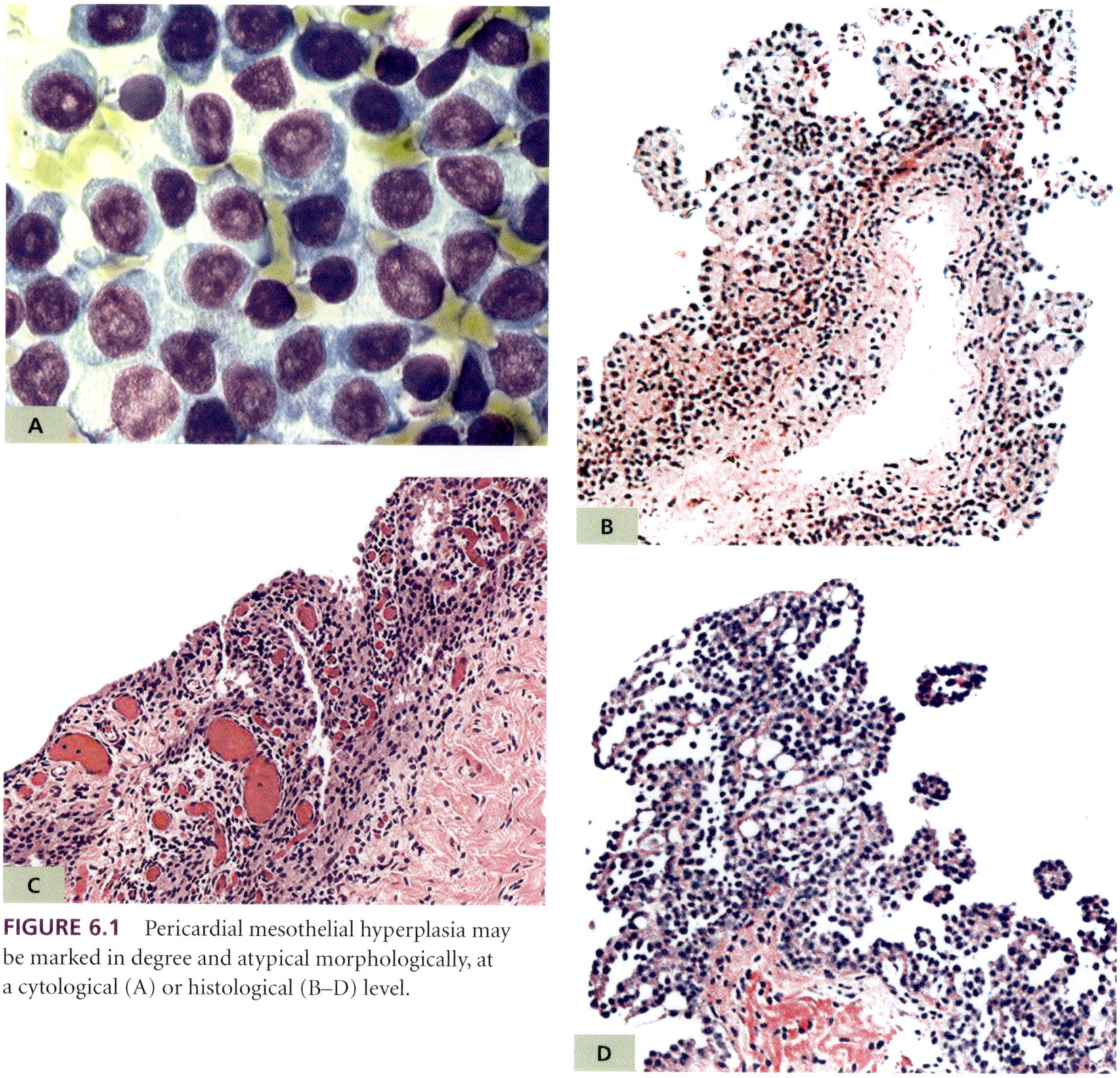

FIGURE 6.1 Pericardial mesothelial hyperplasia may be marked in degree and atypical morphologically, at a cytological (A) or histological (B–D) level.

value, in our opinion. Some authors have suggested that adenocarcinoma and mesothelioma cells express EMA strongly, with the latter showing a "tram-track" pattern of immunoreactivity, whereas reactive mesothelial cells are EMA-negative or only weakly positive (697). Mutant p53 protein has also been used to assist in this distinction, with p53 immunopositivity **(Figure 6.2)** putatively being present in malignant mesotheliomas and absent in reactive processes (698). However, our experience has shown that the stated dichotomy is not absolute, by any means, and we would not recommend sole diagnostic reliance on immunohistologic results in this context.

The clinical history is particularly important to the interpretation of pericardial specimens. Patients may have had idiopathic recurrent benign pericardial effusions for many years, or, conversely, they may have developed recalcitrant effusions only in the very recent past (696,699). Obviously, the first of those scenarios would suggest a benign process, whereas the second is most consonant with a malignancy. Positive immunostains for carcinoembryonic antigen (CEA) (**Figure 6.3**), MOC31, and the CA72.4 antigen

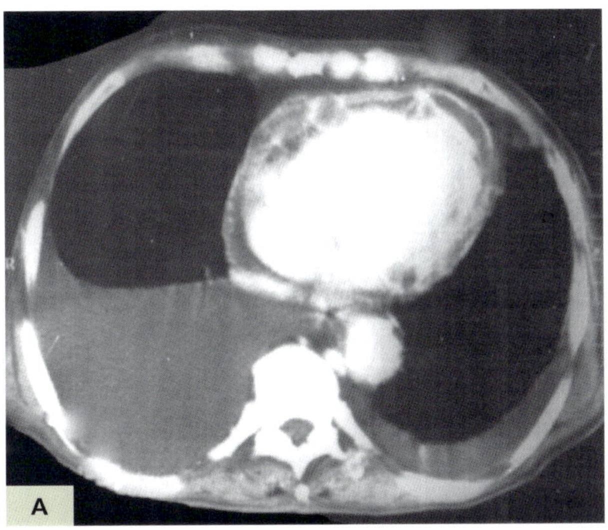

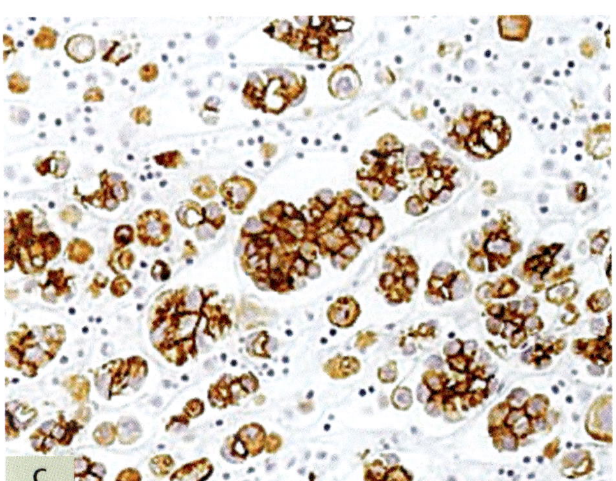

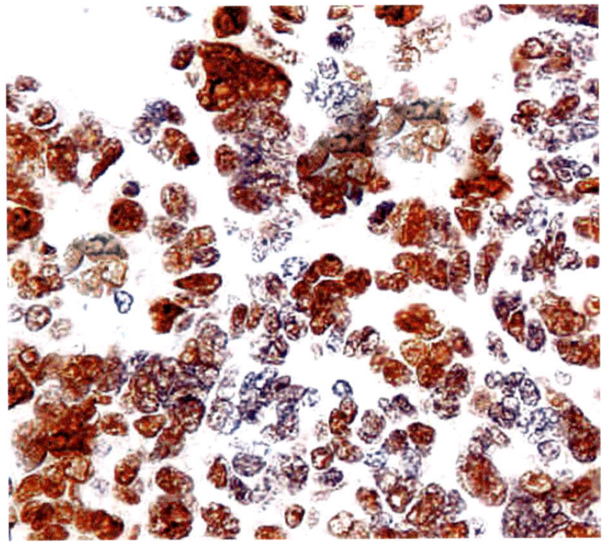

FIGURE 6.2 Immunoreactivity for mutant p53 protein—shown here—has been touted as a discriminant between benign and malignant mesothelial proliferations in the pericardium and elsewhere. However, the authors suggest the use of caution regarding that point.

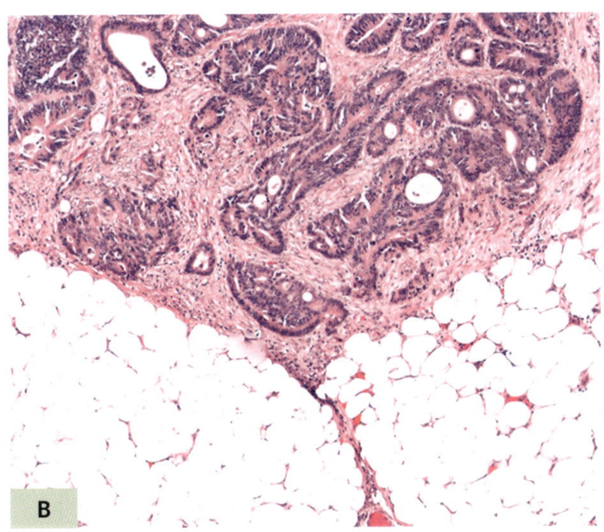

FIGURE 6.3 Metastatic adenocarcinoma (MAC) in the pericardium (A [additionally showing a right pleural effusion] & B) may also be simulated pathologically by florid benign mesothelial proliferations. Immunohistological evaluation of MAC in cytological preparations or in tissue sections demonstrates the presence of glandular epithelial markers such as MOC-31 (C). (*Continued*)

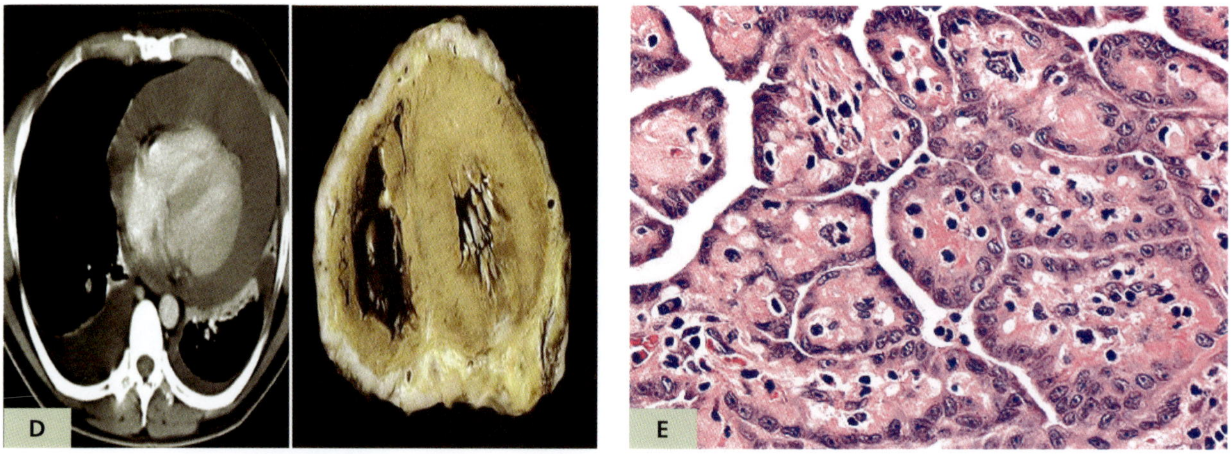

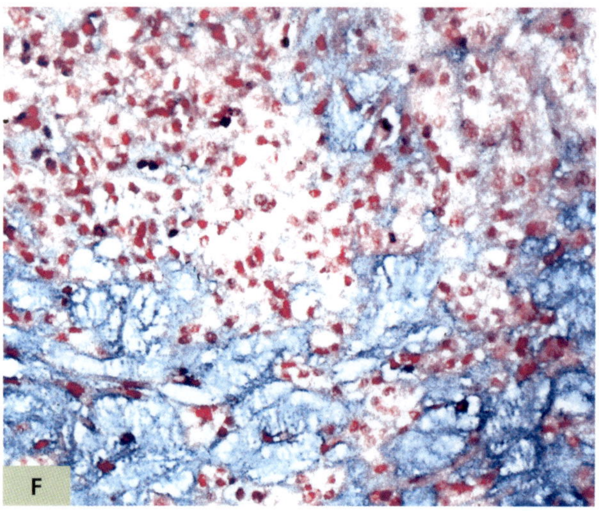

FIGURE 6.3 (*Continued*) Primary pericardial epithelioid mesothelioma (D) cannot be separated from florid mesothelial hyperplasia by any other but morphological means. Mesothelioma shows a higher level of nuclear atypia (E). Both of the latter two processes are comparable histochemically—showing the production of hyaluronidase-sensitive stromal mucin (F, with the alcian blue stain), and they have similar immunoprofiles.

would argue for the presence of another diagnostic alternative; namely, metastatic carcinoma in the pericardium (700). Furthermore, that condition usually assumes a grossly visible and multifocal infiltrate which is detectable radiographically.

ATYPICAL VIRAL PERICARDITIS

Occasional examples of viral pericarditis have been documented in which a lesional lymphoid infiltrate exhibited marked cytological atypia (701) **(Figure 6.4)** and simulated the morphological image of *non-Hodgkin's lymphoma* (702–706) or *myeloma* (707,708). Flow cytometric or immunohistochemical studies in such cases show a polytypic and T-lymphocyte-dominant cell

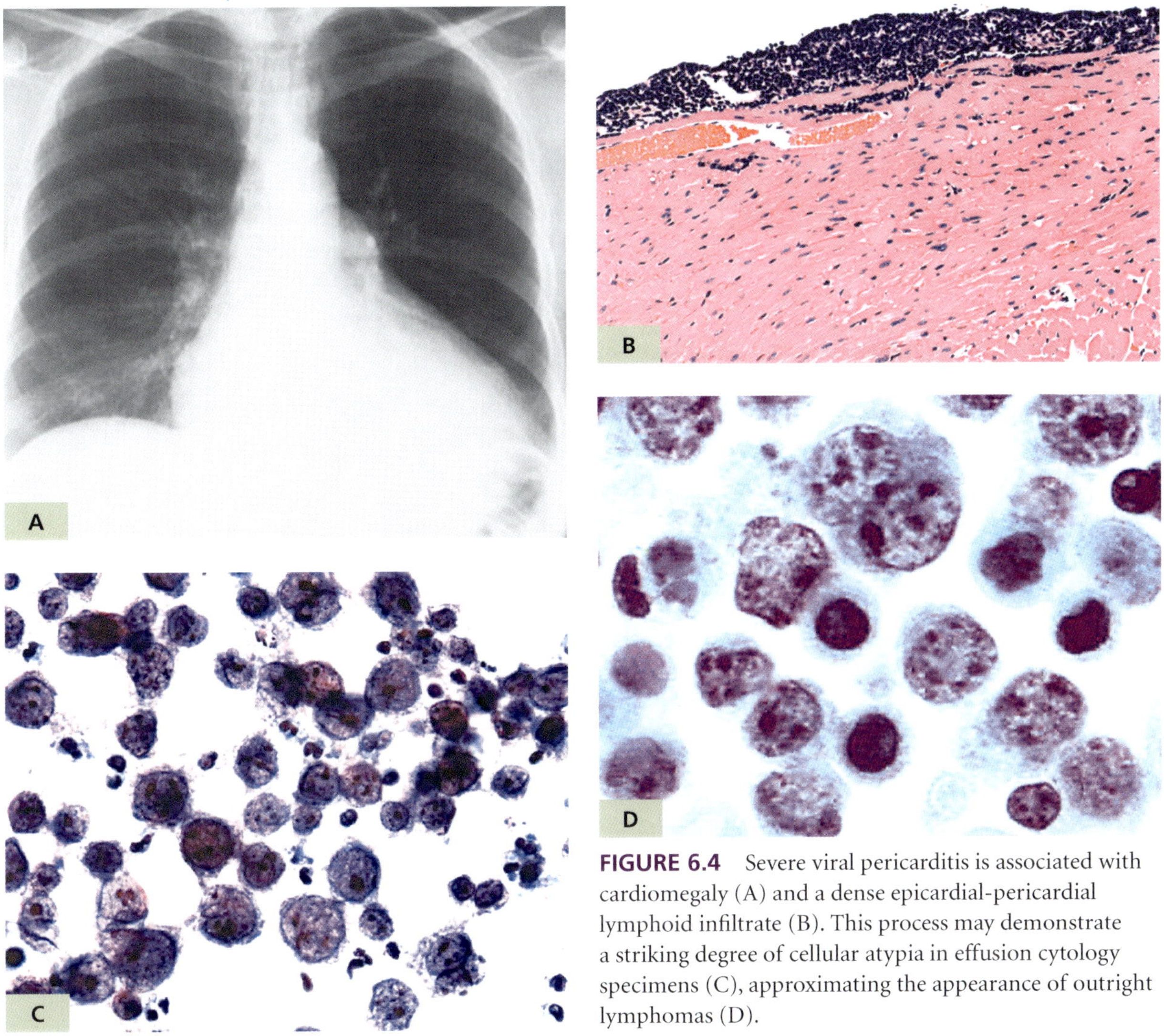

FIGURE 6.4 Severe viral pericarditis is associated with cardiomegaly (A) and a dense epicardial-pericardial lymphoid infiltrate (B). This process may demonstrate a striking degree of cellular atypia in effusion cytology specimens (C), approximating the appearance of outright lymphomas (D).

population, with no evidence of rearranged immunoglobulin or T-cell receptor genes. The infiltrate resolves when the infection is successfully expunged by the host.

ORGANIZING AND VASCULARIZING SUBACUTE PERICARDITIS

Particularly in cases of hemorrhagic pericarditis that are associated with infection or trauma, one may see a significant proliferation of neovascular channels in the pericardial space (**Figure 6.5**) during the organizing phase of a hemopericardium. These may assume a racemose or micropapillary architecture, partially imitating the histologic image of angiosarcoma and paralleling the appearance of papillary endothelial hyperplasia (see above) (**Figure 6.6**).

As discussed above, the endothelial cells in organizing-recanalizing pericardial thrombi are typically bland cytologically, and they mantle a fibrinous—rather than a fibrous—matrix. There is no involvement of the subjacent epicardial stroma, and admixed inflammatory cells are usually present.

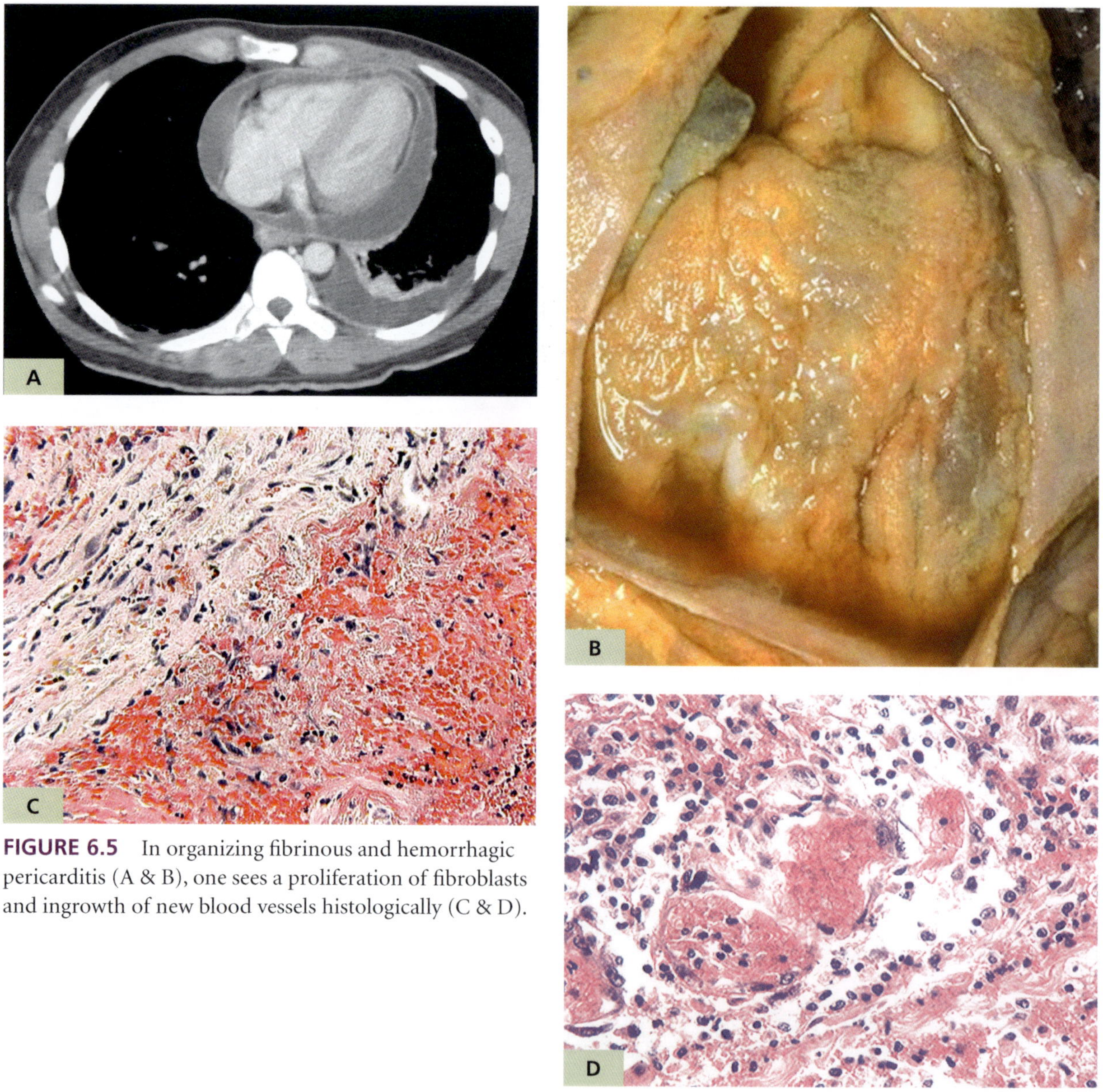

FIGURE 6.5 In organizing fibrinous and hemorrhagic pericarditis (A & B), one sees a proliferation of fibroblasts and ingrowth of new blood vessels histologically (C & D).

Those characteristics differ diametrically from those of true pericardial *angiosarcoma* (709,710) **(Figure 6.7)**, which demonstrates obvious cellular atypia, invasion of adjacent tissues, and a paucity or absence of intralesional inflammation. Moreover, organizing hemorrhagic pericarditis does not form mass lesions, in contrast to true vascular neoplasms.

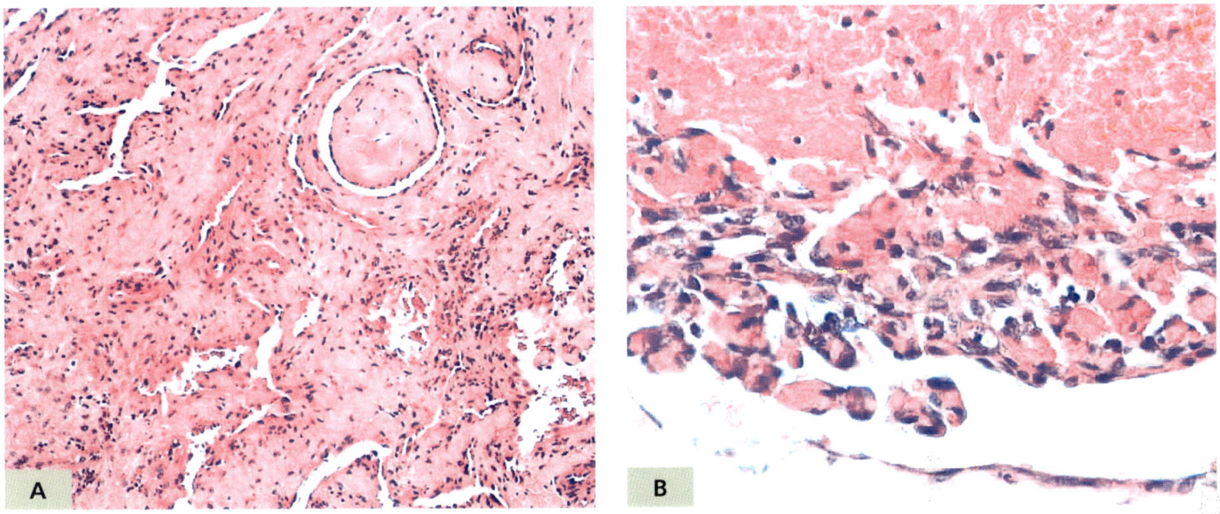

FIGURE 6.6 In the latter stages of organizing hemorrhagic-fibrinous pericarditis, neovascularization of pericardial blood may yield the image of a Masson lesion (A & B) as seen in the lumina of cardiovascular structures elsewhere (also see Figure 5.34).

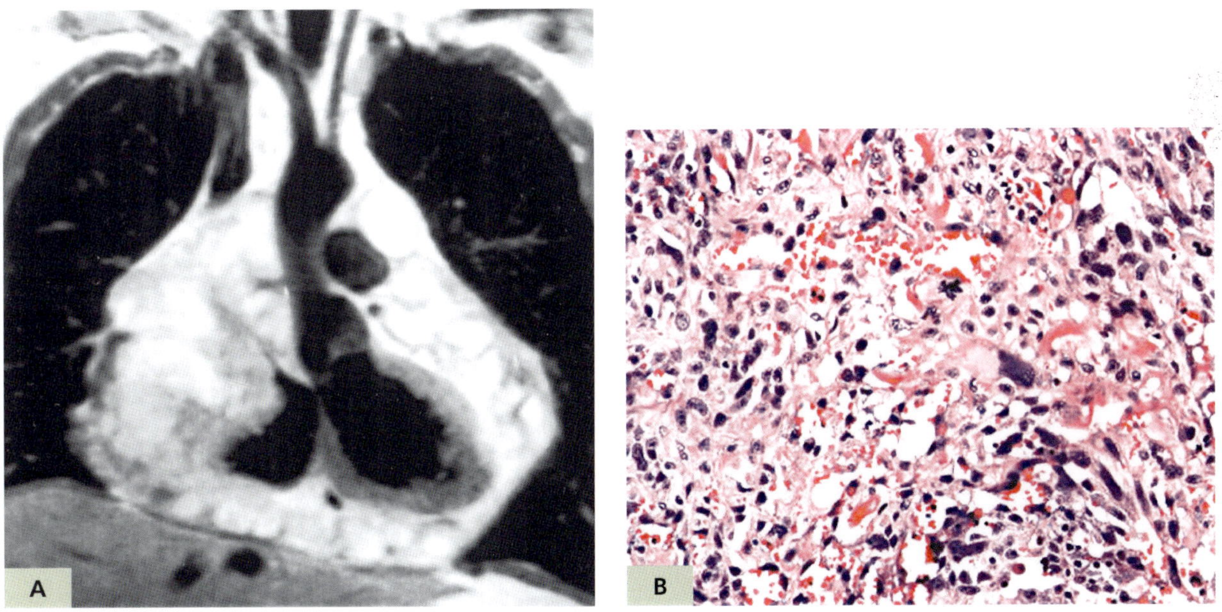

FIGURE 6.7 In contrast to Masson lesions, pericardial angiosarcomas are mass-forming and destructive neoplasms (A) with obvious cellular pleomorphism and nuclear atypicality (B, also see Figure 5.35).

CONSTRICTIVE (FIBROSING) PERICARDITIS

Patients with prior fibrinous pericarditis or those with "IgG4 disease" (711–714) may develop thick circumferential rinds of fibrous tissue that obliterates the pericardial space (**Figure 6.8**). The resulting lesions may closely imitate the clinicopathologic features of *desmoplastic mesothelioma* (DM) (**Figure 6.9**) of the pericardium (693).

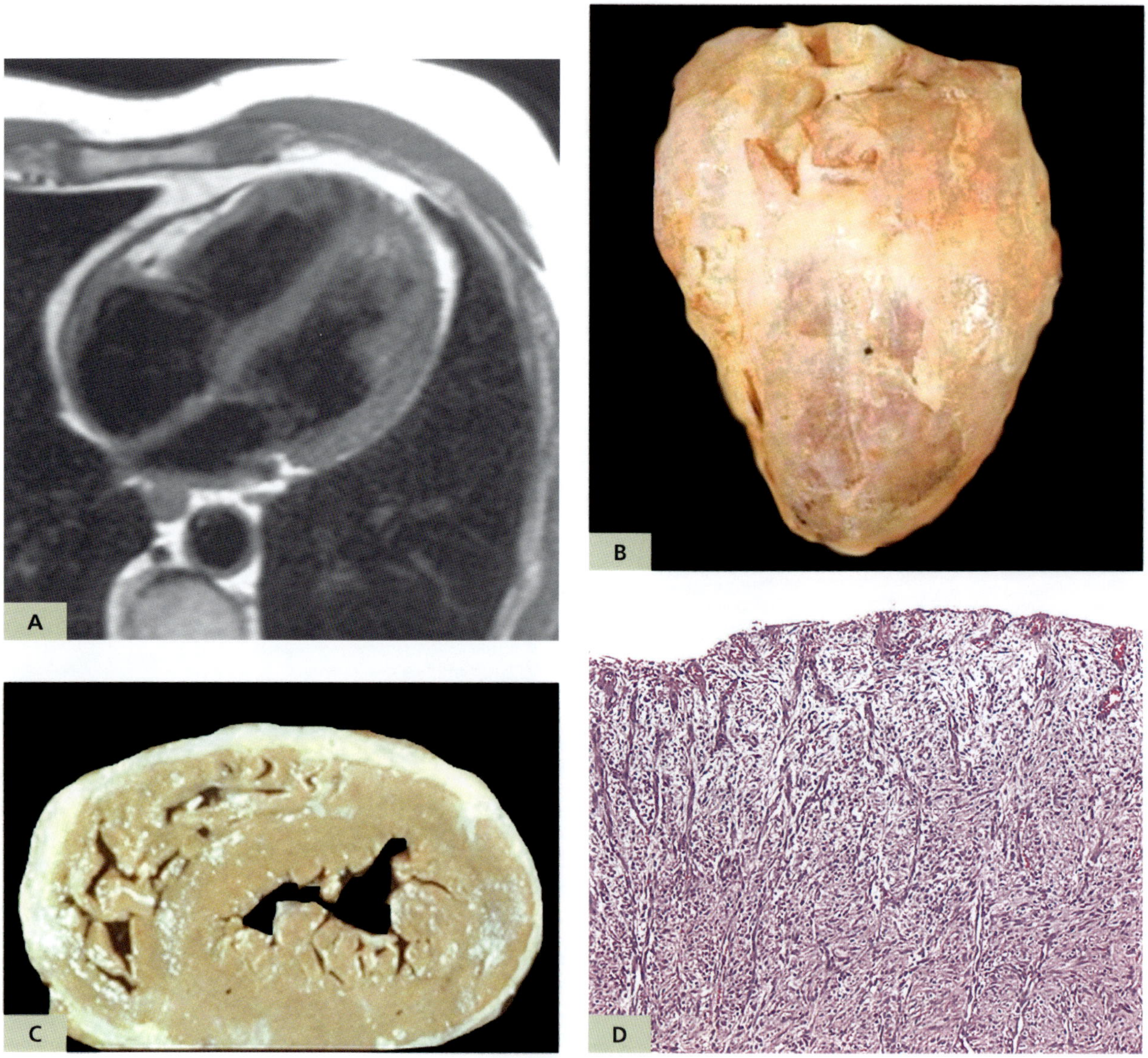

FIGURE 6.8 Constrictive (fibrosing) pericarditis represents the late phase of a foregoing inflammatory pericardial disorder. The pericardium is bound down to the epicardium and greatly thickening by proliferating fibrous tissue (A–C). Microscopically, it may have the appearance of a hypertrophic scar (D) or be represented by mature, lamellated, hypocellular fibrous tissue. In either instance, the possibility of sarcomatoid or desmoplastic mesothelioma may be raised.

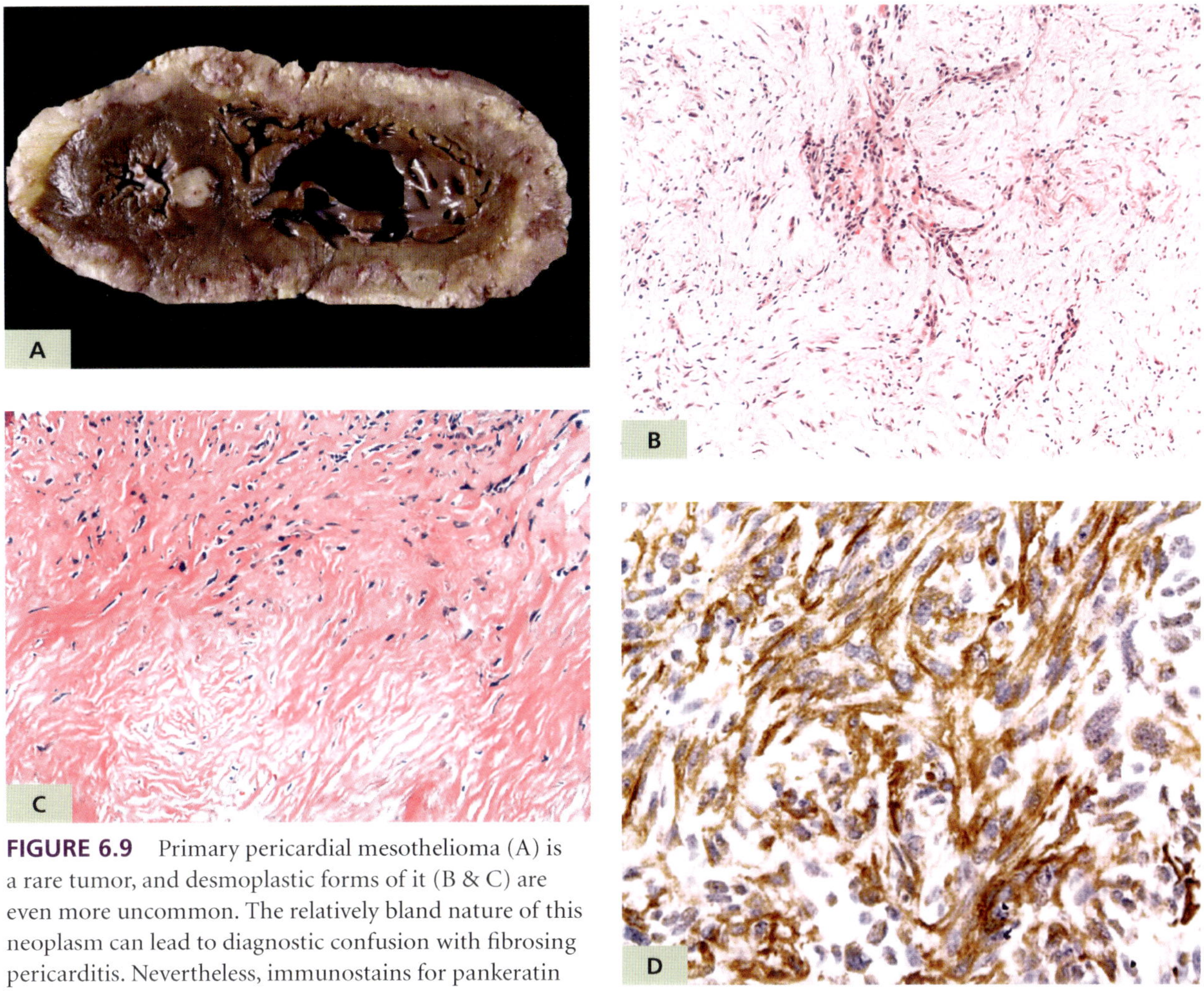

FIGURE 6.9 Primary pericardial mesothelioma (A) is a rare tumor, and desmoplastic forms of it (B & C) are even more uncommon. The relatively bland nature of this neoplasm can lead to diagnostic confusion with fibrosing pericarditis. Nevertheless, immunostains for pankeratin are diffusely reactive in mesothelioma (D) but frequently less so in pericarditis.

Constrictive pericarditis is a fibrosing process with a low cellular density, uniform matrical collagenization, a lack of nuclear atypicality in constituent fibroblasts, and an absence of myocardial involvement. The number of IgG4-immunoreactive plasma cells may also be increased in that condition (**Figure 6.10**) in a proportion of cases (713). In contrast, DM shows irregular areas of cell density, fibromyxoid stroma, **at least focal nuclear atypia**, and invasion of the myocardium. Furthermore, constrictive pericarditis usually is keratin-negative, whereas DM manifests diffuse immunoreactivity for that marker (693) (Figure 6.10).

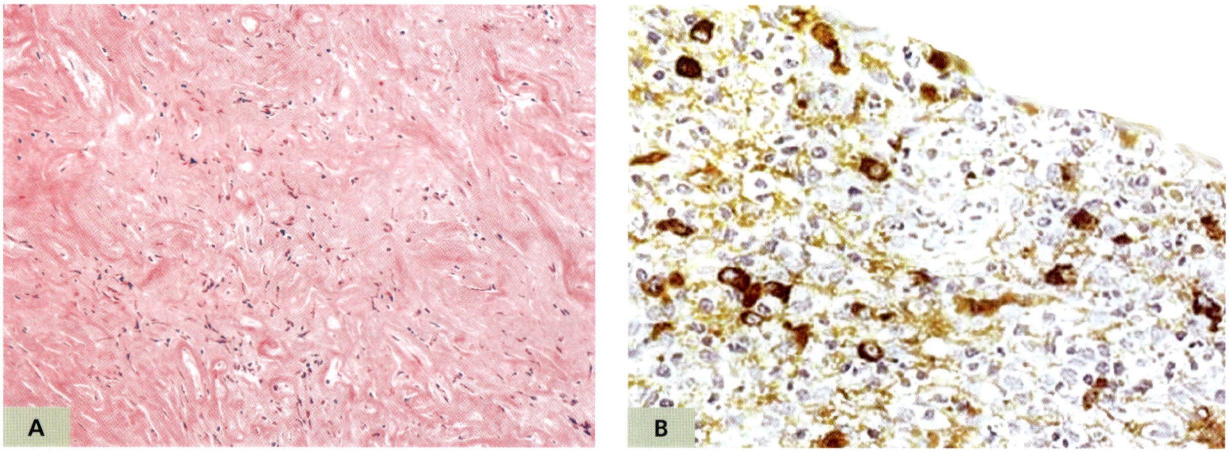

FIGURE 6.10 Some examples of fibrosing pericarditis (A) are part of the spectrum of IgG4-mediated fibroinflammatory lesions. Immunostains for that immunoglobulin (B) can be diagnostically definitive and exclude the possibility of desmoplastic mesothelioma.

Patients with both constrictive pericarditis and DM need surgical removal of the abnormal pericardial tissue in order to improve diastolic filling of the heart. In addition, however, chemotherapy is required in the treatment of DM. Prognosis for the two conditions differs substantially, with virtually all DM patients dying of the disease (693).

PSEUDOTUMORAL PERICARDIAL FAT PADS

In obese patients, fatty investment of the epicardium and pericardium may be prominent **(Figure 6.11)**. Furthermore, fat deposition in those structures can be nonuniform, potentially simulating the radiographic and macroscopic appearances of pericardial *lipoma* (715–720) or *liposarcoma* (716,717,721,722).

The more difficult distinction between hyperplastic fat pads and the latter two neoplasms concerns lipomas and not liposarcomas. That is true because the main morphological difference between lipoma and nonneoplastic fat accumulation is simply the presence of a fibrous capsule in the first but not the second of those lesions. In contrast, liposarcomas contain lipoblasts **(Figure 6.12)** and show higher cellular density, greater stromal fibrosis, myxoid stroma, and nuclear atypia (717,721,722). Cytogenetic assessment demonstrates supernumerary ring and giant rod chromosomes in atypical lipomatous tumors and well-differentiated liposarcoma. In addition, amplification of chromosome 12q13-15, involving the MDM2, CDK4, and CPM genes, can be seen with fluorescent in-situ hybridization techniques in adipocytic tumors (723) but not in exuberant pericardial fat pads.

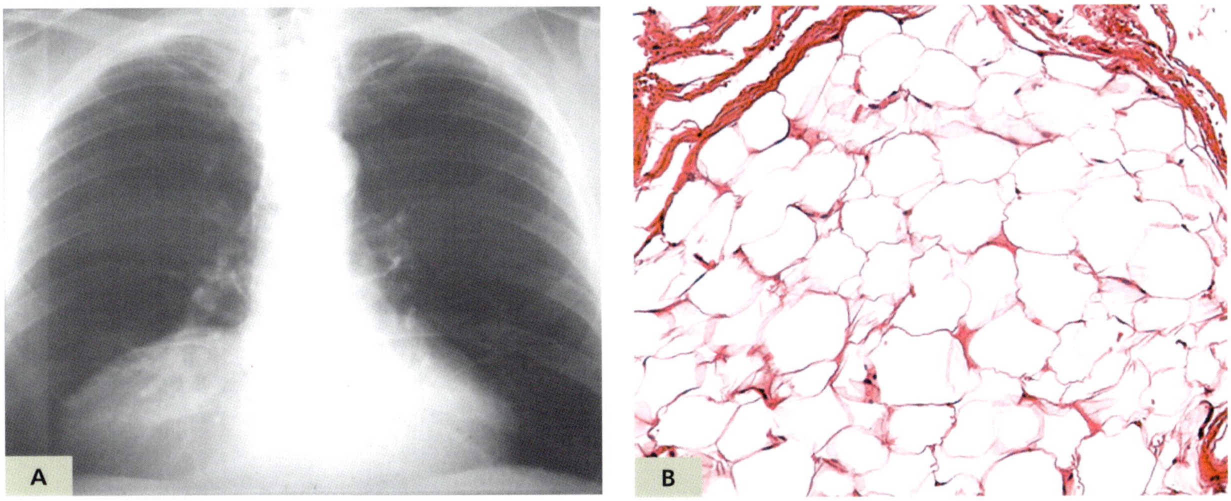

FIGURE 6.11 A & B: In obese individuals, a large epicardial-pericardial fat pad can simulate the appearance of an adipocytic neoplasm.

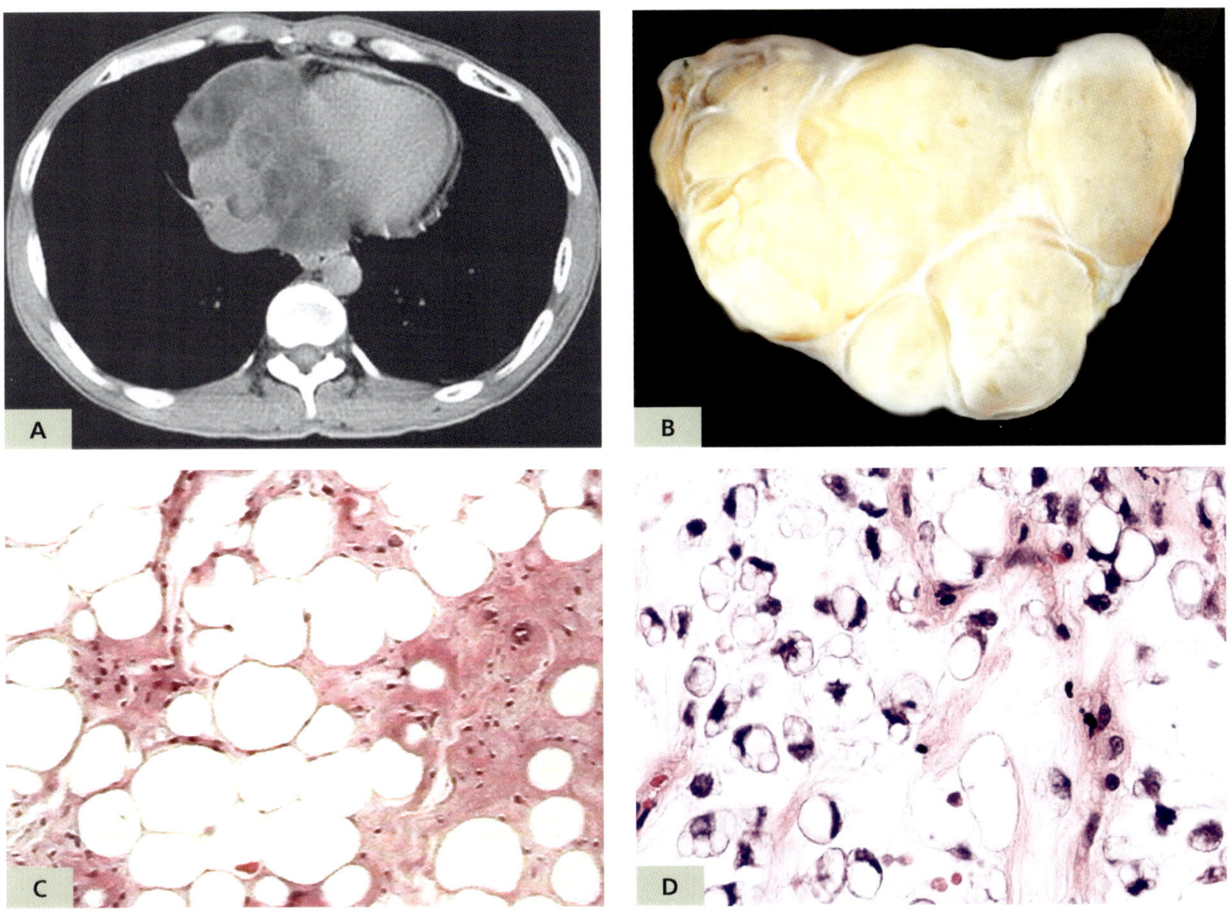

FIGURE 6.12 Liposarcoma of the pericardium is a bulky and infiltrative mass (A & B). It is more cellular than normal adipose tissue, and contains lipoblasts at least focally (C & D).

OTHER NEOPLASTIC MIMICS IN THE PERICARDIUM

Inflammatory pseudotumors (724), ***Castleman's disease*** (725,726), and ***tumefactive extramedullary hematopoiesis*** (727) can be encountered in the pericardium **(Figure 6.13)** as well as the myocardium, as described earlier in this book. Basic diagnostic and differential diagnostic data attending those lesions are identical in the two locations. *Inflammatory myofibroblastic tumor, follicular non-Hodgkin's lymphoma*, and *granulocytic sarcoma* are the principal neoplasms to be excluded, respectively. The attributes of those lesions have been considered in the foregoing discussion.

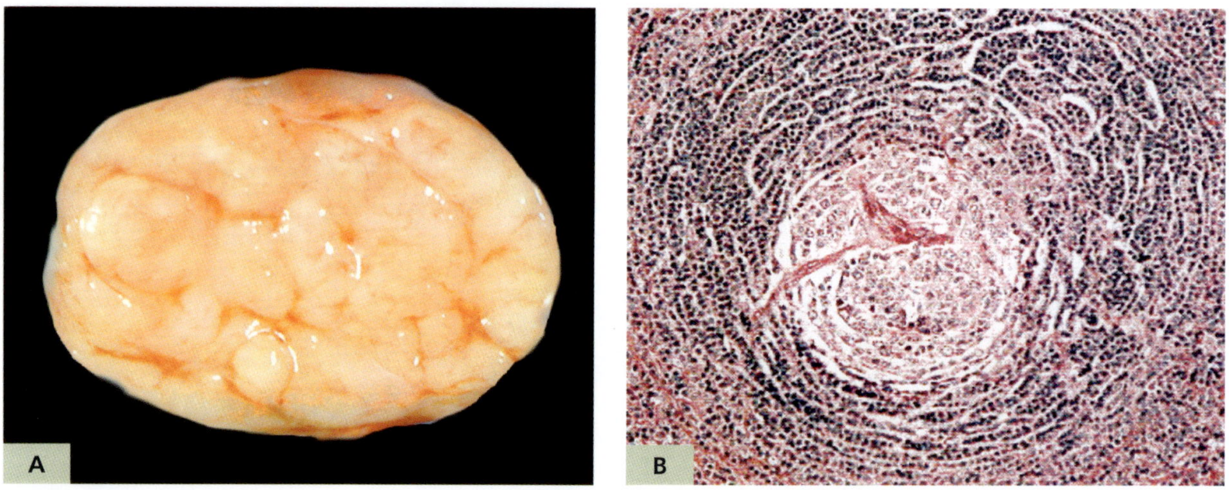

FIGURE 6.13 A & B: Castleman's disease may affect the pericardium as well as the myocardium (also see Figures 5.47 and 5.48), potentially simulating a lymphoma.

7

Pseudoneoplastic Lesions of Blood Vessels

- "INFLAMMATORY" AORTIC ANEURYSMS
- INFLAMMATORY PSEUDOTUMOR OF THE CAROTID ARTERY
- ANEURYSMAL BONE CYST-LIKE LESIONS OF THE CAROTID ARTERY
- TUMEFACTIVE LESIONS CAUSED BY WEGENER'S GRANULOMATOSIS

"INFLAMMATORY" AORTIC ANEURYSMS

In either the thorax or the abdomen, aortic aneurysms in some patients may be accompanied by a dense periadventitial and tumefactive accumulation of fibrous tissue, as well as a chronic inflammatory infiltrate that includes a mixture of lymphocytes and plasma cells **(Figure 7.1)**. Vascular abnormalities in this

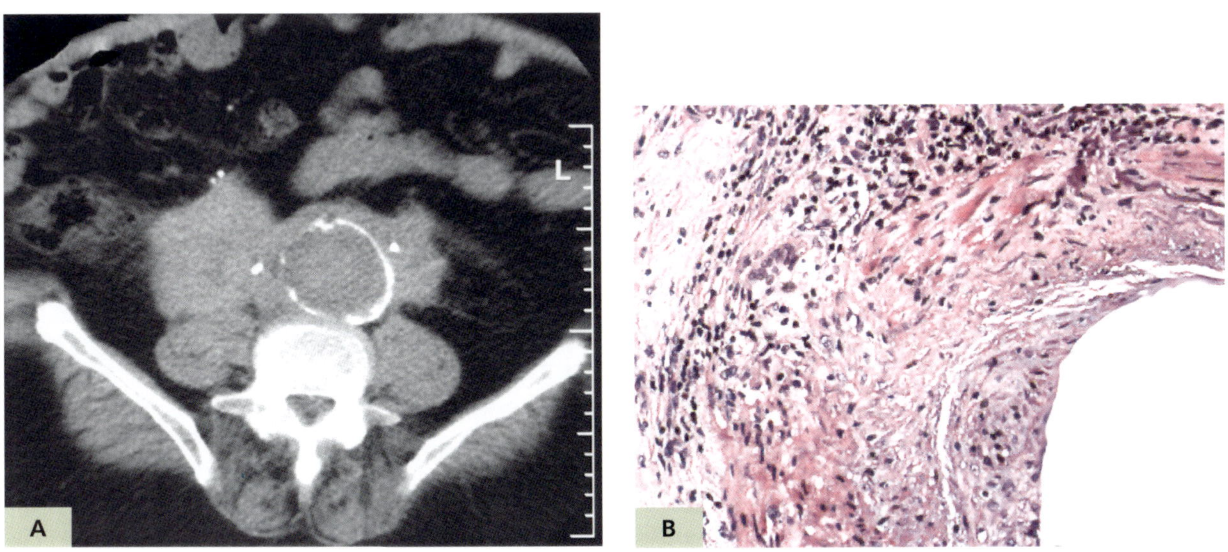

FIGURE 7.1 Inflammatory abdominal aortic aneurysms are associated with a perivascular mass (A), which comprises dense fibrous tissue in which chronic inflammatory cells are dispersed (B and C). *(Continued)*

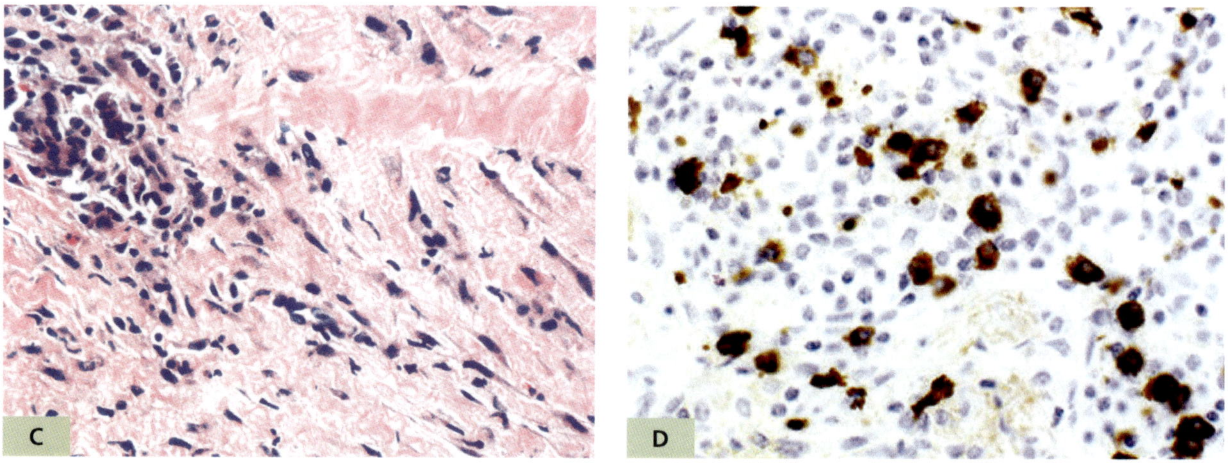

FIGURE 7.1 *(Continued)* Immunostains for IgG4 (D) are positive.

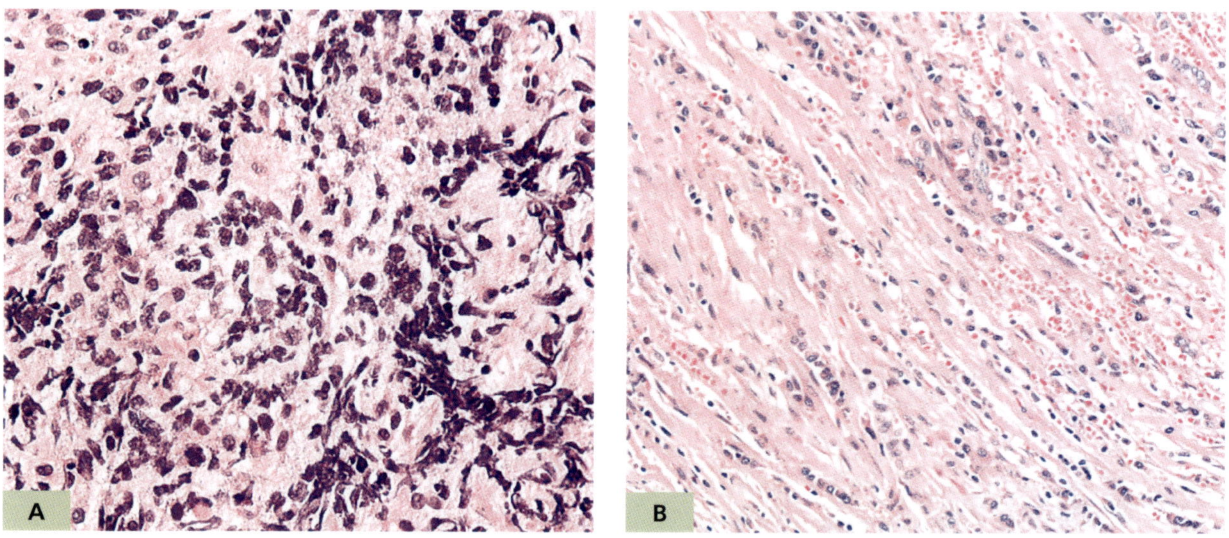

FIGURE 7.2 The differential diagnosis of inflammatory abdominal aortic aneurysms includes sclerosing non-Hodgkin's lymphoma (A) and sclerosing metastatic carcinoma (B; primary site in the stomach).

morphological category have been designated as "inflammatory aneurysms" (IAs) and at least some are thought to be related to systemic IgG4 disease (727–730).

The morphological features of these lesions overlap considerably with those of Ormond's disease. Accordingly, the differential diagnosis in such cases centers mainly on *sclerosing lymphomas* (731,732) **(Figure 7.2)** and *metastatic adenocarcinoma* (especially of mammary or gastric origin) with secondary sclerosis (733). Another consideration is that of *sclerotic desmoid-type fibromatosis*

(734) **(Figure 7.3)**. Those disorders can be excluded by strict morphological analysis and immunohistology. IAs do not contain any cytologically atypical elements, and they are nonreactive for epithelial markers. Moreover, spindle cells in IAs lack intranuclear beta-catenin immunoreactivity, as expected in desmoid tumors (734) **(Figure 7.4)**. A subset of IAs contains an abundance of IgG4+ lymphoplasmacytoid cells, unlike any of the other three differential diagnostic alternatives (729).

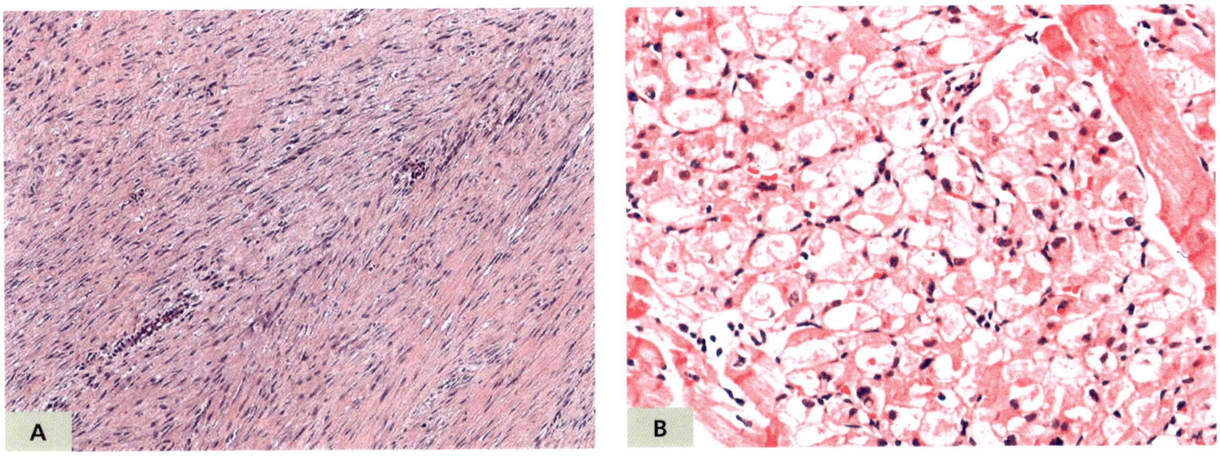

FIGURE 7.3 Retroperitoneal desmoid-type fibromatosis (A) with intratumoral sclerosis (B) also enters into diagnostic consideration in cases of inflammatory abdominal aortic aneurysm.

FIGURE 7.4 Desmoid-type fibromatosis shows intranuclear localization of beta-catenin, as shown here. That finding is not shared by inflammatory aortic aneurysms.

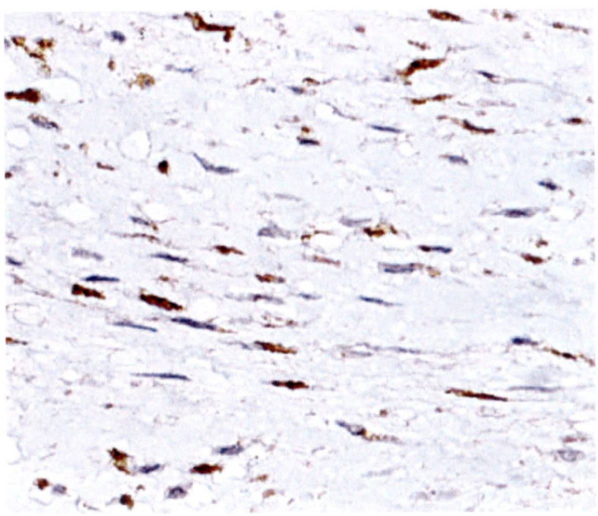

INFLAMMATORY PSEUDOTUMOR OF THE CAROTID ARTERY

Several reports have been made of inflammatory pseudotumors (IPTs; plasma-cell granulomas) of the carotid sheath. In some instances, those mass-forming lesions were responsible for symptoms and signs of vascular stenosis (735–737).

Depending on the particular composition of any given IPT, with more or less fibrous tissue and chronic inflammation, differential diagnostic considerations are focused on *inflammatory myofibroblastic tumor* (IMT), *sclerosing lymphomas, dendritic-cell sarcomas,* and *inflammatory malignant fibrous histiocytoma* (IMFH). The first of those lesions demonstrates clonality in molecular analyses, and is immunoreactive for *ALK*-1 gene product **(Figure 7.5)** in 40% of cases (627,628). The great majority of sclerosing lymphomas are variants of nodular sclerosis-type Hodgkin's disease or B-cell tumors that manifest CD20, CD30, or CD79a (731,732). That profile is unlike the T-cell predominant lymphoid population in IPTs. Dendritic cell tumors are immunoreactive for CD21, CD35, or S100 protein (630), all of which are absent in IPTs. IMFH shows a much higher level of nuclear atypicality **(see Figure 5.30)** and tissue invasiveness than of either IPT or IMT (629).

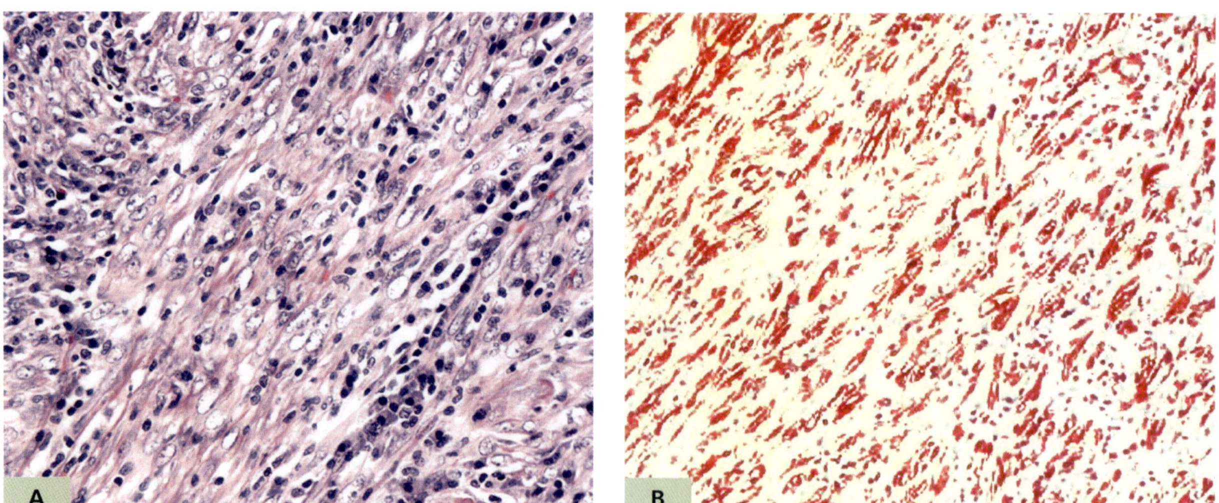

FIGURE 7.5 Retroperitoneal inflammatory myofibroblastic tumor (RIMT) (A) contains a greater number of spindle cells than does inflammatory aortic aneurysm (IAA). In addition, RIMT is immunoreactive for ALK-1 protein in 40% of cases (B), whereas IAA consistently lacks that marker.

ANEURYSMAL BONE CYST-LIKE LESIONS OF THE CAROTID ARTERY

Rare examples have been documented of tumefactive pericarotid lesions (**Figure 7.6**) that resembled aneurysmal bone cysts (ABCs) (738). These masses showed a mixture of compact epithelioid and fusiform cells, punctuated by angiectoid spaces filled with erythrocytes. Osteoclast-like giant cells were concentrated around the peripheral aspects of the blood lakes, and were also scattered randomly throughout the lesions (**Figure 7.7**). Nuclear atypia was minimal, and only physiologic mitotic activity was present.

The main differential diagnostic alternative in such cases is that of *giant-cell tumor of soft parts* (739,740) (**Figure 7.8**), which is likely a "fibrohistiocytic" neoplasm. That tumor is expected to show a uniform dispersal of osteoclast-like cells throughout the lesion, with little or no formation of vascular spaces. On the other hand, ABCs often contain areas of amorphous basophilic stromal material (**Figure 7.9**) that are not seen in giant cell tumors.

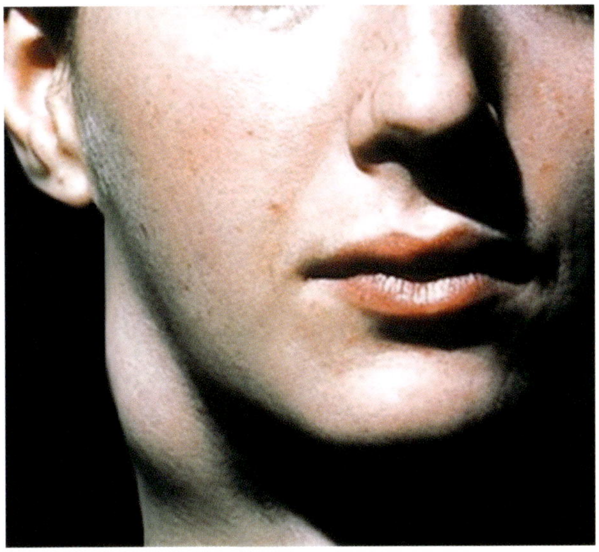

FIGURE 7.6 A rare entity that may simulate vascular neoplasms and other soft tissue tumors is represented by aneurysmal bone cyst-like lesion of the carotid artery sheath. It is seen clinically in this photograph as a mass lesion of the right neck.

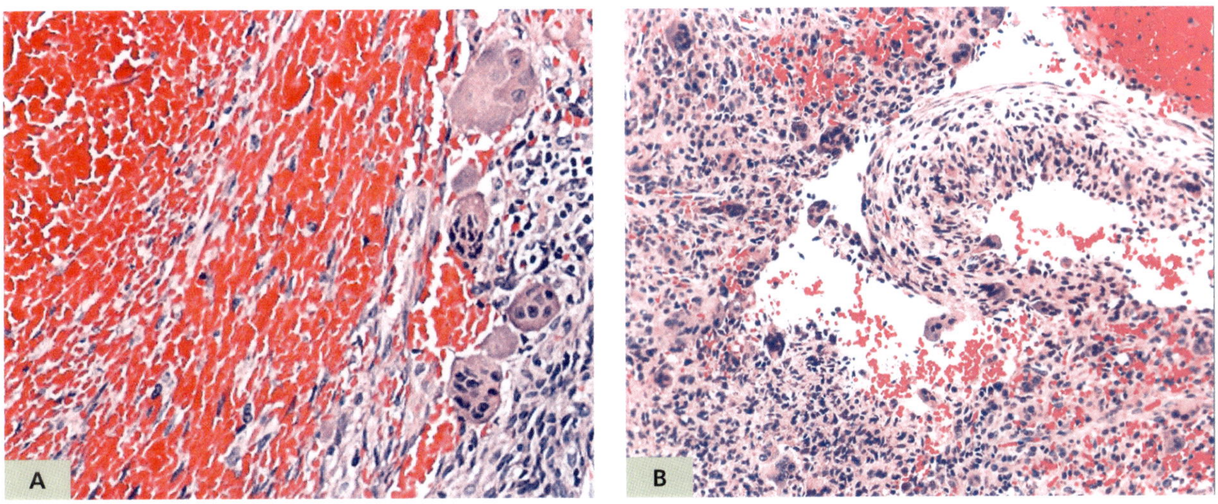

FIGURE 7.7 A & B: Pericarotid aneurysmal bone cyst-like lesion demonstrates the presence of blood lakes, mantled by tissue septa comprising epithelioid mononuclear cells, fibroblasts, and osteoclast-like giant cells.

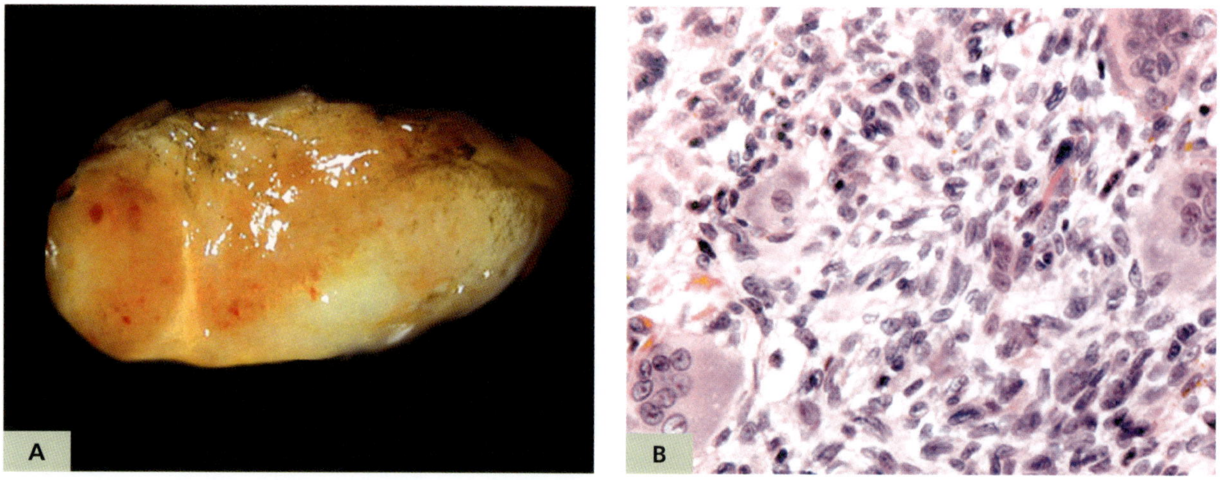

FIGURE 7.8 Giant cell tumor of soft parts (GCTSP) is the principal differential diagnostic alternative to pericarotid aneurysmal bone cyst-like lesion (PABCLL). GCTSP is a solid mass (A) in contrast to PABCLL. The former of those proliferations contains no blood-filled spaces and shows an admixture of mononuclear epithelioid cells and multinucleated giant cells (B).

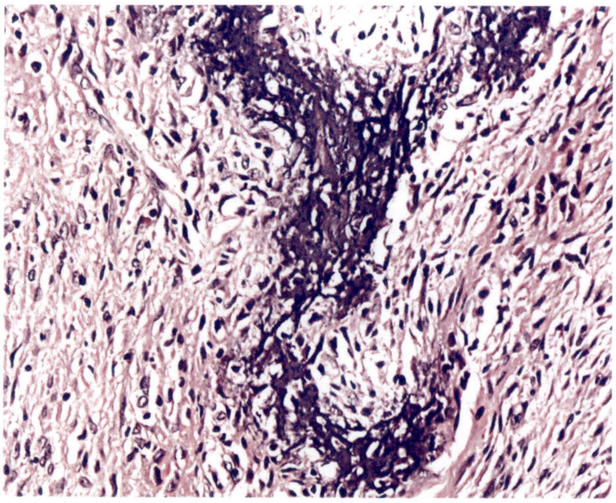

FIGURE 7.9 Pericarotid aneurysmal bone cyst-like lesion may contain amorphous chondrocalcific material, shown here. It is not seen in giant cell tumors of soft parts.

TUMEFACTIVE LESIONS CAUSED BY WEGENER'S GRANULOMATOSIS

Wegener's granulomatosis (WG) is a granulomatous systemic vasculitis that affects small and medium-sized arteries, and which is associated with circulating antibodies to cytoplasmic neutrophil antigens (741). Its principal organ targets are the lungs, kidneys, and upper respiratory mucosa, although several other anatomic locations also may be affected (742). In occasional cases, WG may cause tumefactive lesions in the skin and soft tissues **(Figure 7.10)** that simulate true neoplasms both clinically and pathologically (743,744).

WG has three cardinal histological components. These include *bona fide* arteritis, with or without granulomatous features; extravascular granulomatous inflammation; and geographic zones of tissue necrosis **(Figure 7.11)**. In the background, behind those elements, one also sees a brisk lymphoplasmacytic infiltrate with a modest degree of cytological atypia (742,743). The overall image of WG may closely simulate the appearance of *angiocentric T-cell lymphoma* (745,746) **(Figure 7.12)** with secondary intralesional formation of granulomas,

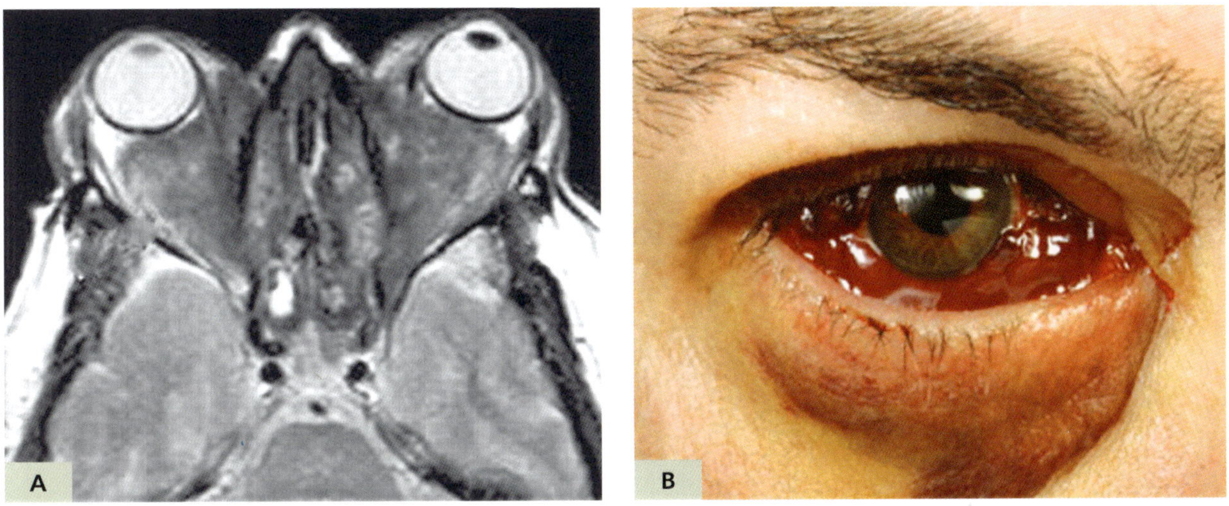

FIGURE 7.10 Wegener's granulomatosis may produce mass-forming pseudoneoplastic extrapulmonary lesions, as shown here in both retrobulbar spaces on a magnetic resonance imaging study (A). Those lesions have produced clinical proptosis and ocular vascular congestion (B).

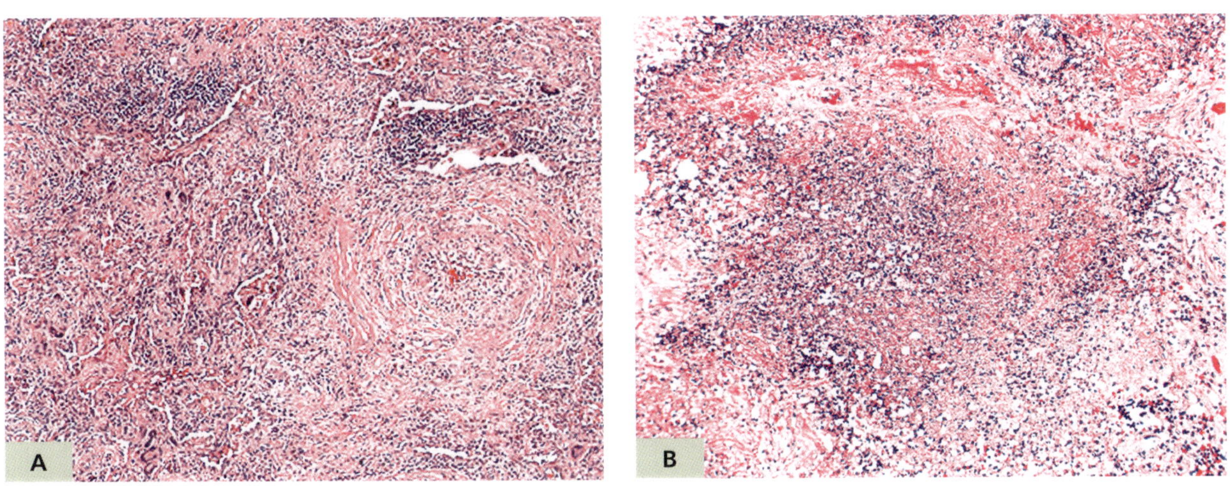

FIGURE 7.11 (A–D) Wegener's granulomatosis is recognized histologically by the concurrent presence of granulomatous inflammation, necrosis, and vasculitis. *(Continued)*

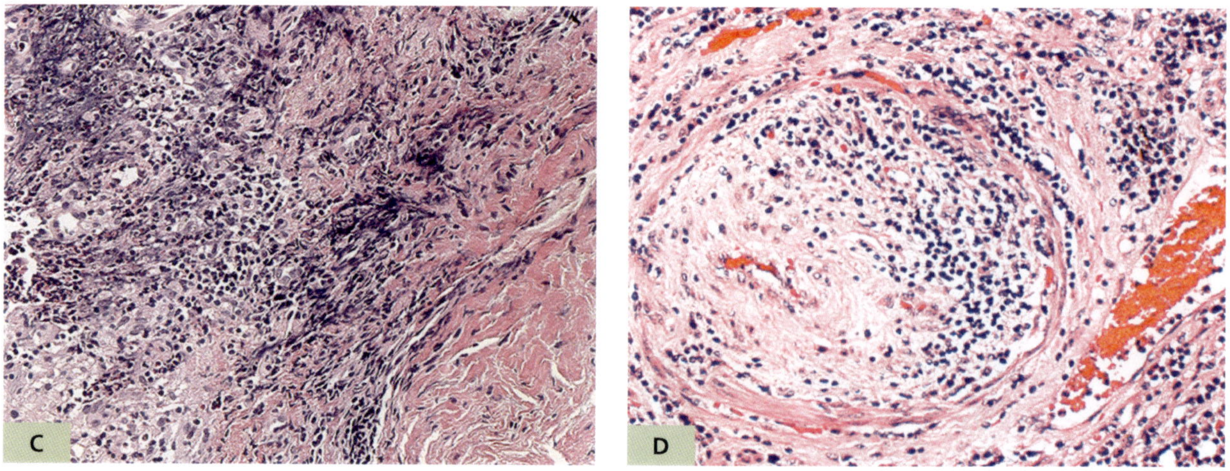

FIGURE 7.11 *(Continued)*

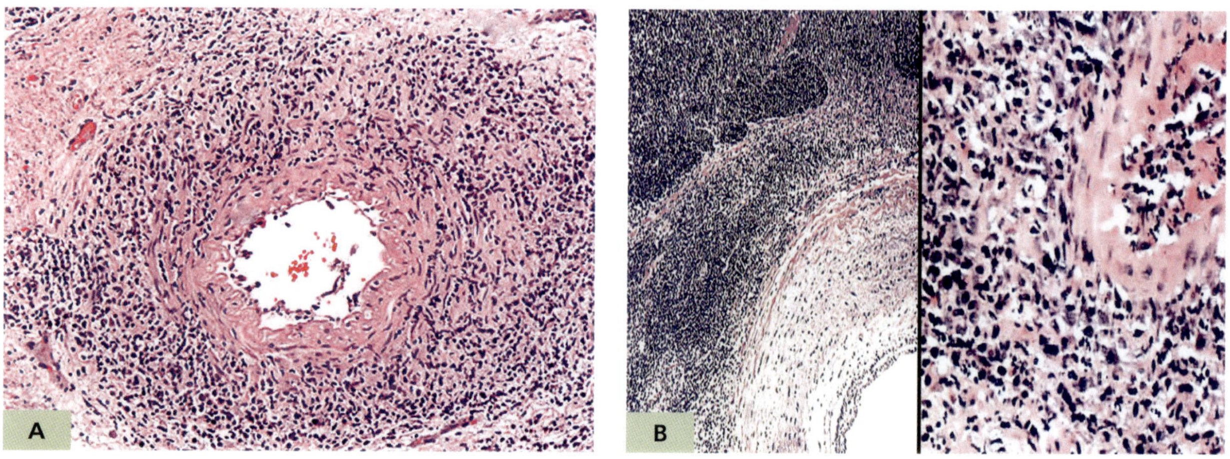

FIGURE 7.12 A & B: Angiocentric T-cell lymphoma (ATCL)—shown here—is an important differential diagnostic consideration in cases of extrathoracic Wegener's granulomatosis that involve medium-sized and large blood vessels. ATCL exhibits a much higher level of cytological atypia and nuclear karryorhexis than that seen in Wegener's disease.

or the peculiar lymphoproliferative disorder known as "*lymphomatoid granulomatosis*" (LYG) (*high-grade angiocentric immunoproliferative lesion*) (747,748) **(Figure 7.13)**. Both of the latter neoplasms are similar to WG immunophenotypically in that they all may comprise a predominant population of T-lymphocytes with admixed plasma cells. However, angiocentric lymphoma also shows the presence of rearranged T-cell receptor genes **(Figure 7.14)**, which are lacking in WG and LYG. With in-situ hybridization studies, LYG typically exhibits integrated Epstein–Barr virus genomes in a proportion of lesional cells (748) **(Figure 7.15)**, but WG and angiocentric T-cell lymphoma do not.

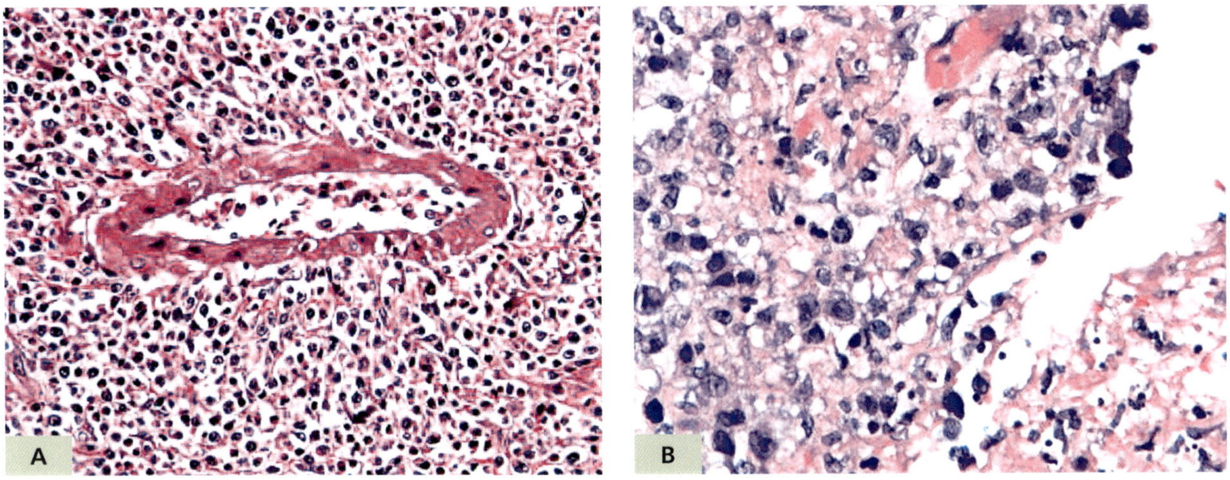

FIGURE 7.13 Another diagnostic alternative to Wegener's granulomatosis is probably the neoplastic condition known as "lymphomatoid granulomatosis" (LYG), particularly in its high-grade form. That disorder is also centered on medium-sized and large blood vessels, with permeation of their walls (A). Cytologic attributes of the lesional cells in LYG show a notable degree of nuclear atypia (B), and granulomas are typically absent.

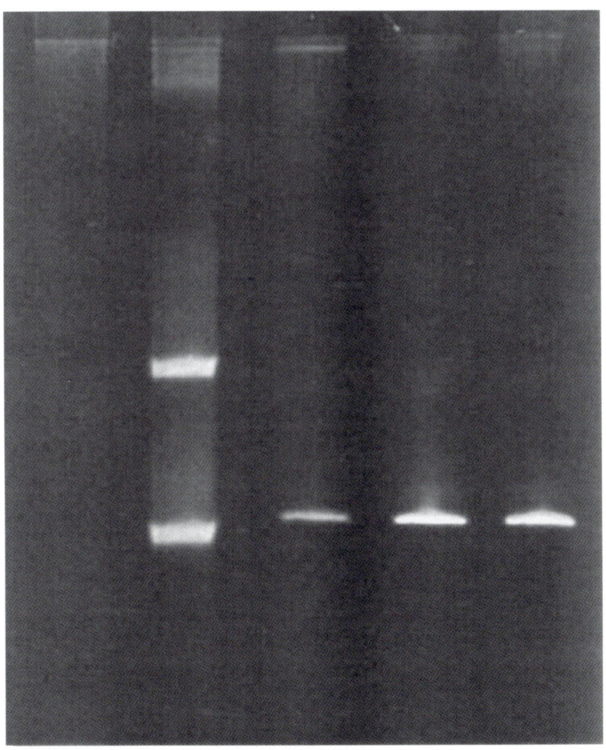

FIGURE 7.14 Angiocentric T-cell lymphomas show rearrangements of T-cell receptor genes in molecular analyses. In this photograph, tumor tissue in lane 2 (lane second from left) demonstrates an obvious new nucleic acid band, relative to controls in other lanes.

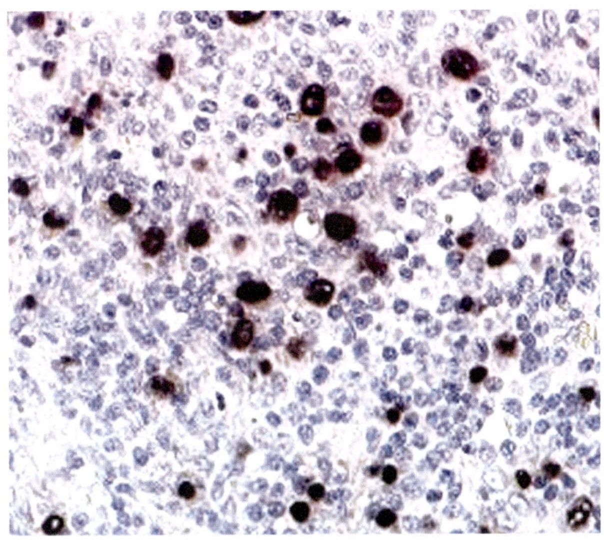

FIGURE 7.15 Lymphomatoid granulomatosis characteristically manifests the presence of Epstein-Barr virus–related nucleic acid in large lesional lymphoid cells, as shown in this in-situ hybridization preparation.

References

1. Ackerman LV. *Surgical Pathology*. 3rd ed. St. Louis, MO: CV Mosby; 1964:407–408.
2. Birch-Hirschfeld A. Die Krankheiten der Orbita. In: Graefe A, Saemisch T, eds. *Handbuch der Gesamten Augenheilkunden*. vol. 9, part 1. Berlin: Springer-Verlag; 1930:111–130.
3. Garner A. Pathology of "pseudotumors" of the orbit: a review. *J Clin Pathol*. 1973;26:639–648.
4. Umiker WO, Iverson L. Postinflammatory "tumors" of the lung. *J Thorac Surg*. 1954;28:55–62.
5. Kuzela DC. Ultrastructural study of a postinflammatory "tumor" of the lung. *Cancer*. 1975;36:149–156.
6. Makela V, Mattila S, Makinen J. Plasma cell granuloma (histiocytoma) of the lung and pleura. *Acta Pathol Microbiol Scand A*. 1972;80:634–640.
7. Bahadori M, Liebow AA. Plasma cell granulomas of the lung. *Cancer*. 1973;31:191–208.
8. Alvarez-Fernandez E, Escalona-Zapata J. Pulmonary plasma cell granuloma: an electron microscopic and tissue culture study. *Histopathology*. 1983;7:279–286.
9. Warter A, Satge D, Roeslin N. Angioinvasive plasma cell granulomas of the lung. *Cancer*. 1987;59:435–443.
10. Sherwin RP, Kern WH, Jones JC. Solitary mast cell granuloma (histiocytoma) of the lung. *Cancer*. 1965;18:634–641.
11. Scott HW Jr, Morrow AG, Payne TP. Solitary xanthoma of the lung. *J Thorac Surg*. 1948;17:821–825.
12. Titus JL, Harrison EG Jr, Clagett OT, Anderson MV, Kuaff LY. Xanthomatous and inflammatory pseudotumor of the lung. *Cancer*. 1962;15:522–538.
13. Wentworth P, Lynch MJ, Fallis JC, Turner JA, Lowden JA, Conen PE. Xanthomatous pseudotumor of lung. *Cancer*. 1968;22:345–355.
14. Buell R, Want N, Seemayer TA, Ahmed MN. Endobronchial plasma cell granuloma (xanthomatous pseudotumor); a light and electron microscopic study. *Hum Pathol*. 1976;7:411–426.
15. Alegre JA, Deust J. Xanthogranuloma as a coin lesion of the lung. *Dis Chest*. 1958;33:427–431.
16. Spencer H. The pulmonary plasma cell-histiocytoma complex. *Histopathology*. 1984;8:903–916.
17. Liebow AA, Hubbel DS. Sclerosing hemangioma (histiocytoma, xanthoma) of the lung. *Cancer*. 1956;9:53–75.
18. Jensen PS, Putnam CE. Hemophilic pseudotumor: diagnosis, treatment, and complications. *Am J Dis Child*. 1975;129:717–719.
19. Hermann G, Yeh HC, Gilbert MS. Computed tomography and ultrasonography of the hemophilic pseudotumor and their use in surgical planning. *Skel Radiol*. 1986;15:123–128.
20. Kelly IM, Lees WR, Russell RC. Tumefactive biliary sludge: a sonographic pseudotumor appearance in the common bile duct. *Clin Radiol*. 1993;47:251–254.
21. Bellamy PR. The mucosal rosette: a periampullary pseudotumor within a duodenal diverticulum. *Clin Radiol*. 1993;47:117–118.
22. Coenen L, Biltjes I. Pseudotumor of the palm due to an anomalous flexor digitorum superficialis muscle belly. *J Hand Surg*. 1991;16A:1046–1051.

23. Meier S, Cagle O. Rounded atelectasis. *Surg Rounds*. 1986;8:85–90.
24. Inoshita T, Boyd W. Rounded atelectasis shown by computed tomography. *South Med J*. 1986;79:764–767.
25. Stark P. Round atelectasis: another pulmonary pseudotumor. *Am Rev Resp Dis*. 1982;125:248–250.
26. Tallroth K, Kiviranta K. Round atelectasis. *Respiration*. 1984;45:71–77.
27. Wick MR, Swanson PE. *Cutaneous Adnexal Tumors: A Guide to Pathologic Diagnosis*. Chicago, IL: ASCP Press; 1991:28.
28. Goldstein N. Ephidrosis (local hyperhidrosis): nevus sudoriferus. *Arch Dermatol*. 1967;96:67–71.
29. Kin JH, Hur H, Lee CW, Kim YT. Apocrine nevus. *J Am Acad Dermatol*. 1988;18:579–581.
30. Amazon K, Robinson MD, Rywlin AM. Ferrugination caused by Monsel's solution: clinical observations and experimentations. *Am J Dermatopathol*. 1980;2:197–205.
31. Olmstead PM, Lund HZ, Leonard DD. Monsel's solution: a histologic nuisance. *J Am Acad Dermatol*. 2980;3:492–498.
32. Tschen JA, Fechner RE. The juxtaoral organ of Chievitz. *Am J Surg Pathol*. 1979;3:147–154.
33. Danforth RA, Baughman RA. Chievitz's organ: a potential pitfall in oral cancer diagnosis. *Oral Surg*. 1979;48:231–235.
34. Ide F, Mishima K, Saito I. Juxtaoral organ of Chievitz presenting clinically as a tumor. *J Clin Pathol*. 2003;56:789–790.
35. Pantanowitz L, Tschen JA. Organ of Chievitz. *Ear Nose Throat J*. 2004;83:230.
36. Kusafuka K, Kameya T. Juxtaoral organ of Chievitz, radiologically suspicious for invasion of lingual squamous cell carcinoma. *Pathol Int*. 2007;57:754–756.
37. McBroom JM, Ramsay AD. The clinicopathological meeting: a means of auditing diagnostic performance. *Am J Surg Pathol*. 1993;17:75–80.
38. Pettinato G, Manivel JC, DeRosa N, Dehner LP. Inflammatory myofibroblastic tumor (plasma cell granuloma): clinicopathologic study of 20 cases with immunohistochemical and ultrastructural observations. *Am J Clin Pathol*. 1990;94:538–546.
39. Berardi RS, Lee SS, Chen HP, Stines GJ. Inflammatory pseudotumors of the lung. *Surg Gynecol Obstet*. 1983;156:89–96.
40. Barbareschi M, Ferrero S, Aldovini D, et al. Inflammatory pseudotumor of the lung: immunohistochemical analysis on four new cases. *Histol Histopathol*. 1990;5:205–211.
41. Cotelingam J, Jaffe ES. Inflammatory pseudotumor of the spleen. *Am J Surg Pathol*. 1984;8:375–380.
42. Monforte-Munoz H, Ro JY, Manning JT Jr, et al. Inflammatory pseudotumor of the spleen: report of two cases with a review of the literature. *Am J Clin Pathol*. 1991;96:491–495.
43. Perrone T, DeWolf-Peeters C, Frizzera G. Inflammatory pseudotumor of lymph nodes: a distinctive pattern of nodal reaction. *Am J Surg Pathol*. 1988;12:351–361.
44. Isaacson P, Buchanan R, Mepham BL. Plasma cell granuloma of the stomach. *Hum Pathol*. 1978;9:355–358.
45. Abrebanel P, Sarfaty S, Gal R, Chaimoff C, Kessler E. Plasma cell granuloma of the pancreas. *Arch Pathol Lab Med*. 1984;108:531–532.
46. Wu JP, Yunis EJ, Fetterman G, et al. Inflammatory pseudotumors of the abdomen: plasma cell granulomas. *J Clin Pathol*. 1973;26:943–948.
47. Day DL, Sane S, Dehner LP. Inflammatory pseudotumor of the mesentery and small intestine. *Pediatr Radiol*. 1986;16:210–215.
48. Chen KT. Inflammatory pseudotumor of the liver. *Hum Pathol*. 1984;15:694–696.
49. Shek TW, Ng IO, Chan KW. Inflammatory pseudotumor of the liver: report of four cases and review of the literature. *Am J Surg Pathol*. 1993;17:231–238.
50. Fish AE, Brodey PA. Plasma cell granuloma of the kidney. *Urology*. 1976;8:89–91.
51. Nochomovitz LE, Orenstein JM. Inflammatory pseudotumor of the urinary bladder: possible relationship to nodular fasciitis. *Am J Surg Pathol*. 1985;9:366–373.

52. Dietrick DD, Kabalin IN, Daniels GF Jr, Epstein AB, Fielding IM. Inflammatory pseudotumor of the bladder. *J Urol.* 1992;148:141–144.
53. Yapp R, Linder J, Schenker JR, Karrer FW. Plasma cell granuloma of the thyroid. *Hum Pathol.* 1985;16:848–850.
54. Earl PD, Lowry JC, Sloan P. Intraoral inflammatory pseudotumor. *Oral Surg Oral Med Oral Pathol.* 1993;76:279–283.
55. Hytiroglou P, Brandwein MS, Strauchen JA, Mirante JP, Urken ML, Biller HF. Inflammatory pseudotumor of the parapharyngeal space. *Head & Neck.* 1992;14:230–234.
56. Pettinato G, Manivel JC, Insabato L, De Chiara A, Petrella G. Plasma cell granuloma (inflammatory pseudotumor) of the breast. *Am J Clin Pathol.* 1988;90:627–632.
57. Eimoto T, Yanaka M, Kurosawa M, Ikeya F. Plasma cell granuloma (inflammatory pseudotumor) of the spinal cord and meninges. *Cancer.* 1978;41:1929–1936.
58. Sitton IE, Harkin IC, Gerber MA. Intracranial inflammatory pseudotumor. *Clin Neuropathol.* 1992;11:36–40.
59. Chang Y, Horoupian DS, Lane B, Fross RD, Smyth LT Jr, Seiling RJ. Inflammatory pseudotumor of the choroid plexus in Sjogren's disease. *Neurosurgery.* 1991;29:287–290.
60. Valdeeswar P, Patwardhan AM, Sathe PA. Cardiac valvular inflammatory pseudotumor. *J Cardiothorac Surg.* 2008;3:53.
61. Tomiyama M, Nakatani S, Ishibashi-Ueda H, Yutani C, Yamagishi M. Inflammatory pseudotumor of the heart. *Ann Intern Med.* 2007;147:351–352.
62. Matsubara O, Tan-Liu NS, Kenney RM, Mark EJ. Inflammatory pseudotumor of the lung: progression from organizing pneumonia to fibrous histiocytoma or to plasma cell granuloma in 32 cases. *Hum Pathol.* 1988;19:807–814.
63. Yi E, Aubry MC. Pulmonary pseudoneoplasms. *Arch Pathol Lab Med.* 2010;134:417–426.
64. Bastlein C, Burlefinger R, Holzberg E, Voeth C, Garbrecht M, Ottenjann R. Common variable immunodeficiency syndrome and nodular lymphoid hyperplasia in the small intestine. *Endoscopy.* 1988;20:272–275.
65. Bejaoui M, Guezmir M, Hamdi M, Mezni F, Gorbel A, Lakhoua R. Lymphoid hyperplasia of the intestine in children: 15 cases. *Ann Pediatrics (Paris).* 1992;39:359–364.
66. Colarian I, Calzada R, Iaszewski R. Nodular lymphoid hyperplasia of the colon in adults: is it common? *Gastrointest Endosc.* 1990;36:421–422.
67. Franchi LM, Chin TW, Nussbaum E, Riker J, Robert M, Talbert WM. Familial pulmonary nodular lymphoid hyperplasia. *J Pediatrics.* 1992;121:89–92.
68. Brodell RT, Santa Cruz DI. Cutaneous pseudolymphomas. *Dermatol Clin.* 1985;3:719–734.
69. Hammer E, Sangueza O, Suwanjindar P, White CR Jr, Braziel RM. Immunophenotypic and genotypic analysis in cutaneous lymphoid hyperplasias. *J Am Acad Dermatol.* 1993;28:426–433.
70. Takano Y, Kato Y, Sugano H. Histopathological and immunohistochemical study of atypical lymphoid hyperplasia and benign lymphoid hyperplasia of the stomach. *Jpn J Cancer Res.* 1992;83:288–293.
71. Samoszuk M, Ramzi E, Ravel I. Disseminated persistent lymphoid hyperplasia containing Epstein–Barr virus and clonal rearrangements of DNA. *Diagn Mol Pathol.* 1993;2:57–60.
72. Cheuk W, Chan JKC. IgG4-related sclerosing disease: a critical appraisal of an evolving clinicopathologic entity. *Adv Anat Pathol.* 2010;17:303–332.
73. Slootweg PI, Panders AK, Nikkels PG. Psammomatoid ossifying fibroma of the paranasal sinuses. *J Craniomaxillofac Surg.* 1993;21:294–297.
74. Chan KW, Khoo US, Ho CM. Fibroosseous pseudotumor of the digits: report of a case with immunohistochemical and ultrastructural studies. *Pathology.* 1993;25:193–196.
75. Bosse A, Niesert W, Wuisman P, Roessner A. Fibrous dysplasia versus osteofibrous dysplasia: morphological, differential diagnostic, and clinical aspects. Experiences from the Westfalen bone tumor registry [in German]. *Z Orthop Ihre Grenzgeb.* 1993;131:42–50.
76. Kearns D, McGill T, Potsic W. Fibrous dysplasia. *Head & Neck.* 1992;14:510–512.

77. Betts NI, Stewart IC, Fonseca RI, ScottRF. Multiple central giant cell lesions with a Noonan-like phenotype. *Oral Surg Oral Med Oral Pathol.* 1993;76:601–607.
78. Wallis MG, Devakumar R, Hosie KB, James KA, Bishop HM. Complex sclerosing lesions (radial scars) of the breast can be palpable. *Clin Radiol.* 1993;48:319–320.
79. Anderson TJ. Battersby S. Radial scars of benign and malignant breasts: comparative features and significance. *J Pathol.* 1985;147:23–32.
80. Farshid G, Rush G. Assessment of 142 stellate lesions with imaging features suggestive of radial scar discovered during population-based screening for breast cancer. *Am J Surg Pathol.* 2004;28:1626–1631.
81. Sohn VY, Causey MW, Steele SR, Keylock JB, Brown TA. The treatment of radial scars in the modern era—surgical excision is not required. *Am Surg.* 2010;76:522–525.
82. Walker AN, Fechner RE, Mills SE, Perry JM. Epithelial polyps of the prostatic urethra: a light microscopic and immunohistochemical study. *Am J Surg Pathol.* 1983;7:351–356.
83. Natsheh A, Prat O, Shenfield OZ, Reinus C, Chertin B. Fibroepithelial polyp of the bladder neck in children. *Pediatr Surg Int.* 2008;24:613–615.
84. Frankendlaler R, Batsakis IG, Suarez PA. Tumefactive fibroinflammatory lesions of the head and neck. *Ann Otol Rhinol Laryngol.* 1993;102:481–482.
85. Savage PD, Wick MR, Thompson RC, Skubitz KM. Tumefactive fibroinflammatory lesion of the extremity. *Arch Pathol Lab Med.* 1991;115:230–232.
86. Klein MH, Rosenberg ZS, Lehman WB. Nonossifying fibroma of bone: a case report. *Bull Hosp Jt Dis Orthop Inst.* 1990;50:64–69.
87. Selby S. Metaphyseal cortical defects in tubular bones of growing children. *J Bone Joint Surg.* 1961;43A:395–404.
88. Bertoni F. Bacchini P, Capanna R, et al. Solid variant of aneurysmal bone cyst. *Cancer.* 1993;71:729–734.
89. Dahlin DC, McLeod RA. Aneurysmal bone cyst and other non-neoplastic conditions. *Skel Radiol.* 1982;8:243–250.
90. Salzer-Kuntschik M. Pitfalls and typical false interpretations in bone tumors, from the viewpoint of long-term consultation [in German]. *Pathologe.* 1996;17:1–5.
91. Sun ZJ, Zhao YF, Yang RL, Zwahlen RA. Aneurysmal bone cysts of the jaws: analysis of 17 cases. *J Oral Maxillofac Surg.* 2010;68:2122–2128.
92. Brastianos P, Gokasian Z, McCarthy EF. Aneurysmal bone cysts of the sacrum: a report of ten cases and review of the literature. *Iowa Orthop J.* 2009;29:74–78.
93. Smith J, Yuppa F, Watson RC. Primary tumors and tumor-like conditions of the clavicle. *Skel Radiol.* 1988;17:235–246.
94. Dahlin DC, Unni KK. *Bone Tumors.* 4th ed. Springfield, IL: Charles C Thomas; 1986:406–481.
95. Jelsma F, Ross PJ. Tumor-like lesions of the calvaria, due to general disease processes. *Am Surg.* 1963;29:247–255.
96. Dromer C, Caulier M, Le Guennec P, et al. Tumor-like bone dystrophy and peripheral joint fusion in a patient with Paget's disease of bone. *Rev Rheum (Engl Ed).* 1995;62:142–146.
97. Hunter SB, Ballinger WE Jr, Rubin JJ. Multiple sclerosis mimicking primary brain tumor. *Arch Pathol Lab Med.* 1987;111:464–468.
98. Takeuchi T, Ogura M, Sato M, et al. Late-onset tumefactive multiple sclerosis. *Radiat Med.* 2008;26:549–552.
99. Chebel S, Rekik O, Boughammoura-Bouatay A, Frih-Ayed M. Pseudotumoral presentation of multiple sclerosis [in French]. *Neurochirurgie.* 2007;53:379–382.
100. Caroli E, Salvati M, Ferrante L. Tumor-like multiple sclerosis: report of four cases and literature review. *Tumori.* 2006;92:559–562.
101. Woolner LB, McConahey WM, Beahrs OH. Stroma lymphomatosa (Hashimoto's thyroiditis) and related disorders. *J Clin Endocrinol Metab.* 1959;19:53–83.
102. LiVolsi VA. The thyroid and parathyroid. In: Sternberg SS, ed. *Diagnostic Surgical Pathology.* 2nd ed. New York, NY: Lippincott-Williams & Wilkins; 1994:523–560.

103. Wick MR, Mills SE, Ritter JH, Lind AC. Postoperative/posttraumatic spindle-cell nodule of the skin: the dermal analogue of nodular fasciitis. *Am J Dermatopathol.* 1999;21:220–224.
104. Stanley MW, Skoog L, Tani EM, Horwitz CA. Nodular fasciitis: spontaneous resolution following diagnosis by fine needle aspiration. *Diagn Cytopathol.* 1993;9:322–324.
105. Lundgren L, Kindblom LG, Willems J, Falkmer U, Angervall L. Proliferative myositis and fasciitis: a light and electron microscopic, cytologic, DNA-cytometric & immunohistochemical study. *APMIS.* 1992;100:437–448.
106. Sarangarajan R, Dehner LP. Cranial and extracranial fasciitis of childhood: a clinicopathologic and immunohistochemical study. *Hum Pathol.* 1999;30:87–92.
107. Silva P, Bruce IA, Malik T, Homer J, Banerjee S. Nodular fasciitis of the head and neck. *J Laryngol Otol.* 2005;119:8–11.
108. Flury D, von Hochstetter AR, Landolt U, Schmid S. Proliferative myositis: a little-known pseudomalignant lesion [in German]. *Schweiz Med Wochenschr.* 1993;123:29–34.
109. Jaffe HL. Giant cell reparative granuloma, traumatic bone cyst, and fibrous (fibro-osseous) dysplasia of the jawbones. *Oral Surg.* 1953;6:159–175.
110. Lorenzo IC, Dorfman HD. Giant cell reparative granuloma of short tubular bones of the hands and feet. *Am J Surg Pathol.* 1980;4:551–563.
111. Sass SM, Pinto MC, Jebahi Y, Bortolon L. Giant cell reparative granuloma in the mandible. *Braz J Otorhinolaryngol.* 2010;76:273.
112. Giusto TJ. Peripheral giant cell granuloma: report of two cases. *J NJ Dent Assoc.* 2010;81:22–24.
113. Hillerdal G. Asbestos-related pleural disease. *Semin Respir Med.* 1987;9:65–74.
114. Stephens M, Gibbs AR, Pooley FD, Wagner JC. Asbestos-induced pleural fibrosis: pathology and mineralogy. *Thorax.* 1987;42:583–588.
115. Howard TJ, Bennion RS, Thompson JE Jr. Xanthogranulomatous cholecystitis: a chronic inflammatory pseudotumor of the gallbladder. *Am Surg.* 1991;57:821–824.
116. Dao AH, Wong SW, Adkins RB Jr. Xanthogranulomatous cholecystitis: a clinical and pathologic study of twelve cases. *Am Surg.* 1989;55:32–35.
117. Malek RS, Elder JS. Xanthogranulomatous pyelonephritis: a critical analysis of 26 cases and of the literature. *J Urol.* 1978;119:589–595.
118. Kuo CC, Wu CF, Huang CC, et al. Xanthogranulomatous pyelonephritis: critical analysis of 30 patients. *Int Urol Nephrol.* 2011;43:15–22.
119. Bair MJ, Lin IT, Chen HL, Wu CH. Xanthogranulomatous pyelonephritis. *Am J Med Sci.* 2010;339:574.
120. Rao RV, Kumar A, Sikora SS, Saxena R, Kapoor VK. Xanthogranulomatous cholecystitis: differentiation from associated gallbladder carcinoma. *Trop Gastroenterol.* 2005;26:31–33.
121. Sommerville J. Pseudoepitheliomatous hyperplasia. *Acta Dermatoven.* 1953;33:236–245.
122. Winer LH. Pseudoepitheliomatous hyperplasia. *Arch Dermatol Syphilol.* 1940;42:856–863.
123. Yi JU, Lee CW. Acroangiodermatitis: a clinical variant of stasis dermatitis. *Int J Dermatol.* 1990;29:515–516.
124. Ackerman LV. Extraosseous localized non-neoplastic bone and cartilage formation (so-called myositis ossificans): clinical and pathological confusion with malignant neoplasms. *J Bone Joint Surg.* 1958;40A:279–298.
125. Goldman AB. Myositis ossificans circumscripta: a benign lesion with a malignant differential diagnosis. *AJR Am J Roentgenol.* 1976;126:32–40.
126. Montgomery EA, Meis JM, Mitchell MS, Enzinger FM. Atypical decubital fibroplasia: a distinctive fibroblastic pseudotumor occurring in debilitated patients. *Am J Surg Pathol.* 1992;16:708–715.
127. Fukunaga M. Atypical decubital fibroplasia with unusual histology. *APMIS.* 2001;109:631–635.
128. Ilaslan H, Joyce M, Bauer T, Sundaram M. Decubital ischemic fasciitis: clinical, pathologic, and MRI features of pseudosarcoma. *AJR Am J Roentgenol.* 2006;187:1338–1341.
129. Liegl B, Fletcher CD. Ischemic fasciitis: analysis of 44 cases indicating an inconsistent association with immobility or debilitation. *Am J Surg Pathol.* 2008;32:1546–1552.

130. Murphy FP, Dahlin DC, Sullivan CR. Articular synovial chondromatosis. *J Bone Joint Surg.* 1962;44A:77–86.
131. Gad A, Willen H, Willen R, Thorstensson S, Ekman L. Necrotizing sialometaplasia of the lip simulating squamous cell carcinoma. *Histopathology.* 1980;4:111–118.
132. Pagni F, Zarate AF, Urbanski SJ. Necrotizing sialometaplasia of bronchial mucosa. *Int J Surg Pathol.* 2010;18:64–65.
133. Carlson DL. Necrotizing sialometaplasia: a practical approach to the diagnosis. *Arch Pathol Lab Med.* 2009;133:692–698.
134. Parisi JE, Scheithauer BW. Glial tumors. In: Nelson JS, Parisi JE, Schochet SS, eds. *Principles & Practice of Neuropathology.* St Louis, MO: CV Mosby, 1993:123–183.
135. Young RH, Scully RE. Nephrogenic adenoma: a report of 15 cases. *Am J Surg Pathol.* 1986;10:268–275.
136. Saul SH. Inflammatory cloacogenic polyp. *Hum Pathol.* 1987;18:1120–1125.
137. Herman AH, Nabseth DC. Colitis cystica profunda: localized, segmental, and diffuse. *Arch Surg.* 1973;106:337–341.
138. Rosai J, Dehner LP. Nodular mesothelial hyperplasia in hernia sacs: a benign reactive condition simulating a neoplastic process. *Cancer.* 1975;35:165–175.
139. Cagle PT, Churg A. Differential diagnosis of benign and malignant mesothelial proliferations on pleural biopsies. *Arch Pathol Lab Med.* 2005;129:1421–1427.
140. Lee A, Baloch ZW, Yu G, Gupta PK. Mesothelial hyperplasia with reactive atypia: diagnostic pitfalls and role of immunohistochemical studies. *Diagn Cytopathol.* 2000;22:113–116.
141. Henderson DW, Shilkin KB, Whitaker D. Reactive mesothelial hyperplasia vs. mesothelioma, including mesothelioma in-situ: a brief review. *Am J Clin Pathol.* 1998;110:397–404.
142. Gambill EE. Pancreatitis associated with pancreatic carcinoma: a study of 26 cases. *Mayo Clin Proc.* 1971;46:174–177.
143. Bostwick DG, Egbert BM, Fajardo CF. Radiation injury of the normal and neoplastic prostate. *Am J Surg Pathol.* 1982;6:541–551.
144. Magi-Galluzzi C, Sanderson H, Epstein JI. Atypia in non-neoplastic prostate glands after radiotherapy for prostate cancer: duration of atypia and relation to type of radiotherapy. *Am J Surg Pathol.* 2003;27:206–212.
145. Civantos F. Difficulties in interpreting specimens after neoadjuvant hormonal therapy and radiation with illustration of neuroendocrine differentiation. *Mol Urol.* 2000;4:117–121.
146. Gaudin PB, Zelefsky MJ, Leibel SA, Fuks Z, Reuter VE. Histopathologic effects of three-dimensional conformal external beam radiation therapy on benign and malignant prostate tissues. *Am J Surg Pathol.* 1999;23:1021–1031.
147. Lane Z, Epstein JI. Polypoid/papillary cystitis: a series of 41 cases misdiagnosed as papillary urothelial neoplasia. *Am J Surg Pathol.* 2008;32:758–764.
148. Bonneau R, Brochu P. Neuromuscular choristoma. *Am J Surg Pathol.* 1983;7:521–528.
149. Daroca PJ Jr, Reed RI, Love GL, Kraus SO. Myoid hamartoma of the breast. *Hum Pathol.* 1985;16:212–219.
150. McDonald JR, Harrington SW, Clagett OT. Hamartoma (often called chondroma) of the lung. *J Thorac Surg.* 1945;14:128–143.
151. Takeyama J, Hayashi T, Sanada T, Shimanuki Y, Saito M, Shirane R. Rhabdomyomatous mesenchymal hamartoma associated with nasofrontal meningocele and dermoid cyst. *J Cutan Pathol.* 2005;32:310–313.
152. Cummings TJ, George TM, Fuchs HE, McLendon RE. The pathology of extracranial scalp and skull masses in young children. *Clin Neuropathol.* 2004;23:34–43.
153. Ferran M, Tribo MJ, Gonzalez-Rivero MA, Alameda F, Pujol RM. Congenital hamartoma of the scalp with meningothelial, sebaceous, muscular, and immature glandular components. *Am J Dermatopathol.* 2007;29:568–572.
154. Merchant WJ, Gale J. Intestinal metaplasia in stilbestrol-induced vaginal adenosis. *Histopathology.* 1993;23:373–376.

155. Antonioli DA, Burke L. Vaginal adenosis: analysis of 325 biopsy specimens from 100 patients. *Am J Clin Pathol.* 1975;64:625–638.
156. Robboy SJ, Hill EC, Sandberg EC, Czernobilsky B. Vaginal adenosis in women born prior to the diethylstilbestrol era. *Hum Pathol.* 1986;17:488–492.
157. Jones MA, Andrews J, Tarraza HM. Mesonephric remnant hyperplasia of the cervix: a clinicopathologic analysis of 14 cases. *Gynecol Oncol.* 1993;49:41–47.
158. Goldman RL. Hamartomatous polyp of Brunner's glands. *Gastroenterology.* 1963;44:57–62.
159. Sibley DA, Cooper PH. Rudimentary meningocele: a variant of "primary cutaneous meningioma." *J Cutan Pathol.* 1989;16:72–82.
160. Karma P, Rasanen O, Karja J. Nasal gliomas: a review and report of two cases. *Laryngoscope.* 1977;87:1169–1179.
161. McCall T, Chin SS, Salzman KL, Fults DW. Tuberous sclerosis: a syndrome of incomplete tumor suppression. *Neurosurg Focus.* 2006;20:E3.
162. Pritchard JE. Fibrous dysplasia of the bones. *Am J Med Sci.* 1951;222:313–332.
163. Regezi JA. Odontogenic cysts, odontogenic tumors, fibroosseous, and giant cell lesions of the jaws. *Mod Pathol.* 2002;15:331–341.
164. Dobbie JW. Adrenal cortical nodular hyperplasia: the aging adrenal. *J Pathol.* 1969;99:1–18.
165. Jones EC, Clement PB, Young RH. Sclerosing adenosis of the prostate gland: a clinicopathological and immunohistochemical study of 11 cases. *Am J Surg Pathol.* 1991;15:1171–1180.
166. Epstein J, Armas OA. Atypical basal cell hyperplasia of the prostate. *Am J Surg Pathol.* 1992;16:1205–1214.
167. Wanless IR, Mawdsley C, Adams R. The pathogenesis of focal nodular hyperplasia of the liver. *Hepatology.* 1985;5:1194–1200.
168. Kim T, Hori M, Onishi H. Liver masses with central or eccentric scar. *Semin Ultrasound CT MR.* 2009;30:418–425.
169. Yan BC, Hart JA. Recent developments in liver pathology. *Arch Pathol Lab Med.* 2009;133:1078–1086.
170. Boss JH, Scully RE, Wegner KH, Cohen RB. Structural variations in the adult ovary: clinical significance. *Obstet Gynecol.* 1965;25:747–763.
171. Silverberg SO. Arias-Stella phenomenon in spontaneous and therapeutic abortion. *Am J Obstet Gynecol.* 1972;112:777–780.
172. Nucci MR. Tumor-like glandular lesions of the uterine cervix. *Int J Gynecol Pathol.* 2002;21:347–359.
173. Arias-Stella J. The Arias-Stella reaction: facts and fancies four decades after. *Adv Anat Pathol.* 2002;12–23.
174. Yokota N, Kuribayashi T, Nagamine M, Tanaka M, Matsukura S, Wakisaka S. Paraplegia caused by brown tumor in primary hyperparathyroidism: case report. *J Neurosurg.* 1989;71:446–448.
175. Bassler T, Wong ET, Brynes RK. Osteitis fibrosa cystica simulating metastatic tumor: an almost-forgotten relationship. *Am J Clin Pathol.* 1993;100:697–700.
176. Verlaan L, van der Wal B, de Maat GJ, Walemkamp G, Nollen-Lopez L, van Ooij A. Primary hyperparathyroidism and pathological fractures: a review. *Acta Orthop Belg.* 2007;73:300–305.
177. Triantaffillidou K, Zouloumis L, Karakinaris G, Kalimeras E, Iordanidis F. Brown tumors of the jaws associated with primary or secondary hyperparathyroidism: a clinical study and review of the literature. *Am J Otolaryngol.* 2006;27:281–286.
178. Al-Gahtany M, Cusimano M, Singer W, Bilbao J, Kovacs K, Marotta T. Brown tumors of the skull base: case report and review of the literature. *J Neurosurg.* 2003;98:417–420.
179. Leslie KO, Silverberg SO. Microglandular hyperplasia of the cervix. *Pathol Annu.* 1982;17:95–114.
180. Proppe KH, Scully RE, Rosai J. Postoperative spindle cell nodules of genitourinary tract resembling sarcomas: a report of eight cases. *Am J Surg Pathol.* 1984;8:101–108.
181. Young RH. Spindle cell lesions of the urinary bladder. *Histol Histopathol.* 1990;5:505–512.

182. Garijo MF, Val-Bernal JF, Vega A, Val D. Postoperative spindle-cell nodule of the breast: pseudosarcomatous myofibroblastic proliferation following endosurgery. *Pathol Int.* 2008;58:787–791.
183. Lott S, Lopez-Beltran A, Maclennan GT, Montironi R, Cheng L. Soft tissue tumors of the urinary bladder, part I: myofibroblastic proliferations, benign neoplasms, and tumors of uncertain malignant potential. *Hum Pathol.* 2007;38:807–823.
184. Micci F, Haugom L, Abeler VM, Bjerkehagen B, Heim S. Trisomy 7 in postoperative spindle cell nodules. *Cancer Genet Cytogenet.* 2007;174:147–150.
185. Spiess PE, Tuziak T, Tibbs RF, et al. Pseudosarcomatous and sarcomatous proliferations of the bladder. *Hum Pathol.* 2007;38:753–761.
186. Harik LR, Merino C, Coindre JM, Amin MB, Pedeutour F, Weiss SW. Pseudosarcomatous myofibroblastic proliferations of the bladder: a clinicopathologic study of 42 cases. *Am J Surg Pathol.* 2006;30:787–794.
187. Sencer SF, Haake RI, Weisdorf DJ. Hemorrhagic cystitis after bone marrow transplantation: risk factors and complications. *Transplantation.* 1993;56:875–879.
188. Murray M. Non-neoplastic alterations of the mammary epithelium can mimic atypia. *Arch Pathol Lab Med.* 2009;133:722–728.
189. Young RH. Tumor-like lesions of the urinary bladder. *Mod Pathol.* 2009;22(suppl):S37–S52.
190. Nash G, Said JW, eds. *Pathology of AIDS & HIV Infection.* Philadelphia, PA: WB Saunders; 1992:5–25.
191. Umlas J, Federman M, Crawford C, O'Hara CJ, Fitzgibbon JS, Modeste A. Spindle cell pseudotumor due to *Mycobacterium avium-intracellulare* in patients with acquired immunodeficiency syndrome (AIDS). *Am J Surg Pathol.* 1991;15:1181–1187.
192. Wood C, Nickoloff BJ, Todes-Taylor NR. Pseudotumor resulting from atypical mycobacterial infection: a "histoid" variety of *Mycobacterium avium-intracellulare* complex infection. *Am J Clin Pathol.* 1985;83:524–527.
193. Chen KT. Mycobacterial spindle cell pseudotumor of lymph nodes. *Am J Surg Pathol.* 1992;16:276–281.
194. Wagner M, Rose VA, Linder R, Schulze HJ, Krueger GR. Human pathogenic virus-associated pseudolymphomas and lymphomas with primary cutaneous manifestation in humans and animals. *Clin Infect Dis.* 1998;27:1299–1308.
195. Chalvardjian A, Picard L, Shaw R, Davey R, Cairns JD. Malakoplakia of the female genital tract. *Am J Obstet Gynecol.* 1980;138:391–394.
196. Lioy-Lupis MT, Quintana RM, Monsalve J, Iotti RM. Testicular malakoplakia. *Arch Esp Urol.* 1993;46:822–824.
197. Kohl SK, Hans CP. Cutaneous malakoplakia. *Arch Pathol Lab Med.* 2008;132:113–117.
198. Yousef GM, Naghibi B, Hamodat MM. Malakoplakia outside the urinary tract. *Arch Pathol Lab Med.* 2007;131:297–300.
199. Srigley JR. Benign mimickers of prostatic adenocarcinoma. *Mod Pathol.* 2004;17:328–348.
200. Mansfield RE. Histoid leprosy. *Arch Pathol.* 1969;87:580–585.
201. Triscott JA, Nappi O, Ferrara G, Wick MR. "Pseudoneoplastic" leprosy. Leprosy revisited. *Am J Dermatopathol.* 1995;17:297–302.
202. Vantrappen G, Agg HO, Geboes K, Ponette E. Yersinia enteritis. *Med Clin North Am.* 1982;66:639–653.
203. Koss MN. Unusual tumor-like conditions of the lung. *Adv Pathol Lab Med.* 1994;7:123–150.
204. Albrecht E. Uber Harmartome. *Verh Dtsch Ges Pathol.* 1904;7:153–157.
205. McDonald JR, Harrington SW, Clagett OT. Hamartoma (often called chondroma) of the lung. *J Thorac Cardiovasc Surg.* 1945;14:128–143.
206. Tomashefski JF Jr. Benign endobronchial mesenchymal tumors: their relationship to parenchymal pulmonary hamartomas. *Am J Surg Pathol.* 1982;6:531–540.
207. Koutras P, Urschel HC, Paulson DL. Hamartoma of the lung. *J Thorac Cardiovasc Surg.* 1971;61:768–776.

208. Carter D, Eggleston JC. Tumors of the lower respiratory tract. In: *Atlas of Tumor Pathology*. Series 2. Washington, DC: Armed Forces Institute of Pathology; 1980:221–231.
209. Carney JA. The triad of gastric epithelioid leiomyosarcoma, functioning extra-adrenal paraganglioma, and pulmonary chondroma. *Cancer*. 1979;43:374–382.
210. Wick MR, Ruebner BH, Carney JA. Gastric tumors in patients with pulmonary chondroma or extra-adrenal paraganglioma: an ultrastructural study. *Arch Pathol Lab Med*. 1981;105:527–531.
211. van den Bosch JM, Wagenaar SS, Corrin B, Elbers JR, Knaepen PJ, Westermann CJ. Mesenchymoma of the lung (so-called hamartoma): a review of 154 parenchymal and endobronchial cases. *Thorax*. 1987;42:790–793.
212. Salminen US. Pulmonary hamartoma. A clinical study of 77 cases in a 21-year period and review of the literature. *Ear J Cardiothorac Surg*. 1990;4:15–18.
213. Hansen CP, Holtveg H, Francis D, Raasch L, Bertelsen S. Pulmonary hamartoma. *J Thorac Cardiovasc Surg*. 1992;104:674–678.
214. Wang SC. Lung hamartoma: a report of 30 cases and review of 477 cases [in Chinese]. *Zhonghua Wai Ke Za Zhi*. 1992;30:540–542.
215. Hamper UM, Khouri NF, Stitik FP, Siegelman SS. Pulmonary hamartoma: diagnosis by transthoracic needle aspiration biopsy. *Radiology*. 1985;155:15–18.
216. Bateson EM. Histogenesis of intrapulmonary and endobronchial hamartomas and chondromas (cartilage-containing tumors): a hypothesis. *J Pathol*. 1970;101:77–83.
217. Bateson EM. So-called hamartoma of the lung: a true neoplasm of fibrous connective tissue of the bronchi. *Cancer*. 1973;31:1458–1467.
218. Bateson EM. Relationship between intrapulmonary and endobronchial cartilage-containing tumors (so-called hamartoma). *Thorax*. 1965;20:447–461.
219. Incze JS, Lui PS. Morphology of the epithelial component of human lung hamartomas. *Hum Pathol*. 1977;8:411–419.
220. Sone FJ, Churg AM. The infrastructure of pulmonary hamartoma. *Cancer*. 1977;39:1064–1070.
221. Perez-Atayde AR. Seller MW. Pulmonary hamartoma: an ultrastructural study. *Cancer*. 1984;53:485–492.
222. Johansson M, Dietrich C, Mandahl N, et al. Recombinations of chromosomal bands 6p21 and 14q24 characterize pulmonary hamartomas. *Br J Cancer*. 1993;67:1236–1241.
223. Fletcher JA, Pinkus GS, Donovan K, et al. Clonal rearrangement of chromosome band 6p21 in the mesenchymal component of pulmonary chondroid hamartoma. *Cancer Res*. 1992;52:6224–6228.
224. Nappi O, Glasner SD, Swanson PE, Wick MR. Biphasic and monophasic sarcomatoid carcinomas of the lung. *Am J Clin Pathol*. 1994;102:331–340.
225. Liebow AA. Tumors of the lower respiratory tract. In: *Atlas of Tumor Pathology*. Series I. Washington, DC: Armed Forces Institute of Pathology; 1952:139–141.
226. Landreneau RJ, Hazelrigg SR, Ferson PF, et al. Thoracoscopic resection of 85 pulmonary lesions. *Ann Thorac Surg*. I992;54:415–420.
227. Nakano M, Fukuda M, Sasayama K, Nakata T, Fujimoto S, Araki J. Nd-YAG laser treatment for central airway lesions. *Nippon Kyoubu Shikkan Gakkai Zasshi*. 1992;30:1007–1015.
228. Su LD, Atayde-Perez A, Sheldon S, Fletcher JA, Weiss SW. Inflammatory myofibroblastic tumor: cytogenetic evidence supporting clonal origin. *Mod Pathol*. 1998;11:364–368.
229. Coffin CM, Dehner LP, Meis-Kindblom JM. Inflammatory myofibroblastic tumor, inflammatory fibrosarcoma, and related lesions: an historical review with differential diagnostic considerations. *Semin Diagn Pathol*. 1998;15:102–110.
230. Spencer H. The pulmonary plasma cell/histiocytoma complex. *Histopathology*. 1984;8:903–916.
231. Matsubara O, Tan-Liu NS, Kenney RM, Mark EJ. Inflammatory pseudotumors of the lung: progression from organizing pneumonia to fibrous histiocytoma or to plasma cell granuloma in 32 cases. *Hum Pathol*. 1988;19:807–814.

232. Pettinato G, Manivel JC, Rosa ND, Dehner LP. Inflammatory myofibroblastic tumor (plasma cell granuloma): clinicopathologic study of 20 cases with immunohistochemical and ultrastructural observations. *Am J Clin Pathol.* 1990;94:538–546.
233. Cavazza Gelli MC, Agostini L, Sgarbi G, De Marco L, Gardini G. Calcified pseudotumor of the pleura: description of a case. *Pathologica.* 2002;94:201–205.
234. Fetsch JF, Montgomery EA, Meis JM. Calcifying fibrous pseudotumor. *Am J Surg Pathol.* 1993;17:502–508.
235. Pinkard NB, Wilson RW, Lawless N, et al. Calcifying fibrous pseudotumor of the pleura: a report of three cases of a newly described entity involving the pleura. *Am J Clin Pathol.* 1996;105:189–194.
236. Pomplun S, Goldstraw P, Davies SE, Burke MM, Nicholson AG. Calcifying fibrous pseudotumor arising within an inflammatory pseudotumor: evidence of progression from one lesion to the other? *Histopathology.* 2000;37:380–382.
237. Suh JH, Shin OR, Kim YH. Multiple calcifying fibrous pseudotumor of the pleura. *J Thorac Oncol.* 2008;3:1356–1358.
238. Bahadori M, Liebow AA. Plasma cell granulomas of the lung. *Cancer.* 1973;31:191–208.
239. Anthony PP. Inflammatory pseudotumor (plasma cell granuloma) of lung, liver, and other organs. *Histopathology.* 1993;23:501–503.
240. Ahn JM, Kim WS, Yeon KM, Kim IO, Im JG, Han MC. Plasma cell granuloma involving the tracheobronchial angle in a child: a case report. *Pediatr Radiol.* 1995;25:204–205.
241. Copin MC, Gosselin BH, Ribet ME. Plasma cell granuloma of the lung: difficulties in diagnosis and prognosis. *Ann Thorac Surg.* 1996;61:1477–1482.
242. Mas Estelles F, Andres V, Vallcanera A, Muro D, Cortina H. Plasma cell granuloma of the lung in childhood: atypical radiologic findings and association with hypertrophic osteoarthropathy. *Pediatr Radiol.* 1995;25:369–372.
243. Monzon CM, Gilchrist GS, Burgert EO, et al. Plasma cell granuloma of the lung in children. *Pediatrics.* 1982;70:268–274.
244. Tomita T, Dixon A, Watanabe I, Mantz F, Richany S. Sclerosing vascular variant of plasma cell granuloma. *Hum Pathol.* 1980;11:197–202.
245. Toccanier MF, Exquis B, Groebli Y. Plasma cell granuloma. Immunohistochemical Investigations about 9 cases. *Ann Pathol.* 1982;2:21–28.
246. Kobashi Y, Fukuda M, Nakata M, Irei T, Oka M. Inflammatory pseudotumor of the lung: clinicopathological analysis in seven adult patients. *Int J Clin Oncol.* 2006;11:461–466.
247. Mohsenifar Z, Bein ME, Mott LJ, Tashkin DP. Cystic organizing pneumonia with elements of plasma cell granuloma. *Arch Pathol Lab Med.* 1979;103:600–601.
248. Cerfolio RJ, Allen MS, Nascimento AG, et al. Inflammatory pseudotumors of the lung. *Ann Thorac Surg.* 1999;67:933–936.
249. Agrons GA, Rosado-de-Cristenson ML, Kirejczyk WM, Conran RM, Stocker JT. Pulmonary inflammatory pseudotumor: radiologic features. *Radiology.* 1998;206:511–518.
250. Kawisawa T, Okamoto A. IgG4-related sclerosing disease. *World J Gastroenterol.* 2008;14:3948–3955.
251. Shrestha B, Sekiguchi H, Colby TV, et al. Distinctive pulmonary histopathology with increased IgG4-positive plasma cells in patients with autoimmune pancreatitis; report of 6 and 12 cases with similar histopathology. *Am J Surg Pathol.* 2009;33:1450–1462.
252. Yamamoto H, Yamaguchi H, Aishima S, et al. Inflammatory myofibroblastic tumor versus IgG4-related sclerosing disease and inflammatory pseudotumor: a comparative clinicopathologic study. *Am J Surg Pathol.* 2009;33:1330–1340.
253. Zen Y, Inoue D, Kitao A, et al. IgG4-related lung and pleural disease: a clinicopathologic study of 21 cases. *Am J Surg Pathol.* 2009;33:1886–1893.
254. Kojima M, Nakamura N, Itoh H, et al. Presence of immunoglobulin heavy-chain rearrangement in so-called "plasma cell granuloma" of the lung. *Pathol Res Pract.* 2010;206:83–87.

255. Park SH, Choe GY, Kim CW, Chi JG, Sung SH. Inflammatory pseudotumor of the lung in a child with Mycoplasma pneumonia. *J Korean Med Sci.* 1990;5:213–223.
256. Harjula A, Mattila S, Kyoesola K, Heikkilae L, Maekinen J. Plasma cell granuloma of lung and pleura. *Scand J Thorac Cardiovasc Surg.* 1986;20:119–121.
257. Loo KT, Seneviratne S, Chan JKC. Mycobacterial infection mimicking inflammatory pseudotumor of the lung. *Histopathology.* 1989;14:217–219.
258. Kim I, Kim WS, Yeon KM, Chi JG. Inflammatory pseudotumor of the lung manifesting as a posterior mediastinal mass. *Ped Radiol.* 1992;22:467–468.
259. Kuhr H, Svane S. Pulmonary pseudotumor caused by *Cryptococcus neoformans* [in Norwegian]. *Tidsskr Norweg Laegeforen.* 1991;111:3288–3290.
260. Bishopric GA, d'Agay MF, Schlemmer B, Sarfati E, Brocheriou C. Pulmonary pseudotumor due to *Corynebacterium equi* in a patient with the acquired immunodeficiency syndrome. *Thorax.* 1988;43:486–487.
261. Yanagisawa K, Traquina DN. Inflammatory pseudotumor: an unusual case of recurrent pneumonia in childhood. *Int J Ped Otorhinolaryngol.* 1993;25:261–268.
262. Freschi P, Pocecco M, Carini C, Silvestri F, Alcaro P. Post-traumatic inflammatory pseudotumor of the lung: Description of a case. *Ped Med e Chir.* 1989;11:93–96.
263. Roikjaer O, Thomsen JK. Plasmacytoma of the lung. *Cancer.* 1986;58:2671–2674.
264. Weiss LM, Yousem SA, Warnke RA. Non-Hodgkin's lymphomas of the lung. *Am J Surg Pathol.* 1985;9:480–490.
265. Toh HC, Ang PT. Primary pulmonary lymphoma—clinical review from a single institution in Singapore. *Leuk Lymphoma.* 1997;27:153–163.
266. Kradin RL, Mark EJ. Benign lymphoid disorders of the lung with a theory regarding their development. *Hum Pathol.* 1983;14:857–867.
267. Michal M, Mukensnabl P. Epithelial plasma cell granuloma-like tumors of the lungs: a hitherto-unrecognized tumor. *Pathol Res Pract.* 2002;198:311–316.
268. Wick MR, Ritter JH, Nappi O. Inflammatory sarcomatoid carcinoma of the lung: report of three cases and comparison with inflammatory pseudotumors in adult patients. *Hum Pathol.* 1995;26:1014–1021.
269. Yousem SA, Hochholzer L. Pulmonary hyalinizing granuloma. *Am J Clin Pathol.* 1987;87:1–6.
270. Alvarez-Fernandez E, Carretero-Albinana L, Menarguez-Palance J. Sclerosing hemangioma of the lung: an immunohistochemical study of intermediate filaments and endothelial markers. *Arch Pathol Lab Med.* 1989;113:121–124.
271. Illei PB, Rosai J, Klimstra DS. Expression of thyroid transcription factor-1 and other markers in sclerosing hemangioma of the lung. *Arch Pathol Lab Med.* 2001;125:1335–1339.
272. Ledet SC, Brown RW, Cagle PT. p53 immunoreactivity in the differentiation of inflammatory pseudotumor from sarcoma involving the lung. *Mod Pathol.* 1995;8:282–286.
273. Doski JJ, Priebe CJ Jr, Driessnack M, Smith T, Kane P, Romero J. Corticosteroids in the management of unresected plasma cell granuloma (inflammatory pseudotumor) of the lung. *J Ped Surg.* 1991;26:1064–1066.
274. Umeki S. A case of plasma cell granuloma which resolved after steroid treatment [in Japanese]. *Nihon Kyoubu Shikkan Gakkai Zasshi.* 1993;31:123–126.
275. Imperato JP, Folkman J, Sagerman RH, Cassady JR. Treatment of plasma cell granuloma of the lung with radiation therapy: a report of two cases and a review of the literature. *Cancer.* 1986;57:2127–2129.
276. Wood C, Nickoloff BJ, Todes-Taylor NR. Pseudotumor resulting from atypical mycobacterial infection: a "histoid" variety of *Mycobacterium avium-intracellulare* complex infection. *Am J Clin Pathol.* 1985;83:524–527.
277. Brandwein M, Choid H-SH, Strauchen J, Stroler M, Jagirdar J. Spindle cell reaction to nontuberculous mycobacteriosis in AIDS mimicking a spindle cell neoplasm: evidence for dual histiocytic and fibroblast-like characteristics of cells. *Virchows Arch Pathol Anat.* 1990;416:281–286.

278. Umlas J, Federman M, Crawford C, O'Hara BAC, Fitzgibbons J, Modeste A. Spindle cell pseudotumor due to *Mycobacterium avium-intracellulare* in patients with acquired immunodeficiency syndrome (AIDS): positive staining of mycobacteria for cytoskeleton filaments. *Am J Surg Pathol.* 1991;15(12):1181–1187.
279. Chen KT. Mycobacterial spindle cell pseudotumor of lymph nodes. *Am J Surg Pathol.* 1992;16(3):276–281.
280. Wade HW. The histoid variety of lepromatous leprosy. *Int Lepr.* 1963;31:129–142.
281. Sekosan M, Cleto M, Senseng C, Farolan M, Sekosan J. Spindle cell pseudotumors in the lungs due to *Mycobacterium tuberculosis* in a transplant patient. *Am J Surg Pathol.* 1992;18:1065–1068.
282. Isaacson PG, Spencer J. Malignant lymphoma of mucosa-associated lymphoid tissue. *Histopathology.* 1987;11:445–462.
283. Addis BJ, Hyjek E, Isaacson PG. Primary pulmonary lymphoma: a reappraisal of its histogenesis and its relationship to pseudolymphoma and lymphoid interstitial pneumonia. *Histopathology.* 1988;13:l–7.
284. Theron S, Andronikou S, George R, et al. Non-infective pulmonary disease in HIV-positive children. *Pediatr Radiol.* 2009;39:555–564.
285. Koss MN. Lymphoproliferative disorders of the lung. In: Marchevsky AM, ed. *Surgical Pathology of Lung Neoplasms.* New York, NY: Marcel Dekker; 1990.
286. Koss MN, Hochholzer L, Langloss JM, Wehunt WD, Lazarus AA. Lymphoid interstitial pneumonia: clinicopathological and immunopathological findings in 18 cases. *Pathology.* 1987;19:178–185.
287. Morris JC, Rosen MJ, Marchevsky AM, Teirstein AS. Lymphocytic interstitial pneumonia in patients at risk for the acquired immune deficiency syndrome. *Chest.* 1987;91:63–67.
288. Strimlan CV, Rosenow EC III, Divertie MB, Harrison EG Jr. Pulmonary manifestations of Sjogren's syndrome. *Chest.* 1976;70:354–361.
289. Liebow AA, Carrington CB. Diffuse pulmonary lymphoreticular infiltration association with dysproteinemia. *Med Clin North Am.* 1973;57:809–843.
290. Kradin RL, Mark EJ. Benign lymphoid disorders of the lung with a theory regarding their development. *Hum Pathol.* 1983;14:857–867.
291. Vath RR, Alexander CB, Fulmer JD. The lymphocytic infiltrative lung diseases. *Clin Chest Med.* 1982;3:619–634.
292. Koss MN, Hochholzer L, Nichols PW, Wehunt WD, Lazarus AA. Primary non-Hodgkin's lymphomas and pseudolymphomas of the lung: a study of 161 patients. *Hum Pathol.* 1983;14:1024–1038.
293. Banerjee D, Dildar A. Malignant lymphomas complicating lymphoid interstitial pneumonia. *Hum Pathol.* 1982;13:780–782.
294. Salhany KG, Pietra GG. Extranodal lymphoid disorders. *Am J Clin Pathol.* 1993;99:472–485.
295. Andiman WA, Eastman R, Martin K, et al. Opportunistic lymphoproliferations associated with Epstein–Barr viral DNA in infants and children with AIDS. *Lancet.* 1985;2:1390–1393.
296. Schooley RT, Carey RW, Miller G, et al. Chronic Epstein–Barr virus infection associated with fever and interstitial pneumonitis. *Ann Intern Med.* 1986;104:636–646.
297. Resnick L, Pitchenik AE, Fisher E, Croney R. Detection of HTLV-111/LAV-specific IgG and antigen in bronchoalveolar lavage fluid from two patients with lymphocytic interstitial pneumonia associated with AIDS-related complex. *Am J Med.* 1987;82:553–556.
298. Keller AR, Hochholzer L, Castleman B. Hyaline-vascular and plasma cell types of giant lymph node hyperplasia of the mediastinum and other locations. *Cancer.* 1972;29:670–676.
299. Ritter JH, Wick MR. Post-transplant lymphoproliferative disorders: immunohistologic differential diagnosis with severe allograft rejection. *Int J Surg Pathol.* 1994;2:105–116.
300. LaCasce AS. Post-transplant lymphoproliferative disorders. *Oncologist.* 2006;11:674–680.
301. Jacobson CA, LaCasce AS. Lymphoma: risk and response after solid organ transplant. *Oncology.* 2010;24:936–944.

302. Orjuela MA, Alobeid B, Liu X, et al. CD20 expression predicts survival in pediatric post-transplant lymphoproliferative disease (PTLD) following solid organ transplantation [published online ahead of print January 30, 2011]. *Br J Haematol.* 2011;152:733–742.
303. Dolcetti R. B-lymphocytes and Epstein–Barr virus: the lesson of post-transplant lymphoproliferative disorders. *Autoimmun Rev.* 2007;7:96–101.
304. Yousem SA, Martin T, Paradis IL, Keenan R, Griffith BP. Can immunohistological analysis of transbronchial biopsy specimens predict responder status in early acute rejection of lung allografts? *Hum Pathol.* 1994;25:525–529.
305. Foucar E, Rosai J, Dorfman R. Sinus histiocytosis with massive lymphadenopathy (Rosai–Dorfman disease): review of the entity. *Semin Diagn Pathol.* 1990;7:19–73.
306. Wang CW, Colby TV. Histiocytic lesions and proliferations in the lung. *Semin Diagn Pathol.* 2007;24:162–182.
307. Wright DH, Richards DB. Sinus histiocytosis with massive lymphadenopathy (Rosai–Dorfman disease): report of a case with widespread nodal and extranodal dissemination. *Histopathology.* 1981;5:697–709.
308. Ratzinger G, Zelger B, Hobling W, Mikuz G, Zelger BW. Sinus histiocytosis with massive lymphadenopathy (Rosai–Dorfman disease): three unusual manifestations. *Virchows Arch.* 2003;443:797–800.
309. Lutterbach J, Henne K, Pagenstecher A, Bohm J. Lung cancer and Rosai–Dorfman disease: a clinicopathological study. *Strahlenther Onkol.* 2003;179:486–492.
310. Castleman B, Iverson L, Menendez VP. Localized mediastinal lymph node hyperplasia resembling thymoma. *Cancer.* 1956;9:822–830.
311. Yeh CM, Chou CM, Wong LC. Castleman's disease mimicking intrapulmonary malignancy. *Ann Thorac Surg.* 2007;84:e6–e7.
312. Nicholson AG. Lymphocytic interstitial pneumonia and other lymphoproliferative disorders in the lung. *Semin Respir Crit Care Med.* 2001;22:409–422.
313. Buckley J, Shaw PJ, Cartledge JD, Miller RF. Multicentric plasma cell variant Castleman's disease mimicking intrapulmonary malignancy. *Sex Transm Infect.* 2002;78:304–305.
314. Barrie JR, English JC, Muller N. Castleman's disease of the lung: radiographic, high-resolution CT, and pathologic findings. *AJR Am J Roentgenol.* 1996;166:1055–1056.
315. Spedini C, Lombardi C, Lanzani G, Di Fabio D, Chiodera PL. Castleman's disease presenting as an asymptomatic solitary pulmonary nodule. *Monaldi Arch Chest Dis.* 1995;50:363–365.
316. Awotedu AA, Otulana BA, Ukoli CD. Giant lymph node hyperplasia of the lung (Castleman's disease) associated with recurrent pleural effusion. *Thorax.* 1990;45:775–776.
317. Epstein DM, Glickstein MF. Pulmonary lymphoproliferative disorders. *Radiol Clin North Am.* 1989;27:1077–1084.
318. Glickstein MF, Kornstein MJ, Pietra GG, et al. Nonlymphomatous lymphoid disorders of the lung. *AJR Am J Roentgenol.* 1986;147:227–237.
319. Joynt GH, Pantalony D. Angiofollicular lymph node hyperplasia of the lung simulating carcinoma: pseudolymphoma with inflammatory changes. *Can J Surg.* 1975;18:536–541.
320. Frizzera G, Banks PM, Massarelli G, Rosai J. A systemic lymphoproliferative disorder with morphologic features of Castleman's disease: pathological findings in 15 patients. *Am J Surg Pathol.* 1983;7:211–231.
321. Frizzera G. Castleman's disease and related disorders. *Semin Diagn Pathol.* 1988;5:346–364.
322. Krishnan J, Danon AD, Frizzera G. Reactive lymphadenopathies and atypical lymphoproliferative disorders. *Am J Clin Pathol.* 1993;99:385–396.
323. Peterson BA, Frizzera G. Multicentric Castleman's disease. *Semin Oncol.* 1993;20:636–647.
324. Keller AR, Hochholzer L, Castleman B. Hyaline-vascular and plasma-cell types of giant lymph node hyperplasia of the mediastinum and other locations. *Cancer.* 1972;29:670–683.
325. Dorfman RF, Cibull M. Castleman's disease. *Recent Results Cancer Res.* 1978;64:284–287.
326. Bartoli E, Massarelli G, Soggia G, Tanda F. Multicentric giant lymph node hyperplasia: a hyperimmune syndrome with a rapidly progressive course. *Am J Clin Pathol.* 1980;73:423–426.

327. Gaba AR, Stein RS, Sweet DL, Variakojis D. Multicentric giant lymph node hyperplasia. *Am J Clin Pathol.* 1978;69:86–90.
328. Ulbright TM, Santa Cruz DJ. Kaposi's sarcoma: relationship with hematologic, lymphoid, and thymic neoplasia. *Cancer.* 1981;47:963–973.
329. Fazakas A, Csire M, Berencsi G, et al. Multicentric plasmacytic Castleman's disease with polyneuropathy, organomegaly, endocrinopathy, M protein, skin changes syndrome and coexistent human herpesvirus-6 infection—a possible relationship. *Leuk Lymphoma.* 2009;50:1661–1665.
330. Bragg DG, Chor PJ, Murray KA, Kjeldsberg CR. Lymphoproliferative disorders of the lung: histopathology, clinical manifestations, and imaging features. *AJR Am J Roentgenol.* 1994;163:273–281.
331. Suster S, Moran CA. Micronodular thymoma with lymphoid B-cell hyperplasia: clinicopathologic and immunohistochemical study of eighteen cases of a distinctive morphologic variant of thymic epithelial neoplasm. *Am J Surg Pathol.* 1999;23:955–962.
332. Tateyama H, Saito Y, Fujii Y, et al. The spectrum of micronodular thymic epithelial tumors with lymphoid B-cell hyperplasia. *Histopathology.* 2001;38:519–527.
333. Strobel P, Marino M, Feuchtenberger M, et al. Micronodular thymoma: an epithelial tumor with abnormal chemokine expression setting the stage for lymphoma development. *J Pathol.* 2005;207:72–82.
334. Chunduri S, Gaitonde S, Ciurea SO, Hoffman R, Rondelli D. Pulmonary extramedullary hematopoiesis in patients with myelofibrosis undergoing allgeneic stem cell transplantation. *Haematologica.* 2008;93:1593–1595.
335. Bowling MR, Cauthen CG, Perry CD, et al. Pulmonary extramedullary hematopoiesis. *J Thorac Imaging.* 2008;23:138–141.
336. Ogus C, Ozdemir T, Kabaalioglu A. Right hilar mass in a patient with beta-thalassemia major. *Respiration.* 2001;68:215–216.
337. Kumar PV, Arasteh M, Musallaye A, Hakshanash M. Fine needle aspiration diagnosis of extramedullary hematopoiesis presenting as a right lung mass. *Acta Cytol.* 2000;44:698–699.
338. Hsu FI, Filippa DA, Castro-Malaspina H, Downey RJ. Extramedullary hematopoiesis mimicking metastatic lung carcinoma. *Ann Thorac Surg.* 1998;66:1411–1413.
339. Schwarz C, Bittner R, Kirsch A, et al. A 62 year-old woman with bilateral pleural effusions and pulmonary infiltrates caused by extramedullary hematopoiesis. *Respiration.* 2009;78:110–113.
340. Nappi O, Boscaino A, Wick MR. Extramedullary hematopoietic proliferations, extraosseous plasmacytomas, and ectopic splenic implants (splenosis). *Semin Diagn Pathol.* 2003;20:338–356.
341. Wandall HH. A study on neoplastic cells in sputum as a contribution to the diagnosis of primary lung cancer. *Acta Chir Scand.* 1944;91(suppl 93):1–143.
342. Koss LG. *Diagnostic Cytology and Its Histologic Basis.* 4th ed. Philadelphia, PA: JB Lippincott; 1992:849–864.
343. Erozan YS. Cytopathologic diagnosis of pulmonary neoplasms in sputum and bronchoscopic specimens. *Semin Diagn Pathol.* 1986;3:188–195.
344. Jay SJ, Wehr K, Nicholson DP, Smith AE. Diagnostic sensitivity and specificity of pulmonary cytology. *Acta Cytol.* 1980;24:304–312.
345. Pearson FG, Thompson DW, Delarue NC. Experience with the cytologic detection, localization, and treatment of radiographically undemonstrable bronchial carcinoma. *J Thorac Cardiovasc Surg.* 1967;54:371–382.
346. Zavala DC. Diagnostic fiberoptic bronchoscopy: techniques and results of biopsy in 600 patients. *Chest.* 1975;68:12–19.
347. Truong LD, Underwood RD, Greenberg SD, McLarty JW. Diagnosis and typing of lung carcinomas by cytopathologic methods: a review of 108 cases. *Acta Cytol.* 1985;29:379–384.
348. Berkheiser JW. Bronchiolar proliferation and metaplasia associated with bronchiectasis, pulmonary infarct, and anthracosis. *Cancer.* 1959;12:499–508.

349. Berkheiser JW. Bronchiolar proliferation and metaplasia associated with thromboembolism: a pathological and experimental study. *Cancer*. 1963;16:205–211.
350. Kawecka M. Cytological evaluation of the sputum in patients with bronchiectasis and the possibility of erroneous diagnosis of carcinoma. *Acta Union Int Cancer*. 1959;15:469–473.
351. Marchevsky AM, Nieburgs HE, Olenko F, Kirschner P, Teirstein A, Kleinerman J. Pulmonary tumorlets in cases of "tuberculoma" of the lung with malignant cells in brush biopsy. *Acta Cytol*. 1982;26:491–494.
352. Johnston WW, Frable WJ, Cytopathology of the respiratory tract: a review. *Am J Pathol*. 1976;84:371–424.
353. Saccomanno G, Archer VE, Auerbach O, Saunders RD, Brennan LM. Development of carcinoma of the lung as reflected in exfoliated cells. *Cancer*. 1974;33:256–270.
354. Koss LG, Richardson HI. Some pitfalls of cytological diagnosis of lung cancer. *Cancer*. 1955;8:937–947.
355. Plamenac P, Nikulin A, Pikula B. Cytologic changes of the respiratory tract in young adults as a consequence of high levels of air pollution exposure, *Acta Cytol*. 1973;17:241–244.
356. Kern WH. Cytology of hyperplastic and neoplastic lesions of terminal bronchioles and alveoli. *Acta Cytol*. 1965;9:372–379.
357. McKee G, Parums DV. False positive cytodiagnosis in fibrosing alveolitis. *Acta Cytol*. 1990;34:105–107.
358. Meyer EC, Liebow AA. Relationship of interstitial pneumonia and honey-combing and typical epithelial proliferation to cancer of the lung. *Cancer*. 1965;18:322–351.
359. Williams JW. Alveolar metaplasia: its relationship to pulmonary fibrosis in industry and development of lung cancer. *Br J Cancer*. 1957;11:30–42.
360. Johnston WW. Type II pneumocytes in cytologic specimens: a diagnostic dilemma. *Am J Clin Pathol*. 1992;97:608–609.
361. Clayton F. The spectrum and significance of bronchioloalveolar carcinoma. *Pathol Annu*. 1988;23(2):361–394.
362. Stanley MW, Henry-Stanley MJ, Gajl-Peczakska KJ, Bitterman PB. Hyperplasia of type II pneumocytes in acute lung injury. *Am J Clin Pathol*. 1992;97:669–677.
363. Grotte D, Stanley MW, Swanson PC, Henry-Stanley MJ, Davies S. Reactive type II pneumocyte in bronchoalveolar lavage fluid from acute respiratory distress syndrome can be mistaken for cells of adenocarcinoma. *Diagn Cytopathol*. 1990;6:317–322.
364. Miura H, Kato H, Hayata V, Ebihara Y, Gonullu U. Solitary bronchial mucosal neuroma. *Chest*. 1989;95:245–247.
365. Rossi G, Marchioni A, Agostini L, Corradini P, Costantini M, Cavazza A. Traumatic neuroma of the bronchi: bronchoscopy and histology of a hitherto-unreported lesion. *Am J Surg Pathol*. 2008;32:640–641.
366. Pagni F, Zarate AF, Urbanski SJ. Necrotizing sialometaplasia of bronchial mucosa. *Int J Surg Pathol*. 2010;18:64–65.
367. Couture C, Colby TV. Histopathology of bronchiolar disorders. *Semin Respir Crit Care Med*. 2003;24:489–498.
368. Fukuoka J, Franks TJ, Colby TV, et al. Peribronchiolar metaplasia: a common histologic finding in diffuse lung disease and a rare cause of interstitial lung disease: clinicopathologic features of 15 cases. *Am J Surg Pathol*. 2005;29:948–954.
369. Kilicgun A, Turna A, Gurses A. Pulmonary malacoplakia. *Acta Chir Belg*. 2006;106:732–733.
370. Pang LC. Pulmonary malakoplakia coexistent with tuberculosis of the hilar lymph node, mimicking malignancy. *Respiration*. 2005;72:95–100.
371. Kumar P, Rassl DM, Hamilton JR, Spencer DA. Pulmonary malakoplakia in an immunocompetent girl: a case report. *Pediatr Pulmonol*. 2003;36:450–452.
372. Guerrero MF, Ramos JM, Renedo G, Gadea I, Alix A. Pulmonary malakoplakia associated with *Rhodococcus equi* infection in patients with AIDS: case report and review. *Clin Infect Dis*. 1999;28:1334–1336.

373. Shin MS, Cooper JA Jr, Ho KJ. Pulmonary malakoplakia associated with *Rhodococcus equi* infection in a patient with AIDS. *Chest.* 1999;115:889–892.
374. Rekhi B, Jambhekar NA. Morphologic spectrum, immunohistochemical analysis, and clinical features of a series of granular cell tumors of soft tissues: a study from a tertiary referral cancer center. *Ann Diagn Pathol.* 2010;14:162–167.
375. Cibas ES. Effusions (pleural, pericardial, and peritoneal) and peritoneal washings. In: Atkinson B, ed. *Atlas of Diagnostic Cytopathology.* 2nd ed. Philadelphia, PA: WB Saunders; 2003.
376. Bibbo M. *Comprehensive Cytopathology.* 2nd ed. Philadelphia, PA: WB Saunders; 1996.
377. Koss LG. *Diagnostic Cytology and its Histopathologic Bases.* 5th ed. Philadelphia, PA: Lippincott-Williams & Wilkins; 2005.
378. McCaughey WT, Al-Jabi M. Differentiation of serosal hyperplasia and neoplasia in biopsies. *Pathol Annu.* 1986;21(1):271–293.
379. Sears D, Hajdu SI. The cytologic diagnosis of malignant neoplasms in pleural and peritoneal effusions. *Acta Cytol.* 1987;31:85–97.
380. Kobayashi TK, Gotoh T, Nakano K, Kanagawa Y, Kimura T, Sato T. Atypical mesothelial cells associated with eosinophilic pleural effusions: nuclear DNA content and immunocytochemical staining reaction with epithelial markers. *Cytopathology.* 1993;4:37–46.
381. Chen CJ, Chang SC, Tseng HH. Assessment of immunocytochemical and histochemical staining in the distinction between reactive mesothelial cells and adenocarcinoma in body effusions. *Chinese Med J.* 1994;54:149–155.
382. Schultenover SJ. Body cavity fluids. In: Ramzi I, ed. *Clinical Cytopathology and Aspiration Biopsy.* East Norwalk, CT: Appleton-Lange; 1990:165–180.
383. Leong AS-Y, Stevens MW, Mukherjee TM. Malignant mesothelioma: cytologic diagnosis with histologic, immunohistochemical, and ultrastructural correlation. *Semin Diagn Pathol.* 1992;9:141–150.
384. Bedrossian CW, Bonsib S, Moran C. Differential diagnosis between mesothelioma and adenocarcinoma: a multimodal approach based on ultrastructure and immunocytochemistry. *Semin Diagn Pathol.* 1992;9:91–96.
385. Kutty CP, Remeniuk E, Varkey B. Malignant-appearing cells in pleural effusion due to pancreatitis. *Acta Cytol.* 1981;25:412–416.
386. Marchevsky AM, Hauptman E, Gil J, Watson C. Computerized interactive morphometry as an aid in the diagnosis of pleural effusions. *Acta Cytol.* 1987;31:131–136.
387. Kwee WS, Veldhuizen RW, Alons CA, Morawetz F, Boon ME. Quantitative and qualitative differences between benign and malignant mesothelial cells in pleural fluid. *Acta Cytol.* 1982;26:401–406.
388. Oberholzer M, Ettlin R, Christen H, et al. The significance of morphometric methods in cytologic diagnostics: differentiation between mesothelial cells, mesothelioma cells, and metastatic adenocarcinoma cells in pleural effusions with special emphasis on chromatin texture. *Analyt Cell Pathol.* 1991;3:25–42.
389. Ranaldi R, Marinelli F, Barbatelli G, et al. Benign and malignant mesothelial lesions of the pleura: quantitative study. *Appl Pathol.* 1986;4:55–64.
390. Battifora H. The pleura. In: Mills SE, ed. *Sternberg's Diagnostic Surgical Pathology.* 5th ed. Philadelphia, PA: Lippincott-Williams & Wilkins; 2009:1096–1119.
391. Roberts GH, Campbell GH. Exfoliative cytology of diffuse mesothelioma. *J Clin Pathol.* 1972;25:557–582.
392. Bolen JW. Tumors of serosal tissue origin. *Clin Lab Med.* 1987;7:31–50.
393. Whitaker D, Henderson DW, Shilkin KB. The concept of mesothelioma in situ: implications for diagnosis and histogenesis. *Semin Diagn Pathol.* 1992;9:151–161.
394. Bolen JW, Hammar SP, McNutt MA. Reactive and neoplastic serosal tissue: a light-microscopic, ultrastructural, and immunocytochemical study. *Am J Surg Pathol.* 1986;10:34–47.
395. Singh HK, Silverman JF, Berns L, Haddad MG, Park HK. Significance of epithelial membrane antigen in the workup of problematic serous effusions. *Diagn Cytopathol.* 1995;13:3–7.

396. Hasteh F, Lin GY, Weidner N, Michael CW. The use of immunohistochemistry to distinguish reactive mesothelial cells from malignant mesothelioma in cytologic effusions. *Cancer Cytopathol*. 2010;118:90–96.
397. Lidang-Jensen M, Johansen P. Immunocytochemical staining of serous effusions: an additional method in routine cytology practice? *Cytopathology*. 1994;5:93–103.
398. Bethwaite PB, Delahunt B. Holloway LJ, Thornton A. Comparison of silver-staining nucleolar organizer region (AgNOR) counts and proliferating cell nuclear antigen (PCN A) expression in reactive mesothelial hyperplasia and malignant mesothelioma. *Pathology*. 1995;27:1–4.
399. Kafiri G, Thomas DM, Shepherd NA, Krasz T, Lane DP, Hall PA. p53 expression is common in malignant mesothelioma. *Histopathologv*. 1992;21:331–334.
400. Cagle PT, Brown RW, Lebovitz RM. p53 immunostaining in the differentiation of reactive processes from malignancy in pleural biopsy specimens. *Hum Pathol*. 1994;25:443–448.
401. Walts AE, Said JW, Koeffler HP. Is immunoreactivity for p53 useful in distinguishing benign from malignant effusions? Localization of p53 gene product in benign mesothelial and adenocarcinoma cells. *Mod Pathol*. 1994;7:462–468.
402. Humphrey PA. p53: mutations and immunohistochemical detection, with a focus on alterations in urologic malignancies. *Adv Pathol Lab Med*. 1994;7:579–596.
403. Hammar SP. Pleural diseases. In: Dail DH, Hammar SP, eds. *Pulmonary Pathology*. 2nd ed. New York, NY: Springer-Verlag; 1994.
404. Westfall DE, Fan X, Marchevsky AM. Evidence-based guidelines to optimize the selection of antibody panels in cytopathology: pleural effusions with malignant epithelioid cells. *Diagn Cytopathol*. 2010;38:9–14.
405. Marchevsky AM. Application of immunohistochemistry to the diagnosis of malignant mesothelioma. *Arch Pathol Lab Med*. 2008;132:397–401.
406. Marchevsky AM, Wick MR. Evidence-based guidelines for the utilization of immunostains in diagnostic pathology: pulmonary adenocarcinoma versus mesothelioma. *Appl Immunohistochem Mol Morphol*. 2007;15:140–144.
407. Husain AN, Colby TV, Ordonez NG, et al. Guidelines for pathologic diagnosis of malignant mesothelioma: a consensus statement from the International Mesothelioma Interest Group. *Arch Pathol Lab Med*. 2009;133:1317–1331.
408. Yaziji H, Battifora H, Barry TS, et al. Evaluation of 12 antibodies for distinguishing epithelioid mesothelioma from adenocarcinoma: identification of a three-antibody immunohistochemical panel with maximal sensitivity and specificity. *Mod Pathol*. 2006;19:514–523.
409. el-Habashi A, el-Morsi B. Freeman SM, el-Didi M, Marrogi AJ. Tumor oncogenic expression in malignant effusions as a possible method to enhance cytologic diagnostic sensitivity. An immunocytochemical study of 87 cases. *Am J Clin Pathol*. 1995;103:206–214.
410. Czader M, Ali SZ. Flow cytometry as an adjunct to cytomorphologic analysis of serous effusions. *Diagn Cytopathol*. 2003;29:74–78.
411. Mihaescu A, Gebhard S, Chaubert P, et al. Application of molecular genetics to the diagnosis of lymphoid-rich effusions: study of 95 cases with concomitant immunophenotyping. *Diagn Cytopathol*. 2002;27:90–95.
412. Sparks JW. Pulmonary asbestosis. *Radiology*. 1931;17:1249–1257.
413. Smith AR. Pleural calcification resulting from exposure to certain dusts. *Am J Roentgenol Radium Ther Nucl Med*. 1952;69:375–382.
414. Churg A. Asbestos fibers and pleural plaques in a general autopsy population. *Am J Pathol*. 1982;109:88–96.
415. Churg A, DePaoli L. Environmental pleural plaques in residents of a Quebec chrysotile mining town. *Chest*. 1988;94:58–60.
416. Craighead JE. Report of the pneumoconiosis committee of the College of American Pathologists and the National Institute for Occupational Safety and Health. *Arch Pathol Lab Med*. 1982;106:544–596.

417. Fondimare A, Duwoos H, Desbordes J, et al. Calcified fibro-hyaline plaques in the liver in asbestosis. *Nouv Presse Med.* 1973;3:893.
418. Hillerdal G. Pleural plaques in a health survey material: frequency, development and exposure to asbestos. *Scand J Respir Dis.* 1978;59:257–263.
419. Hillerdal G. The pathogenesis of pleural plaques and pulmonary asbestosis: possibilities and impossibilities. *Eur J Respir Dis.* 1980;61:129–138.
420. Hourihane DO, Lessof L, Richardson PC. Hyaline and calcified pleural plaques as an index of exposure to asbestos: a study of radiological and pathological features of 100 cases with a consideration of epidemiology. *BMJ.* 1966;1:1069–1074.
421. Kishimoto T, Ono T, Okada K, Ito H. Relationship between numbers of asbestos bodies in autopsy lung and pleural plaques on chest x-ray film. *Chest.* 1989;95:549–552.
422. Kiviluoto R. Pleural calcification as a roentgenologic sign of nonoccupational endemic anthophyllite asbestosis. *Acta Radiol.* 1960;194:1–67.
423. LeBouffant L, Martin JC, Durif S, Daniel H. Structure and composition of pleural plaques. In: Bogovski P, Gilson JC, Timbrell V, Wagner JC, eds. *Biological Effects of Asbestos.* Lyon, France: International Agency for Research on Cancer; 1973:249–257.
424. Mattson S, Ringqvist T. Pleural plaques and exposure to asbestos. *Scand J Respir Dis.* 1970;75:1–41.
425. Meurman L. Asbestos bodies and pleural plaques in a Finnish series of autopsy cases. *Acta Pathol Microbiol Scand.* 1966;181:7–107.
426. Roberts GH. The pathology of parietal pleural plaques. *J Clin Pathol.* 1961;21:348–353.
427. Solomon A. Radiologic features of asbestos-related visceral pleural changes. *Am J Indust Med.* 1991;19:339–355.
428. Wain SL, Roggli VL, Foster WL Jr. Parietal pleural plaques, asbestos bodies and neoplasia: a clinical, pathologic and roentgenographic correlation of 25 consecutive cases. *Chest.* 1985;86:707–713.
429. Warnock ML, Prescott BT, Kuwahara TJ. Numbers and types of asbestos fibers in subjects with pleural plaques. *Am J Pathol.* 1982;109:37–46.
430. Schwartz DA. New developments in asbestos-induced pleural disease. *Chest.* 1991;99:91–98.
431. Ameille J, Brochard P, Brechot JM, et al. Pleural thickening: a comparison of oblique chest radiographs and high resolution computed tomography in subjects exposed to low levels of asbestos pollution. *Int Arch Occup Environ Health.* 1993;64:545–548.
432. Wilson GE, Haselton PS, Chatterjee AK. Desmoplastic mesothelioma: a review of 17 cases. *J Clin Pathol.* 1992;45:295–298.
433. Cantin R, Al-Jabi M, McCaughey WT. Desmoplastic diffuse mesothelioma. *Am J Surg Pathol.* 1982;6:215–222.
434. Epstein JI, Budin RE. Keratin and epithelial membrane antigen immunoreactivity in non-neoplastic fibrous pleural lesions: implications for the diagnosis of desmoplastic mesothelioma. *Hum Pathol.* 1986;17:566–571.
435. Rdzanek M, Fresco R, Pass HI, Carbone M. Spindle-cell tumors of the pleura: differential diagnosis. *Semin Diagn Pathol.* 2006;23:44–55.
436. Travis WD. Sarcomatoid neoplasms of the lung and pleura. *Arch Pathol Lab Med.* 2010;134:1645–1658.
437. Cagle PT, Truong LD, Spencer EJ, Greenberg SD. Immunohistochemical differentiation of sarcomatoid mesotheliomas from other spindle cell neoplasms. *Am J Clin Pathol.* 1989;92:566–571.
438. Dardick I, Srigley JR, McCaughey WT, van Nostrand AW, Richie AC. Ultrastructural aspects of the histogenesis of diffuse and localized mesothelioma. *Virchows Arch A Path Anat.* 1984;402:373–378.
439. Moran CA, Susler S, Koss M. The spectrum of histologic growth patterns in benign and malignant fibrous tumors of the pleura. *Semin Diagn Pathol.* 1992;9:169–180.
440. Liu CC, Wang HW, Li FY, et al. Solitary fibrous tumors of the pleura: clinicopathological characteristics, immunohistochemical profiles, and surgical outcomes with long-term followup. *Thorac Cardiovasc Surg.* 2008;56:291–297.

441. Nascimento AF, Ruiz R, Hornick JL, Fletcher CDM. Calcifying fibrous "pseudotumor": clinicopathologic study of 15 cases and analysis of its relationship to inflammatory myofibroblastic tumor. *Int J Surg Pathol.* 2002;10:189–196.
442. Kilburn KH, Warshaw R. Pulmonary functional impairment associated with pleural asbestos disease: circumscribed and diffuse thickening. *Chest.* 1990;98:965–972.
443. Oury TD. Benign asbestos-related pleural diseases. In: Roggli VL, Oury TD, Sporn TA, eds. *Pathology of Asbestos-Associated Diseases.* 2nd ed. New York, NY: Springer; 2004:169–192.
444. Zen Y, Inoue D, Kitao A, et al. IgG4-related lung and pleural disease: a clinicopathologic study of 21 cases. *Am J Surg Pathol.* 2009;33:1886–1893.
445. Epler GR, McCloud TC, Gaensler EA. Prevalence and incidence of benign asbestos pleural effusion in a working population. *JAMA.* 1982;247:617–622.
446. Gibbs AR, Stephens M, Griffiths DM, Blight BJN, Pooley FD. Fiber distribution in the lungs and pleura of subjects with asbestos-related diffuse pleural fibrosis. *Br J Indust Med.* 1991;48:762–770.
447. Moalli PA, MacDonald JL, Goodglick LA, Kane AB. Acute injury and regeneration of the mesothelium in response to asbestos fibers. *Am J Pathol.* 1987;128:426–445.
448. Stephens M, Gibbs AR, Pooley FD, Wagner JC. Asbestos-induced diffuse pleural fibrosis: pathology and mineralogy. *Thorax.* 1987;42:583–588.
449. Taskinen E, Ahlamn K, Wukeri M. A current hypothesis of the lymphatic transport of inspired dust to the parietal pleura. *Chest.* 1973;64:193–196.
450. Churg A, Colby TV, Cagle PT, et al. The separation of benign and malignant mesothelial proliferations. *Am J Surg Pathol.* 2000;24:1183–1200.
451. Mangano WE, Cagle PT, Churg A, Vollmer RT, Roggli VL. The diagnosis of desmoplastic malignant mesothelioma and its distinction from fibrous pleurisy: a histologic and immunohistochemical analysis of 31 cases including p53 immunostaining. *Am J Clin Pathol.* 1998;110:191–199.
452. Klebe S, Brownlee NA, Mahar A, et al. Sarcomatoid mesothelioma: a clinicopathologic correlation of 326 cases. *Mod Pathol.* 2010;23:470–479.
453. Anton HC, Ferguson JB, Lewis GP. Pleural extramedullary hematopoiesis in myelosclerosis. *Postgrad Med J.* 1967;43:428–432.
454. Bartlett RP, Greipp PR, Tefferi A, Cupps RE, Mullan BP, Trastek VF. Extramedullary hematopoiesis manifesting as a symptomatic pleural effusion. *Mayo Clin Proc.* 1995;70:1161–1164.
455. Santini M, Fiorelli A, Vicidomini G, Napolitano F. Intrathoracic extramedullary hematopoiesis manifested as a neoplastic lesion within anterior mediastinum. *Ann Thorac Surg.* 2009;88:2001–2004.
456. Ohori NP, Yu J, Landreneau RJ, Thaete FL, Kane K. Rosai–Dorfman disease of the pleura: a rare extranodal presentation. *Hum Pathol.* 2003;34:1210–1211.
457. Chen J, Tang H, Li B, Xiu Q. Rosai-Dorfman disease of multiple organs, including the epicardium: an unusual case with poor prognosis [published online ahead of print April 8, 2010]. *Heart Lung.* 2011;40:168–171.
458. Calore EE, Vazquez CR, Perez NM, et al. Empyema with malakoplakic-like lesions by *Rhodococcus equi* as a presentation of HIV infection. *Pathologica.* 1995;87:525–527.
459. O'Driscoll J. Giant lymph node hyperplasia presenting as a pleural mass. *Ir Med J.* 1985;78:132–133.
460. Reynolds SP, Gibbs AR, Weeks R, Adams H, Davies BH. Massive pleural effusion: an unusual presentation of Castleman's disease. *Eur Respir J.* 1992;5:1150–1153.
461. Ko SF, Ng SH, Hsieh MJ, et al. Castleman disease of the pleura: experience with eight surgically-proven cases. *Ann Thorac Surg.* 2003;76:219–224.
462. Marchevsky AM. Mediastinal tumor-like conditions and tumors that can simulate thymic neoplasms. In: Givel J-C, ed. *Surgery of the Thymus.* Berlin: Springer-Verlag; 1990:151–162.
463. Tazzioli G, Fontana G, De Santis M, Drei B, Melita V, Casolo P. Plasma-cell granuloma of the mediastinum. *Minerva Chir.* 1998;53:549–551.

464. Wick MR, Rosai J. Epithelial tumors; neuroendocrine, germ cell, and nonepithelial tumors. In: Givel J-C, ed. *Surgery of the Thymus*. Berlin: Springer-Verlag; 1990:79–150.
465. Miller JB, Variakojis D, Bitran JD, et al. Diffuse histiocytic lymphoma with sclerosis: a clinicopathologic entity frequently causing superior vena caval obstruction. *Cancer*. 1981;47:748–756.
466. Perrone TA, Frizzera G, Rosai J. Mediastinal diffuse large-cell lymphoma with sclerosis: a clinicopathologic study of 60 cases. *Am J Pathol*. 1986;10:176–191.
467. Baum GL, Green RA, Schwarz J. Enlarging pulmonary histoplasmoma. *Am Rev Respir Dis*. 1960;82:721–726.
468. Schowwengerdt CG. Suyemoto R, Main FB. Granulomatous and fibrous mediastinitis: a review and analysis of 180 cases. *J Thorac Cardiovasc Surg*. 1969;57:365–379.
469. Light AM. Idiopathic fibrosis of the mediastinum: a discussion of three cases and review of the literature. *J Clin Pathol*. 1978;31:78–88.
470. Dines DE, Payne WS, Bernatz PE, Pairolero PC. Mediastinal granulomas and fibrosing mediastinitis. *Chest*. 1979;75:320–324.
471. Strimlan CV, Dines DE, Payne WS. Mediastinal granuloma. *Mayo Clin Proc*. 1975;50:702–705.
472. Ferguson TB, Burford TH. Mediastinal granuloma: a 15-year experience. *Ann Thorac Surg*. 1965;l:125–141.
473. Kunkel WM Jr, Clagett OT, McDonald JR. Mediastinal granulomas. *J Thorac Surg*. 1954;27:565–574.
474. Salyer JM, Harrison HN, Winn DF Jr, Taylor RR. Chronic fibrous mediastinitis and superior vena caval obstruction due to histoplasmosis. *Dis Chest*. 1959;35:364–377.
475. Wieder S, Rabinowitz JG. Fibrous mediastinitis: a late manifestation of mediastinal histoplasmosis. *Radiology*. 1977;125:305–312.
476. Tecce PM, Fishman EK, Kuhlman JE. CT evaluation of the anterior mediastinum: spectrum of disease. *Radiographics*. 1994;14:973–990.
477. Yi E, Aubry MC. Pulmonary pseudoneoplasms. *Arch Pathol Lab Med*. 2010;134:417–425.
478. Cheuk W, Chan JKC. IgG4-relating sclerosing disease: a critical appraisal of an evolving clinicopathologic entity. *Adv Anat Pathol*. 2010;17:303–332.
479. Zen Y, Sawazaki A, Miyayama S, Notsumata K, Tanaka N, Nakanuma Y. A case of retroperitoneal and mediastinal fibrosis exhibiting elevated levels of IgG4 in the absence of sclerosing pancreatitis (autoimmune pancreatitis). *Hum Pathol*. 2006;37:239–243.
480. Flannery MT, Espino M, Altus P, Messina J, Wallach PM. Hodgkin's disease masquerading as sclerosing mediastinitis. *South Med J*. 1994;87:921–923.
481. Dehner LP, Coffin CM. Idiopathic fibrosclerotic disorders and other inflammatory pseudotumors. *Semin Diagn Pathol*. 1998;15:161–173.
482. DasGupta TK, Brasfield RD, O'Hara J. Extra-abdominal desmoids: a clinicopathological study. *Ann Surg*. 1969;170:109–117.
483. Yokoyama R, Tsuneyoshi M, Enjoji M. Extra-abdominal desmoid tumors: correlations between histologic features and biologic behavior. *Surg Pathol*. 1989;2:292.
484. Bhattacharya B, Dilworth HP, Iacobuzio-Donahue C, et al. Nuclear beta-catenin expression distinguishes deep fibromatosis from other benign and malignant fibroblastic and myofibroblastic lesions. *Am J Surg Pathol*. 2005;29:653–659.
485. Wold LE, Weiland LH. Tumefactive fibroinflammatory lesions of the head and neck. *Am J Surg Pathol*. 1983;7:477–482.
486. Olsen KD, DeSanto LW, Wold LE, Weiland LH. Tumefactive fibroinflammatory lesions of the head and neck. *Laryngoscope*. 1986;96:940–944.
487. Savage PD, Wick MR, Thompson RC, Skubitz KM. Tumefactive fibroinflammatory lesion of the extremity. *Arch Pathol Lab Med*. 1991;115:230–232.
488. De Boer WA. Riedel's thyroiditis, retroperitoneal fibrosis, and sclerosing cholangitis: diseases with one pathogenesis? *Gut*. 1993;34:714.
489. Kelly JK, Hwang WS. Idiopathic retractile (sclerosing) mesenteritis and its differential diagnosis. *Am J Surg Pathol*. 1989;13:513–521.

490. Ormond JK. Bilateral ureteral obstruction due to envelopment and compression by an inflammatory retroperitoneal process. *J Urol.* 1948;59:1072–1079.
491. Osborne BM, Butler JJ, Bloustein P, Sumner G. Idiopathic retroperitoneal fibrosis (sclerosing retroperitonitis). *Hum Pathol.* 1987;18:735–739.
492. Ross DS, Daniels GH. Riedel's thymiditis associated with Hashimoto's thyroiditis. *J Endocrinol Invest.* 1992;107:591–595.
493. Turner-Warwick R, Nabarro JD, Domach D. Riedel's thyroiditis and retroperitoneal fibrosis. *Proc R Soc Med.* 1966;59:596–598.
494. Zimmerman-Belsing T, Feldi-Rasmussen U. Riedel's thyroiditis: an autoimmune or primary fibrotic disease? *J Intern Med.* 1994;235:271–274.
495. Mitchinson MJ. The pathology of idiopathic retroperitoneal fibrosis. *J Clin Pathol.* 1970;23:681–689.
496. Rutty GN, Lauder I. Mesothelial inclusions within mediastinal lymph nodes. *Histopathology.* 1994;25:483–487.
497. Brooks JSJ, LiVolsi VA, Pietra GG. Mesothelial cell inclusions in mediastinal lymph nodes mimicking metastatic carcinoma. *Am J Clin Pathol.* 1990;93:741–748.
498. Sion-Vardy N, Diomin V, Benharroch D. Hyperplastic mesothelial cells in subpleural lymph nodes, mimicking metastatic carcinoma. *Ann Diagn Pathol.* 2004;8:373–374.
499. Parkash V, Vidwans M, Carter D. Benign mesothelial cells in mediastinal lymph nodes. *Am J Surg Pathol.* 1999;23:1264–1269.
500. Krech WG, Storey CF, Umiker WC. Thymic cysts: a review of the literature and report of two cases. *J Thorac Cardiovasc Surg.* 1954;27:477–493.
501. Ovrum E, Birkeland S. Mediastinal tumors and cysts: a review of 91 cases. *Scan J Thorac Cardiovasc Surg.* 1979;13:161–168.
502. Bieger RC, McAdams AJ. Thymic cysts. *Arch Pathol.* 1966;82:535–541.
503. Suster S, Rosai J. Multilocular thymic cyst: an acquired reactive process. Study of 18 cases. *Am J Surg Pathol.* 1991;15:388–398.
504. Choi YW, McAdams HP, Jeon SC, et al. Idiopathic multilocular thymic cyst: CT features with clinical and histopathologic correlation. *AJR Am J Roentgenol.* 2001;177:881–885.
505. Wick MR. Cystic lesions of the mediastinum. *Semin Diagn Pathol.* 2005;22:241–253.
506. Suster S, Barbuto D, Carlson G, et al. Multilocular thymic cysts with pseudoepitheliomatous hyperplasia. *Hum Pathol.* 1991;22:455–460.
507. Sau P, Graham JH, Helwig EB. Proliferating epithelial cysts. Clinicopathological analysis of 96 cases. *J Cutan Pathol.* 1995;22:394–406.
508. Leong AS, Brown JH. Malignant transformation in a thymic cyst. *Am J Surg Pathol.* 1984;8:471–475.
509. Hattori H. High-grade thymic carcinoma other than basaloid or mucoepidermoid type could be associated with multilocular thymic cyst: report of two cases. *Histopathology.* 2003;43:501–502.
510. Iezzoni JC, Nass LB. Thymic basaloid carcinoma: a case report and review of the literature. *Mod Pathol.* 1996;9:21–25.
511. Kondo K, Miyoshi T, Sakiyama S, Shimosato Y, Monden Y. Multilocular thymic cyst associated with Sjogren's syndrome. *Ann Thorac Surg.* 2001;72:1367–1369.
512. Chhieng DC, Demaria S, Yee HT, Yang GC. Multilocular thymic cyst with follicular lymphoid hyperplasia in a male infected with HIV: a case report with fine needle aspiration cytology. *Acta Cytol.* 1999;43:1119–1123.
513. Kontny HU, Sleasman JW, Kingma DW, et al. Multilocular thymic cysts in children with human immunodeficiency virus infection: clinical and pathologic aspects. *J Pediatr.* 1997;131:264–270.
514. Avila NA, Mueller BU, Carrasquillo JA, Kontny HU, Jaffe ES, Pizzo PA. Multilocular thymic cysts: imaging features in children with human immunodeficiency virus infection. *Radiology.* 1996;201:130–134.
515. Leonidas JC, Berdon WE, Valderrama E, et al. Human immunodeficiency virus infection and multilocular thymic cysts. *Radiology.* 1996;198:377–379.

516. Baron RL, Sagel SS, Baglan RJ. Thymic cysts following radiation therapy for Hodgkin's disease. *Radiology*. 1981;141:593–597.
517. Kin HC, Nosher J, Haas A, Sweeney W, Lewis R. Cystic degeneration of thymic Hodgkin's disease following radiation therapy. *Cancer*. 1985;55:354–356.
518. Lewis CR, Manoharan A. Benign thymic cysts in Hodgkin's disease: report of a case and review of published cases. *Thorax*. 1987;42:633–634.
519. Borgna-Pignatti C, Andreis IB, Rugolotto S, Balter R, Bontempini L. Thymic cyst appearing after treatment of mediastinal non-Hodgkin lymphoma. *Med Pediatr Oncol*. 1994;22:70–72.
520. Veeze-Kuijpers B, Van Andel JG, Stiegelis WF, Boldewijn JK. Benign thymic cyst following mantle radiotherapy for Hodgkin's disease. *Clin Radiol*. 1987;38:289–290.
521. Kaesberg PR, Foley DB, Pellett J, Hafez GR, Ershler WB. Concurrent development of a thymic cyst and mediastinal Hodgkin's disease. *Med Pediatr Oncol*. 1988;16:293–294.
522. Suster S, Rosai J. Cystic thymomas: a clinicopathologic study of ten cases. *Cancer*. 1992;69:92–97.
523. Moran CA, Suster S. Thymoma with prominent cystic and hemorrhagic changes and areas of necrosis and infarction: a clinicopathologic study of 25 cases. *Am J Surg Pathol*. 2001;25:1086–1090.
524. Moran CA, Suster S. Mediastinal seminomas with prominent cystic changes: a clinicopathologic study of 10 cases. *Am J Surg Pathol*. 1995;19:1047–1053.
525. Moran CA, Suster S. Cystic well-differentiated neuroendocrine carcinoma (carcinoid tumor): a clinicopathologic and immunohistochemical study of two cases. *Am J Clin Pathol*. 2006;126:377–380.
526. Moran CA, Suster S, Silva EG. Low-grade serous carcinoma of the ovary metastatic to the anterior mediastinum simulating multilocular thymic cysts: a clinicopathologic and immunohistochemical study of 3 cases. *Am J Surg Pathol*. 2005;29:496–499.
527. Grant RP, Van Ordstrand HS. Sarcoidosis—recent progress in etiology and pathogenesis. *Cleve Clin Q*. 1967;34:205–216.
528. James DG. Sarcoidosis. *Dis Mon*. 1970;Feb:1–43.
529. Koessler A, Grosshans E, Samain F, Runser C, Bernard F, Heid E. Tumoral sarcoidosis. *Ann Dermatol Venereol*. 1995;122:783–785.
530. Louzir B, Beji M, Souissi Z, Mehiri N, el Mekki F, Dagfous J. Pseudotumor presentation of pulmonary sarcoidosis apropos of 3 cases. *Rev Pneumonol Clin*. 1997;53:144–148.
531. Dumitrescu SM, Schwartz RA, Baredes S, et al. Mutilating facial sarcoidosis. *Dermatology*. 1999;199:265–267.
532. Sacks EL, Donaldson SS, Gordon J, Dorfman RF. Epithelioid granulomas associated with Hodgkin's disease: clinical correlations in 55 previously-untreated patients. *Cancer*. 1978;41:562–567.
533. Trier H, Christensen M. Hodgkin's disease in sarcoidosis: a case report and a review of the literature. *Acta Med Scand*. 1985;218:137–140.
534. Merchant TE, Filippa DA, Yahalom J. Sarcoidosis following chemotherapy for Hodgkin's disease. *Leuk Lymphoma*. 1994;13:339–347.
535. Laurberg P. Sarcoid reactions in pulmonary neoplasms. *Scand J Respir Dis*. 1975;56:20–27.
536. Steinfort DP, Irving LB. Sarcoidal reactions in regional lymph nodes of patients with non-small-cell lung cancer: incidence and implications for minimally-invasive staging with endobronchial ultrasound. *Lung Cancer*. 2009;66:305–308.
537. Singla S, Litzky LA, Kaiser LR, Shrager JB. Should asymptomatic enlarged thymus glands be resected? *J Thorac Cardiovasc Surg*. 2010;140:977–983.
538. Regal MA. Gigantic enlargement of the thymus gland. *Saudi Med J*. 2007;28:1587–1589.
539. Woywodt A, Verhaart S, Kiss A. Massive true thymic hyperplasia. *Eur J Pediatr Surg*. 1999;9:331–333.
540. Yamanaka K, Nakayama H, Watanabe K, Kameda Y. Anterior mediastinal mass in a patient with Graves' disease. *Ann Thorac Surg*. 2006;81:1904–1906.

541. Hofmann WJ, Moller P, Otto HF. Hyperplasias. In: Givel J-C, ed. *Surgery of the Thymus*. New York, NY: Springer; 1990:59–70.
542. Mlika M, Ayadi-Kaddour A, Marghli A, Ismail O, Kilani T, El Mezni F. True thymic hyperplasia versus follicular thymic hyperplasia: a retrospective analysis of 13 cases. *Pathologica*. 2009;101:175–179.
543. Wick MR. The mediastinum. In: Mills SE, ed. *Sternberg's Diagnostic Surgical Pathology*. 5th ed. Philadelphia, PA: Lippincott-Williams & Wilkins; 2009:1120–1177.
544. Becroft DM, Dix MR, Gillman JC, MacGregor BJ, Shaw RL. Benign sinus histiocytosis with massive lymphadenopathy: transient immunological defects in a child with mediastinal involvement. *J Clin Pathol*. 1973;26:463–469.
545. Costa AL, Silva NO, Motta MP, Athanazio RA, Athanazio DA, Athanazio PR. Soft tissue Rosai–Dorfman disease of the posterior mediastinum. *J Bras Pneumonol*. 2009;35:717–720.
546. Lim R, Wittram C, Ferry JA, Shepard JA. FDG-PET of Rosai–Dorfman disease of the thymus. *AJR Am J Roentgenol*. 2004;182:514–515.
547. Srivastava AK, Agrawal RL. Mediastinal masses due to extramedullary hematopoiesis. *Indian J Chest Dis Allied Sci*. 1990;32:39–41.
548. Moran CA, Suster S, Fishback N, Koss MN. Extramedullary hematopoiesis presenting as a posterior mediastinal mass: a study of four cases. *Mod Pathol*. 1995;8:249-251.
549. Roger T. Mediastinal extramedullary hematopoiesis. *J Belge Radiol*. 1998;81:248–249.
550. Psichoglou H, Malagarl K, Spanomichos G. Mediastinal extramedullary hematopoiesis in hemolytic anemia. *JBR-BTR*. 2004;87:150–151.
551. Gogia P, Goel R, Nayar S. Extramedullary paraspinal hematopoiesis in hereditary spherocytosis. *Ann Thorac Med*. 2008;3:64–66.
552. Pulsoni A, Ferrazza G, Malagnino F, et al. Mediastinal extramedullary hematopoiesis as first manifestation of hereditary spherocytosis. *Ann Hematol*. 1992;65:196–198.
553. Hanfling SM. Metastatic cancer to the heart. *Circulation*. 1960;22:474–483.
554. Thurber DL, Edwards JE, Achor RW. Secondary malignant tumors of the pericardium. *Circulation*. 1962;26:228–241.
555. Burnett RC, Shimkin MB. Secondary neoplasms of the heart. *Arch Intern Med*. 1954;93:205–218.
556. McAllister HA Jr, Fenoglio JJ Jr. Tumors of the cardiovascular system. In: *Atlas of Tumor Pathology*. Series 2. Fascicle 15. Washington, DC: Armed Forces Institute of Pathology; 1978.
557. Fine G. Primary tumors of the pericardium and heart. *Cardiovasc Clin*. 1973;5:207–238.
558. Prichard RW. Tumors of the heart: review of the subject and report of one hundred and fifty cases. *Arch Pathol*. 1951;51:98–128.
559. Tazelaar HD, Locke TJ, McGregor CG. Pathology of surgically excised primary cardiac tumors. *Mayo Clin Proc*. 1992;67:957–965.
560. Wiatrowska BA, Walley VM, Masters RG, Goldstein W, Keon WJ. Surgery for cardiac tumors: the university of ottawa heart institute experience. *Can J Cardiol*. 1993;9:65–72.
561. Lund JT, Ehman RL, Julsrud PR, Sinak LJ, Tajik AJ. Cardiac masses: assessment by MR imaging. *AJR Am J Roentgenol*. 1989;152:469–473.
562. Burke AP, Virmani R. Cardiac myxoma: a clinicopathologic study. *Am J Clin Pathol*. 1993;100:671–680.
563. Fenoglio JJ Jr, McAllister HA Jr, Ferrans VJ. Cardiac rhabdomyoma: a clinicopathologic and electron microscopic study. *Am J Cardiol*. 1976;38:241–251.
564. Taber RE, Lam CR. Diagnosis and surgical treatment of intracardiac myxoma and rhabdomyoma. *J Thorac Cardiovasc Surg*. 1960;40:337–354.
565. Silverman JF, Kay S, McCue CM, Lower RR, Brough AJ, Chang CH. Rhabdomyomas of the heart: ultrastructural study of three cases. *Lab Invest*. 1976;35:596–606.
566. Dehner LP, Enzinger FM, Font RL. Fetal rhabdomyoma: an analysis of nine cases. *Cancer*. 1972;30:160–166.
567. Kapadia SB, Meis JM, Frisman DM, Ellis GL, Heffner DK. Fetal rhabdomyoma of the head and neck: a clinicopathologic and immunophenotypic study of 24 cases. *Hum Pathol*. 1993;24:754–765.

568. Crotty PL, Nakhleh RE, Dehner LP. Juvenile rhabdomyoma: an intermediate form of skeletal muscle tumor in children. *Arch Pathol Lab Med.* 1993;117:43–47.
569. Viscardi F, Errico G, Schiavo N, Biban P, Mazzucco A, Luciani GB. Familial fetal-type rhabdomyoma of the tricuspid valve in the neonate: malignant course for a benign disease. *J Thorac Cardiovasc Surg.* 2009;137:751–753.
570. Gao BH, Xie LW, Zhao ZG, Wang ZM, Wang SL. Huge right ventricular fetal-type rhabdomyoma in an infant—a case report. *Chin J Pathol.* 2004;33:302–303.
571. Miller DV, Edwards WD. Cardiovascular tumor-like conditions. *Semin Diagn Pathol.* 2008;25:54–64.
572. Fresneau B, Oberlin O, Brugieres L, Valteau-Couanet D, Patte C. Malignant primary cardiac tumors in childhood and adolescence. *Arch Pediatr.* 2010;17:495–501.
573. Lima RC, Mendes A, Bezerra E, Oliveira W. Surgical treatment of primary cardiac rhabdomyosarcoma. *Rev Bras Cir Cardiovasc.* 2009;24:242–244.
574. Fraternali-Orcioni G, Ravetti JL, Gaggero G, Bocca B, Bisceglia M. Primary embryonal spindle-cell cardiac rhabdomyosarcoma: case report. *Pathol Res Pract.* 2010;206:325–330.
575. Neragi-Miandoab S, Kim J, Vlahakes GJ. Malignant tumors of the heart: a review of tumor type, diagnosis, and therapy. *Clin Oncol.* 2007;19:748–756.
576. Scott RS, Jagirdar J. Right atrial botryoid rhabdomyosarcoma in an adult patient with recurrent pleomorphic rhabdomyosarcoma following doxorubicin therapy. *Ann Diagn Pathol.* 2007;11:274–276.
577. Thomas-de-Montpreville V, Nottin R, Dulmet E, Serraf A. Heart tumors in children and adults: clinicopathologic study of 59 patients from a surgical center. *Cardiovasc Pathol.* 2007;16:22–28.
578. Vujin B, Bene D, Srdic S, Bikicki M, Vuckovic D, Dodic S. Rhabdomyosarcoma of the heart. *Herz.* 2006;31:798–800.
579. Wang JN, Yao CT, Chen JS, Yang YJ, Tsai YC, Wu JM. Cardiac tumors in infants and children. *Acta Paediatr Taiwan.* 2003;44:215–219.
580. Odim J, Reehal V, Laks H, Mehta U, Fishbein MC. Surgical pathology of cardiac tumors: two decades at an urban institution. *Cardiovasc Pathol.* 2003;12:267–270.
581. Talukder MQ, Deo SV, Maleszewski JJ, Park SJ. Late isolated metastasis of renal cell carcinoma in the left ventricular myocardium. *Interact Cardiovasc Thorac Surg.* 2010;11:814–816.
582. Chrissos DN, Stougiannos PN, Mytas DZ, Katsaros AA, Andrikopoulos GK, Kallikazaros IE. Multiple cardiac metastases from malignant melanoma. *Eur J Echocardiogr.* 2008;9:391–392.
583. Ngaage DL, Mullany CJ, Daly RC, et al. Surgical treatment of cardiac papillary fibroelastoma: a single center experience with eighty-eight patients. *Ann Thorac Surg.* 2005;80:1712–1718.
584. Rubin MA, Snell J, Tazelaar HD, Lack EE, Austenfeld MD, Azumi N. Cardiac papillary fibroelastoma: an immunohistochemical investigation and unusual clinical manifestations. *Mod Pathol.* 1995;8:402–407.
585. Raeburn C. Papillary fibroelastic hamartoma of the heart valves. *J Pathol.* 1953;65:371–375.
586. Dobrilovic N, Singh AK, LeGolvan M, Sellke FW. Massive cardiac fibroma [published online ahead of print February 15, 2011]. *J Card Surg.* 2011;26:159–161.
587. Nwachukwu H, Li A, Nair V, Nguyen E, David TE, Butany J. Cardiac fibroma in adults [published online ahead of print October 8, 2010]. *Cardiovasc Pathol.* 2011;20:e146–e152.
588. Tavora F, Li L, Burke A. Sudden coronary death in children. *Cardiovasc Pathol.* 2010;19:336–339.
589. Jain D, Maleszewski JJ, Halushka MK. Benign cardiac tumors and tumorlike conditions. *Ann Diagn Pathol.* 2010;14:215–230.
590. Oster M, Kogon B, Shehata B, Fyfe D. Right atrial fibroma requiring emergent intervention in an 8-week-old infant. *Congenit Heart Dis.* 2009;4:190–192.
591. Bradshaw SH, Hendry P, Boodhwani M, Dennie C, Veinot JP. Left ventricular mesenchymal hamartoma, a new hamartoma of the heart [published online ahead of print September 17, 2010]. *Cardiovasc Pathol.* 2011;20:307–314.

592. Coelho PN, Banazol NG, Soares RJ, Fragata JI. Long-term survival with heart transplantation for fibrosarcoma of the heart. *Ann Thorac Surg*. 2010;90:635–636.
593. Heletz I, Abramson SV. Large obstructive cardiac myxofibrosarcoma is nearly invisible on transthoracic echocardiogram. *Echocardiography*. 2009;26:847–851.
594. Van Veer H, Meuris B, Verbeken E, Herijgers P. Primary atrial fibrosarcoma of the heart. *Cardiovasc Pathol*. 2008;17:325–328.
595. Lazaros GA, Matsakas EP, Madas JS, et al. Primary myxofibrosarcoma of the left atrium: case report and review of the literature. *Angiology*. 2008;59:632–635.
596. Fine G, Morales AR. Mesothelioma of the atrioventricular node. *Arch Pathol*. 1971;92:402–408.
597. Fenoglio JJ Jr, Jacobs DW, McAllister HA Jr. Ultrastructure of the mesothelioma of the atrioventricular node. *Cancer*. 1977;40:721–727.
598. Manion WC, Nelson WP, Hall RJ, Brierty RE. Benign tumor of the heart causing complete heart block. *Am Heart J*. 1972;83:535–542.
599. Burke AP, Anderson PG, Virmani R, James TN, Herrera GA, Ceballos R. Tumor of the atrioventricular nodal region: a clinical and immunohistochemical study. *Arch Pathol Lab Med*. 1990;114:1057–1062.
600. Balasundaram S, Halees SA, Duran C. Mesothelioma of the atrioventricular node: first successful follow-up after excision. *Eur Heart J*. 1992;13:718–719.
601. Monzon-Munoz FJ, Aguilera-Tapia B, Martinez-Penuela-Virseda JM, Oliva-Aldamiz H. Polycystic endodermal heterotopia of the atrioventricular node. *Med Clin*. 1995;104:257–261.
602. Matturri L, Nappo A, Varesi C, Rossi L. Cardiac block caused by metastasis of lung adenocarcinoma to the bundle of His. *Minerva Med*. 1993;84:141–144.
603. Cunningham KS, Veinot JP, Feindel CM, Butany J. Fatty lesions of the atria and interatrial septum. *Hum Pathol*. 2006;37:1245–1251.
604. Kitamura A, Ozaki N, Mukohara N, Yoshida M, Shida T. Primary cardiac liposarcoma causing cardiac tamponade: report of a case. *Surg Today*. 2007;37:974–976.
605. Pollono DG, Drut R. Cardiac liposarcoma and bilateral ovarian mature teratoma in a patient with congenital heart disease and f-anisosplenia. *Pediatr Blood Cancer*. 2008;51:304–305.
606. Dettrick AJ. Lipomatous hypertrophy of the interatrial septum: report of an unusual case. *Histopathology*. 2009;54:777–779.
607. Basu S, Folliguet T, Anselmo M, et al. Lipomatous hypertrophy of the interatrial septum. *Cardiovasc Surg*. 1994;2:229–231.
608. Shirani J, Roberts WC. Clinical, electrocardiographic, and morphologic features of massive fatty deposits ("lipomatous hypertrophy") in the atrial septum. *J Am Coll Cardiol*. 1993;22:226–238.
609. Smith CE, Teague SM, Ameredes T, Peerless JR, Snow NJ. Atrial septal lipomatous hypertrophy and ischemic heart disease: an unusual presentation. *J Clin Anesth*. 1993;5:73–75.
610. Koehler U, Bittinger A. Lipomatous hypertrophy of the atrial septum: cardiac-induced syncope in hamartoma of the right heart atrium [in German]. *Dtsch Med Wochenschr*. 1991;116:1393–1396.
611. Okel BB. The Wolff-Parkinson–White syndrome: report of a case with fatal arrhythmia and autopsy findings of myocarditis, interatrial lipomatous hypertrophy, and prominent right moderator band. *Am Heart J*. 1968;75:673–678.
612. Roberts WC, Roberts JD. The floating heart or the heart too fat to sink: analysis of 55 necropsy patients. *Am J Cardiol*. 1983;52:1286–1289.
613. Burke AP, Litovsky S, Virmani R. Lipomatous hypertrophy of the atrial septum presenting as a right atrial mass. *Am J Surg Pathol*. 1996;20:678–685.
614. Lam KY, Dickens P, Chan AC. Tumors of the heart: a 20 year experience with a review of 12,485 consecutive autopsies. *Arch Pathol Lab Med*. 1993;117:1027–1031.
615. Veinot JP, Tazelaar HD, Edwards WD, Colby TV. Mesothelial/monocytic incidental cardiac excrescences: cardiac MICE. *Mod Pathol*. 1994;7:9–16.

616. Luthringer DJ, Virmani R, Weiss SW, Rosai J. A distinctive cardiovascular lesion resembling histiocytoid (epithelioid) hemangioma. *Am J Surg Pathol.* 1990;14:993–1000.
617. Rosai J, Gold S, Landy R. The histiocytoid hemangioma: a unifying concept embracing several previously described entities of skin, soft tissue, large vessels, bone, and heart. *Hum Pathol.* 1979;10:707–730.
618. Courtice RW, Stinson WA, Walley VM. Tissue fragments recovered at cardiac surgery masquerading as tumoral proliferations: evidence suggesting iatrogenic or artefactual origin and common occurrence. *Am J Surg Pathol.* 1994;18:167–174.
619. Miller DV, Tazelaar HD. Cardiovascular pseudoneoplasms. *Arch Pathol Lab Med.* 2010;134:362–368.
620. Bando Y, Kitagawa T, Uehara H, et al. So-called mesothelial/monocytic incidental cardiac excrescences obtained during valve replacement surgery. *Virchows Arch.* 2000;437:331–335.
621. Wu M, Anderson A, Kahn LB. A report of mesothelial/monocytic incidental cardiac excrescences and a literature review. *Ann Diagn Pathol.* 2000;4:39–43.
622. Brown RW, Campagna LB, Dunn JK, Cagle PT. Immunohistochemical identification of tumor markers in metastatic adenocarcinoma: a diagnostic adjunct in the determination of primary site. *Am J Clin Pathol.* 1997;107:12–19.
623. Vaideeswar P, Patwardhan AM, Sathe PA. Cardiac valvular inflammatory pseudotumor. *J Cardiothorac Surg.* 2008;3:53–58.
624. Adler A, Fimbres A, Marcinak J, et al. Inflammatory pseudotumor of the heart caused by *Listeria monocytogenes* infection. *J Infect.* 2009;58:161–163.
625. Tomiyama M, Nakatani S, Ishibashi-Ueda H, Yutani C, Yamagishi M. Inflammatory pseudotumor of the heart. *Ann Intern Med.* 2007;147:351–352.
626. Stark P, Sandbank JC, Rudnicki C, Zahavi I. Inflammatory pseudotumor of the heart with vasculitis and venous thrombosis. *Chest.* 1992;102:1884–1885.
627. Burke A, Li L, Kling E, Kutys R, Virmani R, Miettinen M. Cardiac inflammatory myofibroblastic tumor: a "benign" neoplasm that may result in syncope, myocardial infarction, and sudden death. *Am J Surg Pathol.* 2007;31:1115–1122.
628. Cessna MH, Zhou H, Sanger WG, et al. Expression of *ALK-1* and p80 in inflammatory myofibroblastic tumor and its mesenchymal mimics: a study of 135 cases. *Mod Pathol.* 2002;15:931–938.
629. Hsieh SC, Chen CY, Chan WP. Malignant fibrous histiocytoma of the heart: a case report. *Acta Cardiol.* 2010;65:85–87.
630. Pileri SA, Grogan TM, Harris NL, et al. Tumors of histiocytes and accessory dendritic cells: an immunohistochemical approach to classification from the International Lymphoma Study Group, based on 61 cases. *Histopathology.* 2002;41:1–29.
631. Ikeda H, Nakamura S, Nishimaki H, et al. Primary lymphoma of the heart: case report and literature review. *Pathol Int.* 2004;54:187–195.
632. Curtsinger CR, Wilson MJ, Yoneda K. Primary cardiac lymphoma. *Cancer.* 1989;64:521–525.
633. Champeaux AL, Blaser JL, Myers JB, Schachter DT. Multiple myeloma involving the myocardium and coronary vessels. *Arch Pathol Lab Med.* 2000;124:910–912.
634. Bothe W, Goebel H, Kunze M, Beyersdorf F. Right atrial solitary fibrous tumor—a new cardiac neoplasm? *Interact Cardiovasc Thorac Surg.* 2005;4:396–397.
635. Iqbal MB, Stravri G, Mittal T, Khaghani A. A calcified cardiac mass [published online ahead of print November 28, 2006]. *Int J Cardiol.* 2007;115:e126–e128.
636. Kirby PA, Sato Y, Tannous R, Dehner LP. Calcifying fibrous psesudotumor of the myocardium. *Pediatr Dev Pathol.* 2006;9:384–387.
637. Masson P. Hemangioendotheliome vegetant intravasculaire. *Bull Soc Anat.* 1923;93:517–523.
638. Koniari I, Tsigkas G, Apostolakis E, Dougenis D. Cardiac papillary endothelial hyperplasia: a current assessment. *Interact Cardiovasc Thorac Surg.* 2008;7:1206–1207.
639. Modi A, Moorjani N, Pontefract D, Livesay S. Isolated papillary endothelial hyperplasia in the left atrial appendage. *Interact Cardiovasc Thorac Surg.* 2008;7:1204–1206.

640. Goldman RL. Papillary endothelial hyperplasia. *Hum Pathol.* 1993;24:1264–1265.
641. Stewart M, Smoller BR. Multiple lesions of intravascular papillary endothelial hyperplasia (Masson's lesions). *Arch Pathol Lab Med.* 1994;118:315–316.
642. Bansal M, Mehrota R, Agrawal V, Kasliwal RR, Trehan N. Primary tumor of the heart: angiosarcoma. *Indian Heart J.* 2009;61:383–384.
643. Edwards WD, Holmes DR Jr, Reeder GS. Diagnosis of active lymphocytic myocarditis by endomyocardial biopsy. *Mayo Clin Proc.* 1982;57:419–428.
644. Aretz HT, Billingham ME, Edwards WD, et al. Myocarditis: a histopathologic definition and classification. *Am J Cardiovasc Pathol.* 1987;1:3–10.
645. Aretz HT. Myocarditis: the Dallas classification. In: Virmani R, Atkinson JB, Fenoglio JJ Jr, eds. *Cardiovascular Pathology*. Philadelphia, PA: WB Saunders; 1991:246–256.
646. Fenoglio JJ Jr, Marboe CC. Endomyocardial biopsy. In: Stemberg SS, ed. *Diagnostic Surgical Pathology*. New York, NY: Raven Press; 1989:877–895.
647. Tazelaar HD. Surgical pathology of the heart: endomyocardial biopsy, valvular heart disease, and cardiac tumors. In: Schoen FJ, Gimbrone MA Jr, eds. *Cardiovascular Pathology: Clinicopathologic Correlations and Pathogenetic Mechanisms.* Baltimore, MD: Williams and Wilkins, 1995:81–107.
648. Flipse TR, Tazelaar HD, Holmes DR Jr. Diagnosis of malignant cardiac disease by endomyocardial biopsy. *Mayo Clin Proc.* 1990;65:1415–1422.
649. Billingham ME. Cardiac transplant pathology. In: Hammond EH, ed. *Solid Organ Transplantation*. Philadelphia, PA: WB Saunders; 1994:69–91.
650. Abu-Farsakh H, Cagle PT, Buffone GJ, Bruner JM, Weilbaecher D, Greenberg SD. Heart allograft involvement with Epstein–Barr virus-associated posttransplant lymphoproliferative disorder. *Arch Pathol Lab Med.* 1992;116:93–95.
651. Eisen HJ, Hicks D, Kant JA, et al. Diagnosis of posttransplantation lymphoproliferative disorder by endomyocardial biopsy in a cardiac allograft *recipient. J Heart Lung Transplant.* 1994;13:241–245.
652. Jost E, Lorenzen J, Haage P, et al. Heart and muscle involvement by extramedullary myeloid leukemia: a case report and review of the literature. *Leuk Lymphoma.* 2005;46:1819–1824.
653. Al-Gwaiz LA, Bassioni W. Immunophenotyping of acute lymphoblastic leukemia using immunohistochemistry in bone marrow biopsy specimens. *Histol Histopathol.* 2008;23:1223–1228.
654. Cleary ML, Nalesnik MA, Shearer WT, Sklar J. Clonal analysis of transplant-associated lymphoproliferations based on the structure of the genomic termini of the Epstein–Barr virus. *Blood.* 1988;72:349–352.
655. Ritter JH, Wick MR. Posttransplant lymphoproliferative disorders: immunohistochemical differential diagnosis with severe allograft rejection. *Int J Surg Pathol.* 1994;2:105–116.
656. Ward JM, O'Leary TJ, Baskin GB, et al. Immunohistochemical localization of human and simian immunodeficiency viral antigens in fixed tissue sections. *Am J Pathol.* 1987;127:199–205.
657. Joshi A, Masek MA, Brown BW Jr, Weiss LM, Billingham ME. "Quilty" revisited: a 10-year perspective. *Hum Pathol.* 1995;26:547–557.
658. Lozano MD, Pardo-Mindan FJ. Significance of endocardial infiltrates (Quilty effect) in the transplanted heart. *J Heart Lung Transplant.* 1994;13:733–734.
659. Luthringer DJ, Yamashita JT, Czer LS, Trento A, Fishbein MC. Nature and significance of epicardial lymphoid infiltrates in cardiac allografts. *J Heart Lung Transplant.* 1995;14:537–543.
660. Richter JT, Strange RG Jr, Fisher SI, Miller DV, Delvecchio DM. Extranodal Rosai-Dorfman disease presesenting as a cardiac mass in an adult: report of a unique case and lack of relationship to IgG4-related sclerosing lesions. *Hum Pathol.* 2010;41:297–301.
661. Maleszewski JJ, Hristov AC, Halushka MK, Miller DV. Extranodal Rosai–Dorfman disease involving the heart: report of two cases. *Cardiovasc.* 2010;19:380–384.
662. Buchino JJ, Byrd RP, Kmetz DR. Disseminated sinus histiocytosis with massive lymphadenopathy: its pathologic aspects. *Arch Pathol Lab Med.* 1982;106:13–16.

663. Foucar E, Rosai J, Dorfman R. Sinus histiocytosis with massive lymphadenopathy (Rosai–Dorfman disease): review of the entity. *Semin Diagn Pathol.* 1990;7:19–73.
664. Morgan NV, Morris MR, Cangul H, et al. Mutations in SLC29A3, encoding an equilibrative nucleoside transporter ENT3, cause a familial histiocytosis syndrome (Faisalabad histiocytosis) and familial Rosai–Dorfman disease. *PLoS Genet.* 2010;6:e1000833–e1000834.
665. Eisen RN, Buckley PJ, Rosai J. Immunophenotypic characterization of sinus histiocytosis with massive lymphadenopathy (Rosai–Dorfman disease). *Semin Diagn Pathol.* 1990;7:74–82.
666. Botelho A, Antunes A, Almeida JC, et al. A rare histiocytosis with severe cardiac involvement: Erdheim-Chester disease. *Rev Port Cardiol.* 2008;27:727–740.
667. Just PA, Cazes A, Goebel H, Mousseaux E, Fabiani JN, Bruneval P. A case of pericoronary pseudotumor due to localized Castleman's disease. *Cardiovasc Pathol.* 2009;18:375–378.
668. Malaisrie SC, Loebe M, Walkes JC, Reardon MJ. Coronary pseudoaneurysm: an unreported complication of Castleman's disease. *Ann Thorac Surg.* 2006;82:318–320.
669. Frizzera G. Castleman's disease and related disorders. *Semin Diagn Pathol.* 1988;5:346–364.
670. Peterson BA, Frizzera G. Multicentric Castleman's disease. *Semin Oncol.* 1993;20:636–647.
671. Menke DM, Dewald GW. Lack of cytogenetic abnormalities in Castleman's disease. *South Med J.* 2001;94:472–474.
672. Schulte KM, Talat N. Castleman's disease—a two-compartment model of HHV8 infection. *Nat Rev Clin Oncol.* 2010;7:533–543.
673. Kojima M, Shimizu K, Ikota H, et al. Follicular variant of hyaline-vascular type of Castleman's disease: histopathological and immunohistochemical study of 11 cases. *J Clin Exp Hematopathol.* 2008;48:39–45.
674. Freeman RK, Howden FM, Gable PS, Bethel KJ. Extramedullary hematopoiesis presenting as an intraatrial mass in a patient with chronic myelogenous leukemia. *J Thorac Cardiovasc Surg.* 1995;110:552–554.
675. Audouin J, Comperat E, LeTourneau A, et al. Myeloid sarcoma: clinical and morphologic criteria useful for diagnosis. *Int J Surg Pathol.* 2003;11:271–282.
676. Goldman BI, Wurzel J. Hematopoiesis/erythropoiesis in myocardial infarcts. *Mod Pathol.* 2001;14:589–594.
677. Hill DA, Swanson PE. Myocardial extramedullary hematopoiesis: a clinicopathologic study. *Mod Pathol.* 2000;13:779–787.
678. Chin JY, Chung MH, Kim JJ, et al. Extensive primary cardiac lymphoma diagnosed by percutaneous endomyocardial biopsy. *J Cardiovasc Ultrasound.* 2009;17:141–144.
679. Cohoon KP, Howe W, McKiernan T. Primary cardiac diffuse large B-cell lymphoma in an immunocompetent patient. *J Invasive Cardiol.* 2008;20:e59–e60.
680. Nascimento AF, Winters GL, Pinkus GS. Primary cardiac lymphoma: clinical, histologic, immunophenotypic, and genotypic features of 5 cases of a rare disorder. *Am J Surg Pathol.* 2007;31:1344–1350.
681. Butany J, Leong SW, Carmichael K, Komeda M. A 30-year analysis of cardiac neoplasms at autopsy. *Can J Cardiol.* 2005;21:675–680.
682. Chalabreysse L, Berger F, Loire R, Devouassoux G, Cordier JF, Thivolet-Bejui F. Primary cardiac lymphoma in immunocompetent patients: a report of three cases and review of the literature. *Virchows Arch.* 2002;441:456–461.
683. Lynch M, Cobbs W Jr, Miller RL, Martin RP. Massive cardiac involvement by malignant lymphoma. *Cardiology.* 1996;87:566–568.
684. Holladay AO, Siegel RJ, Schwartz DA. Cardiac malignant lymphoma in acquired immune deficiency syndrome. *Cancer.* 1992;70:2203–2207.
685. Lee A, Baloch ZW, Yu G, Gupta PK. Mesothelial hyperplasia with reactive atypia: diagnostic pitfalls and role of immunohistochemical studies—a case report. *Diagn Cytopathol.* 2000;22:113–116.
686. Sandhyamani S, Kartha CC, Pattankar VL, Mohan Singh MP, Valiathan MS. Reactive mesothelial nodule of the pericardium. *Ind Heart J.* 1984;36:169–172.

687. Rosai J, Dehner LP. Nodular mesothelial hyperplasia in hernia sacs: a benign reactive condition simulating a neoplastic process. *Cancer.* 1975;35:165–175.
688. Chikkamuniyappa S, Herrick J, Jagirdar JS. Nodular histiocytic-mesothelial hyperplasia: a potential pitfall. *Ann Diagn Pathol.* 2004;8:115–120.
689. Leong AS, Stevens MW, Mukherjee TM. Malignant mesothelioma: cytologic diagnosis with histologic, immunohistochemical, and ultrastructural correlation. *Semin Diagn Pathol.* 1992;9:141–150.
690. Horie M, Noguchi S, Tanaka W, et al. Primary malignant pericardial mesothelioma mimicking pericardial metastasis from adenocarcinoma. *J Thorac Oncol.* 2010;5:2012–2014.
691. Sakuraba M, T, Hirama M, Ogura K. Malignant pericardial mesothelioma. *Eur J Cardiothorac Surg.* 2011;39:420–421.
692. Patel J, Sheppard MN. Primary malignant mesothelioma of the pericardium. *Cardiovasc Pathol.* 2011;2:107–109.
693. Terada T. Primary sarcomatoid malignant mesothelioma of the pericardium. *Med Oncol.* 2012;29:1345–1346.
694. Bendek M, Ferenc M, Freudenberg N. Post-irradiation pericardial malignant mesothelioma: an autopsy case and review of the literature. *Cardiovasc Pathol.* 2010;19:377–379.
695. Yazdi HM, Hajdu SI, Melamed MR. Cytopathology of pericardial effusions. *Acta Cytol.* 1980;24:401–412.
696. Wiener HG, Kristensen IB, Haubek A, Kristensen B, Baandrup U. The diagnostic value of pericardial cytology: an analysis of 95 cases. *Acta Cytol.* 1991;35:149–153.
697. Singh HK, Silverman JF, Berns L, Haddad ME, Park HK. Significance of epithelial membrane antigen in the workup of problematic serous effusions. *Diagn Cytopathol.* 1995;13:3–7.
698. Cagle PT, Brown RW, Lebovitz RM. p53 immunostaining in the differentiation of reactive processes from malignancy in pleural biopsy specimens. *Hum Pathol.* 1994;25:443–448.
699. Fazekas T, Ungi I, Tiszlavicz L. Primary malignant mesothelioma of the pericardium. *Am Heart J.* 1992;124:227–231.
700. Mason MR, Bedrossian CW, Fahey CA. Value of immunocytochemistry in the study of malignant effusions. *Diagn Cytopathol.* 1987;3:215–221.
701. Maeder M, Spieler P, Krapf R, Diethelm M. Cytologically-malignant lymphoid pericardial effusion with benign clinical outcome. *Swiss Med Wkly.* 2005;135:377–381.
702. Cay S, Durak A, Aydogdu S, Turhan N. Massive pericardial effusion as the primary manifestation of high-grade malignant lymphoma. *Turk Kardiyol Dern Ars.* 2009;37:578–579.
703. Carbone A, Gloghini A. KSHV/HHV8-associated lymphomas. *Br J Haematol.* 2008;140:13–24.
704. Bashir H, Hudson MM, Kaste SC, Howard SC, Krasin M, Metzger ML. Pericardial involvement at diagnosis in pediatric Hodgkin lymphoma patients. *Pediatr Blood Cancer.* 2007;49:666–671.
705. Grebenc ML, Rosado-de-Christenson ML, Burke AP, Green CE, Galvin JR. Primary cardiac and pericardial neoplasms: radiologic-pathologic correlation. *Radiographics.* 2000;20:1073–1103.
706. Pavlidis NA, Elisaf M, Bai M, Tolis C, Papadimitriou C. Primary lymphoma of the pericardium: report of a "cured" case and review of the literature. *Med Pediatr Oncol.* 1994;22:287–291.
707. Franzese MG, Ieva R, Correale M, Palumbo G, Capalbo SF, Di Biase M. An extramedullary lesion in multiple myeloma: voluminous pericardial mass. *Clin Cardiol.* 2009;32:e73.
708. Serefhanoglu S, Sayinalp N, Haznedaroglu IC, et al. Extramedullary plasmacytomas of the thyroid and pericardium as initial presentation of multiple myeloma. *Ann Hematol.* 2008;87:853–854.
709. Bhattacharya P, Singh P, Bahal A, et al. Angiosarcoma of the pericardium: a report of two cases. *Indian J Pathol Microbiol.* 2007;50:777–779.
710. Yaho H, Mihamoto T, Mukai S, Yamamura M, Nakagawa T, Ryomoto M. Angiosarcoma of the pericardium: review of 9 reports from Japan. *Jpn J Thorac Cardiovasc Surg.* 2003;51:65–67.
711. Zen Y, Nakanuma Y. IgG4-related disease: a cross-sectional study of 114 cases. *Am J Surg Pathol.* 2010;34:1812–1819.

712. Iberti C. Retroperitoneal fibroses: etiopathogenesis and taxonomic assessment. *Eur Rev Med Pharmacol Sci.* 2007;11:375–382.
713. Sugimoto T, Morita Y, Isshiki K, et al. Constrictive pericarditis as an emerging manifestation of hyper-IgG4 disease [published online ahead of print August 28, 2007]. *Int J Cardiol.* 2008;130:e100–e101.
714. Neild GH, Rodriguez-Justo M, Wall C, Connolly JO. Hyper-IgG4 disease: report and characterization of a new disease. *BMC Med.* 2006;4:23–24.
715. Pressman G, Verma N. Pericardial fat masquerading as a tumor. *Echocardiography.* 2010;27:e18–e20.
716. Vander Salm TJ. Unusual primary tumors of the heart. *Semin Thorac Cardiovasc Surg.* 2000;12:89–100.
717. Molina JE, Edwards JE, Ward HB. Primary cardiac tumors: experience at the University of Minnesota. *Thorac Cardiovasc Surg.* 1990;38(suppl):183–191.
718. Durak D, Eren B. Pericardial lipoma: an autopsy case and review of the literature. *J Forensic Sci.* 2007;52:949–950.
719. Yamamoto T, Nejima J, Ino T, et al. A case of massive left atrial lipoma occupying pericardial space. *Jpn Heart J.* 2004;45:715–721.
720. Gaerte SC, Meyer CA, Winer-Muram HT, Tarver RD, Conces DJ Jr. Fat-containing lesions of the chest. *Radiographics.* 2002;22:S61–S78.
721. Kendall SW, Williams EA, Hunt JB, Petch MC, Wells FC, Milstein BB. Recurrent primary liposarcoma of the pericardium: management by repeated resections. *Ann Thorac Surg.* 1993;56:560–562.
722. Can C, Arpaci F, Celasun B, Gunhan O, Finci R. Primary pericardial liposarcoma presenting with cardiac tamponade and multiple organ metastases. *Chest.* 1993;103:328–329.
723. Nishio J. Contributions of cytogenetics and molecular cytogenetics to the diagnosis of adipocytic tumors [published online ahead of print January 11, 2011]. *J Biomed Biotechnol.* 2011;2011:524067.
724. Agarwala BN, Ruschhaupt DG, Sand ME. Pseudotumor of the pericardium. *Pediatr Cardiol.* 1997;18:429–431.
725. Virmani R, Bewtra C, McAllister HA, Schulte RD. Intrapericardial giant lymph node hyperplasia. *Am J Surg Pathol.* 1982;6:475–481.
726. Carvalho N, Eiras D, Martins T, Ramos S, Abecasis M, Anjos R. Castleman disease with pericardial location: third case of the literature. *Rev Port Cir Cardiothorac Vasc.* 2009;16:139–141.
727. Shih LY, Lin FC, Kuo TT. Cutaneous and pericardial extramedullary hematopoiesis with cardiac tamponade in chronic myeloid leukemia. *Am J Clin Pathol.* 1988;89:693–697.
728. Kasashima S, Zen Y, Kawashima A, et al. Inflammatory abdominal aortic aneurysm: close relationship to IgG4-related periaortitis. *Am J Surg Pathol.* 2008;32:197–204.
729. Kasashima S, Zen Y. IgG4-related inflammatory abdominal aortic aneurysm. *Curr Opin Rheumatol.* 2011;23:18–23.
730. Stone JR. Aortitis, periaortitis, and retroperitoneal fibrosis, as manifestations of IgG4-related systemic disease. *Curr Opin Rheumatol.* 2011;23:88–94.
731. Kendall AR, Lakey WH. Sclerosing Hodgkin's disease versus idiopathic retroperitoneal fibrosis. *J Urol.* 1961;86:217–221.
732. Waldron JA Jr, Newcomer LN, Katz ME, Cadman E. Sclerosing variants of follicular center-cell lymphomas presenting in the retroperitoneum. *Cancer.* 1983;52:712–720.
733. Yousef GM, Gabril MY, Al-Haddad S, Mulligan AM, Honey RJ. Invasive lobular carcinoma of the breast presenting as retroperitoneal fibrosis: a case report. *J Med Case Reports.* 2010;4:175–176.
734. Ferenc T, Sygut J, Kopcszynski J, et al. Aggressive fibromatosis (desmoids tumors): definition, occurrence, pathology, diagnostic problems, clinical behavior, and genetic background. *Pol J Pathol.* 2006;57:5–15.
735. Okamoto M, Takahashi H, Yamanaka J, Nemoto S, Kuno K, Ishii T. Sclerosing inflammatory pseudotumor arising from the carotid artery region. *Auris Nasus Larynx.* 1997;24:315–320.

736. Kim GE, Cho YP, Chung DH, Kwon TW, Kim OJ. Inflammatory pseudotumor of carotid artery: a case report. *Cardiovasc Surg*. 1999;7:342–347.
737. Lee HK, Kim EJ, Ro JY, Kwon Y, Kim GE. Inflammaory pseudotumor of the carotid artery: radiologic findings. *J Comput Assist Tomogr*. 2003;27:253–256.
738. Petrik PK, Findlay JM, Sherlock RA. Aneurysmal cyst, bone type, primary in an artery. *Am J Surg Pathol*. 1993;17:1062–1066.
739. Rys J, Kruczak A, Marczyk E, et al. Primary soft tissue giant cell tumor of the neck: cytological and histological characteristics of the tumor and differential diagnosis. *Pol J Pathol*. 2009;60:98–104.
740. Holst VA, Elenitsas R. Primary giant cell tumor of soft tissue. *J Cutan Pathol*. 2001;28:492–495.
741. Wilde B, Van Paassen P, Witzke O, Tervaert JW. New pathophysiological insights and treatment of ANCA-associated vasculitis. *Kidney Int*. 2011;79:599–612.
742. El-Zammar OA, Katzenstein AL. Pathological diagnosis of granulomatous lung disease: a review. *Histopathology*. 2007;50:289–310.
743. Goulart RA, Mark EJ, Rosen S. Tumefactions as an extravascular manifestation of Wegener's granulomatosis. *Am J Surg Pathol*. 1995;19:145–153.
744. Chua J, Lim L. Systemic Wegener's granulomatosis with severe orbito-ocular involvement. *Singapore Med J*. 2008;49:e259–e262.
745. Mayou SC, Anstey A, Norton AJ, Kirby JD. Angiocentric T-cell lymphoma in skin. *J R Soc Med*. 1991;84:683–684.
746. Ferry JA, Fung CY, Zukerberg L, et al. Lymphoma of the ocular adnexa: a study of 353 cases. *Am J Surg Pathol*. 2007;31:170–184.
747. Tong MM, Cooke B, Barnetson RS. Lymphomatoid granulomatosis. *J Am Acad Dermatol*. 1992;27:872–876.
748. Katzenstein AL, Doxtrader E, Narender S. Lymphomatoid granulomatosis: insights gained over 4 decades. *Am J Surg Pathol*. 2010;34:e35–e48.

Index